Legal Essentials of Health Care Administration

George D. Pozgar, MBA, CHE
Consultant
GP Health Care Consulting, International
Annapolis, Maryland
Surveyor
The Joint Commission
Oakbrook Terrace, Illinois

Legal Review
Nina M. Santucci
General Counsel
Essex Corporation
Columbia, Maryland

JONES AND BARTLETT PUBLISHERS
Sudbury, Massachusetts
BOSTON TORONTO LONDON SINGAPORE

World Headquarters
Jones and Bartlett Publishers
40 Tall Pine Drive
Sudbury, MA 01776
978-443-5000
info@jbpub.com
www.jbpub.com

Jones and Bartlett Publishers Canada
6339 Ormindale Way
Mississauga, Ontario L5V 1J2
Canada

Jones and Bartlett Publishers International
Barb House, Barb Mews
London W6 7PA
United Kingdom

Jones and Bartlett's books and products are available through most bookstores and online booksellers. To contact Jones and Bartlett Publishers directly, call 800-832-0034, fax 978-443-8000, or visit our website www.jbpub.com.

Substantial discounts on bulk quantities of Jones and Bartlett's publications are available to corporations, professional associations, and other qualified organizations. For details and specific discount information, contact the special sales department at Jones and Bartlett via the above contact information or send an email to specialsales@jbpub.com.

Production Credits
Publisher: Michael Brown
Production Director: Amy Rose
Associate Editor: Katey Birtcher
Production Editor: Tracey Chapman
Marketing Manager: Sophie Fleck
Manufacturing and Inventory Control Supervisor: Amy Bacus
Composition: Publishers' Design and Publishers' Services, Inc.
Cover Design: Brian Moore
Cover Image: © Artifan/ShutterStock, Inc.; Photos.com
Printing and Binding: Malloy, Inc.
Cover Printing: Malloy, Inc.

Library of Congress Cataloging-in-Publication Data
Pozgar, George D.
Legal essentials of health care administration / George D. Pozgar ; Legal review, Nina M. Santucci.
p. cm.
Includes bibliographical references and index.
ISBN-13: 978-0-7637-6130-1 (pbk.)
ISBN-10: 0-7637-6130-3 (pbk.)
1. Medical care—Law and legislation—United States. I. Santucci, Nina M. II. Title.
KF3821.P694 2008
344.7304'1—dc22

2008014755

6048
Printed in the United States of America
12 11 10 09 08 10 9 8 7 6 5 4 3 2 1

Contents

Chapter 6 Civil Procedure and Trial Practice 69

Chapter 7 Corporate Structure and Liability 93

Chapter 8 Medical Staff 107

Acknowledgments

I am grateful to the very special people in the more than 650 hospitals in 40 states with whom I have consulted, surveyed, and provided education over the past 15 years. Their shared experiences have served to remind me of the importance to make this book more valuable in the classroom and as a reference for practicing health care professionals.

To my students in health care law classes at the New School for Social Research, Molloy College, Long Island University, C.W. Post College, Saint Francis College, Saint Joseph's College, my intern from Brown University, and my resident in hospital administration, while I was an on-site faculty member of the George Washington University, as well as those I have instructed through the years at various seminars, I will always be indebted for your inspiration.

Many thanks are also extended to all those special people at the National Library of Medicine and the Library of Congress for their guidance over the years in locating research materials.

The author especially acknowledges the staff at Jones and Bartlett Publishers whose guidance and assistance was so important in making this book a reality.

Preface

This book is an abridged version of *Legal Aspects of Health Care Administration, 10th Edition*, which has been widely used by health care professionals and students in both undergraduate and graduate health care programs. The legal topics presented in the following chapters lay a strong foundation in health law. Although this book is a must for students taking introductory legal courses, it is of particular value as a supplemental reading in other courses as well. It is a sound reference book for those who wish to become more informed about how the law, ethics, and health care intersect.

Essentials provides an understanding as to what steps the providers of care, legislative bodies, patients, patients' families, and patient advocates can take to help prevent the wide variety of harmful events surrounding patient care. It presents a review of health law topics in an interesting and understandable format, leading the reader through the complicated maze of the legal system.

To assist the reader in applying the substantive material in this book, actual court cases are presented. The decisions in cases discussed are generally governed both by applicable state and federal statutes and common-law principles. When reviewing a case, the reader must keep in mind that the case law and statutes of one state are not binding in another state.

The first chapter begins with an historical perspective on the development of hospitals, illustrating both their progress and failures through the centuries. As the book progresses, there is broad discussion of the legal system, including the sources of law and government organization. The text continues with a basic review of tort law, criminal issues, contracts, civil procedure and trial practice, and a wide range of real-life legal and ethical dilemmas that caregivers have faced as they wound their way through the courts. The final chapters provide an overview of various ways to improve the quality and delivery of health care.

The content of this book serves as a reminder to its readers that they must learn from the mistakes and tragedies experienced by others in order to avoid repeating them. The legal cases and resulting headlines should be a reminder of the responsibility the caregiver has to the profession he or she has chosen and that the knowledge gained from studying this book should be heeded to help prevent becoming the next headline:

- **Medicare Won't Pay Hospitals for Errors**

  Beginning Oct. 1, Medicare no longer will pay those extra costs for eight preventable errors, including catheter-caused urinary tract infections, injuries from falls, and leaving objects in the body after surgery. Nor can hospitals bill the injured patient for those extra costs.

  —*The Associated Press, 2008*

- **Robert Courtney Pleads Guilty to 20 Felony Counts**

  Ultimately investigators discover he has diluted 72 different medications in

98,000 prescriptions for 4,200 patients since 1992. As a result civil suits are named and hundreds of families will never know if adequate dosages could have saved their loved ones. Courtney is sentenced to 30 years in federal prison for his crime. This episode truly looks at the darkest side of greed, Robert Courtney, a man who preyed on the weakest of victims and took away their only weapon in the fight against cancer.[i]

—*American Greed, February 27, 2008*

- **Health Insurer Fined for Dropping Breast Cancer Patient**

Patsy Bates, 52, a hairdresser from Lakewood, had been left with more than $129,000 in unpaid medical bills when Health Net Inc. canceled her policy in 2004. On Friday, arbitration judge Sam Cianchetti ordered Health Net to repay that amount while providing $8.4 million in punitive damages and $750,000 for emotional distress.

• • •

"It's hard to imagine a policy more reprehensible than tying bonuses to encourage the recision of health insurance that helps keep the public well and alive," Cianchetti wrote in the Bates decision.

—*Baltimore Sun, February 23, 2008*

- **Incubator Fire Critically Burns Newborn**

Oxygen ignited inside a special hood worn by a newborn infant in a hospital, burning the boy's head and face and leaving him in critical condition.

—*THE CAPITAL, January 24, 2008*

Note: i. http://www.cnbc.com/id/23291456.

- **John Ritter's Doctors Cleared of Negligence in Actor's Death**

A jury cleared a cardiologist and a radiologist Friday of negligence in the diagnosis and treatment of actor John Ritter, who died of a torn aorta in 2003. Jurors found that the radiologist advised Ritter to follow up with treatment by a physician after a body scan two years before his death. Ritter didn't follow the order.

—*The Huffington Post, March 14, 2008*

- **Doctor Charged with Stealing 94-Year-Old Mother's Savings**

A physician was accused yesterday of stealing his 94-year-old mother's life savings of more than $800,000 after taking control of her finances through a power of attorney, leaving her virtually impoverished.

—*THE CAPITAL, January 24, 2008*

- **Mature Human Embryos Created from Adult Skin Cells**

. . . opponents of research on human embryos lashed out at the approach.

—*The Washington Post, January 18, 2008*

- **Hospitals Delay Cardiac Arrest Action**

No one knows precisely how many patients go through cardiac arrest and resuscitation. Estimates range from 370,000 to 750,000, the researchers report. Only about 30% survive long enough to go home.

—*U.S.A. Today, January 3, 2008*

- **Half of Doctors Mum About Medical Mistakes**

Washington—Nearly half of all U.S. doctors fail to report incompetent or unethical colleagues, even though they agree that such mistakes should be reported, researchers said on Monday.

They found that 46 percent of physicians surveyed admitted they knew of a serious medical error that had been made but did not tell authorities about it.

—*Reuters, December 3, 2007*

- **Nursing Home Citations Climb 22%**

  More nursing homes are being cited for serious violations as inspectors face increasing pressure to crack down on dangerous conditions . . . .

  —*U.S.A. Today, November 28, 2007*

- **R.I. Hospital Fined for Brain Surgery Errors**

  Rhode Island Hospital has been fined $50,000 and reprimanded by the state Department of Health after its third instance this year of a doctor performing brain surgery on the wrong side of a patient's head.

  —*U.S.A. Today, November 28, 2007*

- **The Quaid Twins: Fighting for Their Lives**

  At the hospital on Nov. 18, they were allegedly among three patients given 1,000 times the recommended dose of heparin, a drug used to prevent IV catheters from clotting.

  —*People, December 10, 2007*

- **Infant's Family Speaks Out Following Hospital Deaths**

  Hospital officials said six premature babies were accidentally given adult doses of heparin at Methodist's newborn intensive care unit. The mistake was caught and the six were treated, but two of them . . . died . . . officials said.

  —*Indiana News, September 19, 2006*

When reviewing the various cases in this book, the reader should consider what happened, why things went wrong, what the relevant ethical and legal issues are, and how the event could have been prevented. The reader should also consider if one fact in a particular case changed, how the outcome might be different. What would the fact be? The cases presented in the text have been chosen because of their continuing frequency of occurrence.

*Author's Note: This text is educational in nature and should not be considered a substitute for legal advice on any particular issue. Moreover, each chapter presents an overview, rather than an exhaustive treatment, of the various topics.

The author, legal reviewers, and/or publisher cannot be responsible for any errors or omissions, including: additions to, interpretations of, and/or changes in the regulations presented in this book.

1

Historical Perspective

This chapter provides the reader with a brief overview of the advance of civilization as disclosed in the history of hospitals. A study of the past often reveals errors that can be avoided, customs that persist only because of tradition, and practices that have been superseded by others that are more effectual. The past can also bring to light some long-abandoned procedures, which can be revived to some advantage. The story of the birth and evolution of the hospital portrays the triumph of civilization over barbarism and the progress of civilization toward an ideal characterized by an interest in the welfare of the community.

EARLY HINDU AND EGYPTIAN HOSPITALS

Two ancient civilizations, India and Egypt, had crude hospitals. Hindu literature reveals that in the 6th century BC, Buddha appointed a physician for every 10 villages and built hospitals for the crippled and the poor. His son, Upatiso, built shelters for the diseased and for pregnant women. These examples probably moved Buddha's devotees to erect similar hospitals. Historians agree that hospitals existed in Ceylon as early as 437 BC.

During his reign from 273 to 232 BC, King Asoka built hospitals that hold historical significance because of their similarities to the modern hospital. Attendants gave gentle care to the sick, provided patients with fresh fruits and vegetables, prepared their medicines, gave massages, and maintained their personal cleanliness. Hindu physicians, adept at surgery, were required to take daily baths, keep their hair and nails short, wear white clothes, and promise that they would respect the confidence of their patients. Although bedside care was outstanding for those times, medicine was only beginning to find its way.

Egyptian physicians were probably the first to use drugs such as alum, peppermint, castor oil, and opium. In surgery, anesthesia consisted of hitting the patient on the head with a wooden mallet to render the patient unconscious. Surgery was largely limited to fractures, and medical treatment was usually given in the home. Therapy away from home was often available in temples, which functioned as hospitals.

GREEK AND ROMAN HOSPITALS

The term "hospital" derives from the Latin word *hospitalis*, which relates to guests and their treatment. The word reflects the early use of these institutions not merely as places of healing but as havens for the poor and weary travelers. Hospitals first appeared in Greece as *aesculapia*, named after the Greek god of medicine, Aesculapius. For many centuries, hospitals developed in association with religious institutions, such as the Hindu hospitals opened in Sri Lanka in the 5th century BC and the monastery-based European hospitals of the Middle Ages (5th century to 15th century). The Hotel-Dieu in Paris, a monastic hospital founded in 660, is still in operation today.

In early Greek and Roman civilization, when medical practices were rife with mysticism and superstitions, temples were also used as hospitals. Every sanctuary had a sacred altar before which the patient, dressed in white, was required to present gifts and offer prayers. If a patient was healed, the cure was credited to miracles and divine visitations.

Greek temples provided refuge for the sick. One of these sanctuaries, dedicated to Aesculapius, is said to have existed as early as 1134 BC at Titanus. Ruins attest to the existence of another, more famous Greek temple built several centuries later in the Hieron, or sacred grove, at Epidaurius. Here physicians ministered to the sick holistically in body and soul. They prescribed medications such as salt, honey, and water from a sacred spring. They gave patients hot and cold baths to promote speedy cures and encouraged long hours of sunshine and sea air, combined with pleasant vistas, as an important part of treatment. The temple hospitals housed libraries and rooms for visitors, attendants, priests, and physicians. The temple at Epidaurius even boasted what might be described as the site of the first clinical records. The columns of the temple were inscribed with the names of patients, brief histories of their cases, and comments as to whether or not they were cured.

The aesculapia spread rapidly throughout the Roman Empire as well as through the Greek world. Although some hospitals were simply spas, others followed the therapy outlined by the leading physicians of the day. Hippocrates, for example, a physician born about 460 BC, advocated medical theories, which have startling similarity to those of the present day. He employed the principles of percussion and auscultation, wrote intelligently on fractures, performed numerous surgical operations, and described such conditions as epilepsy, tuberculosis, malaria, and ulcers. He also kept detailed clinical records of many of his patients. Physicians like Hippocrates not only cared for patients in the temples but also gave instruction to young medical students.

HOSPITALS OF THE EARLY CHRISTIAN ERA

Christianity and the doctrines preached by Jesus stressing the emotions of love and pity gave impetus to the establishment of hospitals, which, with the advance of Christianity, became integral parts of the church institution. These Christian hospitals replaced those of Greece and Rome and were devoted entirely to care of the sick, and they accommodated patients in buildings outside the church proper.

The decree of Constantine in 335 closed the aesculapia and stimulated the building of Christian hospitals. By the year 500, most large towns in the Roman empire had erected hospitals. Nursing, inspired by religion, was gentle and considerate. The medical precepts of Hippocrates, Antyllus, and other early Greek physicians soon began to be discarded because of their pagan origins. Instead, health care turned toward mysticism and theurgy (the working of a divine agency in human affairs) as sources of healing.

Hospitals rarely succeeded during the centuries leading to the Middle Ages; only a few existed outside Italian cities. Occasional almshouses in Europe sheltered some of the sick, while inns along the Roman roads housed others.

MOHAMMEDAN HOSPITALS

The followers of Mohammed were almost as zealous as the Christians in caring for the sick. In Baghdad, Cairo, Damascus, Cordova, and many other cities under their control, luxurious hospital accommodations were frequently provided. Harun al-Rashid, the glamorous caliph (a title for a religious or civil ruler claiming succession from Muhammad) of Baghdad (786 to 809), built a system of hospitals. Medical care in these hospitals was free. About four centuries later, in 1160, a Jewish traveler reported that he had found as many as 60 dispensaries and infirmaries in Baghdad alone. The Persian physician Rhazes, who lived from about 850 to 923, was skilled in surgery. He was probably the first to use the intestines of sheep for suturing and cleansing patient wounds with alcohol.

Mohammedan physicians like Rhazes received much of their medical knowledge from the persecuted Christian sect known as the Nestorians. Nestorius, driven into the desert with his followers after having been appointed patriarch of Constantinople, took up the study of medicine. The school at Edessa in Mesopotamia, with its two large hospitals, eventually came under the control of the Nestorians in which they established a remarkable teaching institution. Eventually driven out of Mesopotamia by the orthodox bishop Cyrus, they fled to Persia, establishing the famous school at Gundishapur, which is conceded to be the true starting point of Mohammedan medicine. Gundishapur was home to the world's oldest known teaching hospital and also contained a library and a university. It was located in the present-day province of Khuzistan, in the southwest of Iran, not far from the Karun river.

Mohammedan medicine flourished up to about the 15th century. Mohammedan physicians were acquainted with the possibilities of inhalation anesthesia. They instituted precautions against adulteration of drugs and developed a vast number of new drugs. Mohammedan countries also built asylums for the mentally ill a thousand years before such institutions appeared in Europe. The people of Islam made a brilliant start in medicine but never fulfilled the great promise that glowed in their early work in medical arts and hospitalization. Wars, politics, superstitions, and a nonprogressive philosophy stunted the growth of a system that had influenced the development of hospitals.

EARLY MILITARY HOSPITALS

Engraved on a limestone pillar dating back to the Sumerians (2920 BC) are pictures, which, among other military procedures, show the assemblage of the wounded. The book of Deuteronomy records that Moses laid down outstanding rules of military hygiene. Out of the urgency of care for the wounded in battle came much of the impetus for medical progress. Hippocrates is quoted as saying that "war is the only proper school for a surgeon." Under the Romans, surgery advanced largely because of experience gained through gladiatorial and military surgery.

MEDIEVAL HOSPITALS

Religion continued to dominate the establishment of hospitals during the Middle Ages. Although physicians cared for physical ailments to afford relief, they rarely attempted to cure the sick. Dissection of a human body would have been sacrilege because the body was created in the image of God.

Religion continued to be the most important factor in the establishment of hospitals during the Middle Ages. A number of religious orders created travelers' rests and infirmaries adjacent to monasteries that provided food and temporary shelter for weary travelers and pilgrims.

The hospital movement grew rapidly during the Crusades, which began in 1096. Military hospital orders sprang up, and accommodations for sick and exhausted crusaders were provided along all traveled roads. One body of crusaders organized the Hospitalers of the Order of St. John, which in 1099 established in the Holy Land a hospital capable of caring for 2000 patients. Knights of this order took personal charge of service to patients and often denied themselves so that the sick might have food and medical care.

Finally, an active period of hospital growth came during the late 12th and early 13th centuries. In 1198, Pope Innocent III urged that hospitals of the Holy Spirit be subscribed for by the citizenry of many towns. He set an example by founding a model hospital in Rome, known as Santo Spirito in Sassia. Built in 1204, it survived until 1922, when it was destroyed by fire. In Rome, nine other hospitals were founded shortly after completion of the one in Sassia. It is estimated that in Germany alone 155 towns had hospitals of the Holy Spirit during early medieval times.

Although most hospitals erected during the Middle Ages were associated with monasteries or founded by religious groups, a few cities, particularly in England, built municipal institutions. Like all hospitals of the period, the buildings were costly, often decorated with colorful tapestries and stained glass windows, but the interiors often consisted of large, drafty halls with beds lining each side.

With the spread of leprosy during the 12th and 13th centuries, lazar houses sprang up, supplying additional hospital facilities. Crude structures, lazar houses were usually built on the outskirts of towns and maintained for the segregation of lepers rather than for their treatment. Special groups of attendants, including members of the Order of St. Lazar, nursed the patients. The group represented an important social and hygienic movement because their actions served to check the spread of epidemics through isolation. The group is credited for virtually stamping out leprosy.

During the same period of hospital growth, three famous London institutions were established: St. Bartholomew's in 1137, St. Thomas's before 1207, and St. Mary of Bethlehem in 1247. St. Bartholomew's cared for the sick poor, but unlike like many hospitals of that day, it was well organized. St. Thomas's Hospital was founded by a woman, later canonized as St. Mary Overie. It burned in 1207, was rebuilt six years later, and constructed again on a new site in 1228. St. Mary of Bethlehem was the first English hospital to be used exclusively for the mentally ill.

The Hotel-Dieu of Paris was probably typical of the better hospitals of the Middle Ages. Built at the beginning of the 13th century, the hospital provided four principal rooms for patients in various stages of disease, as well as a room for convalescents and another for maternity patients. Illustrations by artists of the time show that two persons generally shared one bed. Heavy curtains sometimes hung from canopies over the bed to afford privacy, but this advantage was more than offset by the fact that the draperies, never washed, spread infection and prevented free ventilation. The institution was self-contained, maintaining a bakery, herb garden, and farm. Often, patients who had fully recovered remained at the hospital to work on the farm or in the garden for several days in appreciation for the care they had received.

THE "DARK AGE" OF HOSPITALS

Most hospitals during the Middle Ages, however, were not as efficiently managed as the Hotel-Dieu of Paris. Pictures and records prove that many hospitals commonly crowded several patients into one bed regardless of the type or seriousness of illness. A mildly ill patient might be placed in the same bed as an occupant suffering from a contagious disease. A notable exception to the general deterioration in medicine during this era was the effort of those monks who copied by hand and preserved the writings of Hippocrates and other ancient physicians.

The great Al-Mansur Hospital, built in Cairo in 1276, struck a contrast to the European institutions of the Middle Ages. It was equipped with separate wards for the more serious diseases and outpatient clinics. The handful of hospitals like Al-Mansur would lay the groundwork for hospital progress to come in later centuries.

HOSPITALS OF THE RENAISSANCE

During the revival of learning around the close of the 14th century, hundreds of medical hospitals in Western Europe received the new, more inquiring surgeons that the Renaissance produced. New drugs were developed, and anatomy became a recognized study. Ancient Greek writings were printed, and dissection was performed by such masters as Leonardo da Vinci, known as the originator of cross-sectional anatomy, and Vesalius. Hospitals also became more organized. Memoranda from 1569 describe the duties of the medical staff in the civil hospital of Padua, a city that was home to the most famous medical school during the 16th century. These read:

> There shall be a doctor of physic upon whom rests the duty of visiting all the poor patients in the building, females as well as males; a doctor of surgery whose duty it is to apply ointments to all the poor people in the hospital who have wounds of any kind; and a barber who is competent to do, for the women as well as the men, all the other things that a good surgeon usually does.

The practice of surgery during the Renaissance became more scientific. Surgery was practiced by the long-robe surgeons, a small group who were educated in the universities and permitted to perform all types of operations, and by the short-robe surgeons, the barbers who in most communities were allowed only to leech and shave the patient, unless permission was granted to extend the scope of treatment. Both groups were regarded as inferior to physicians.

In 1506, a band of long-robe surgeons organized the Royal College of Surgeons of Edinburgh. By 1540, both the long- and the short-robe surgeons in England joined to form the Company of Barber-Surgeons of London. In 1528, English physicians were organized by Thomas Linacre, physician to Henry VIII, as the Royal College of Physicians of England.

During the 16th century, Henry VIII of England ordered that hospitals associated with the Catholic church be given over to secular uses or destroyed. The sick were turned into the streets. Conditions in hospitals became so intolerable that the king was petitioned to return one or two buildings for the care of patients. Henry consented and restored St. Bartholomew's in 1544. Practically the only hope for the sick poor among outlying towns was to journey many miles to London.

The dearth of hospitals in England continued throughout the 17th century, when the medical school was developed. The French and the English quickly accepted what had originated in Italy: the first attempt to make medical instruction practical. St. Bartholomew's took the lead in education by establishing a medical library in 1667 and permitted apprentices to walk the wards for clinical teaching under experienced surgeons.

In 1634, an outstanding contribution was made to nursing by the founding of the order of the Daughters of Charity of St. Vincent de Paul. Originating at the Hotel-Dieu of Paris as a small group of village girls who were taught nursing by the nuns, the order grew rapidly and was transplanted to the United States by Mother Seton in 1809.

HOSPITALS OF THE 18TH CENTURY

During the 18th century, the building of hospitals revived partially. Because of poverty, at first the movement made slow progress in England, but a few hospitals were built and supported jointly by parishes. By 1732, there were 115 such institutions in England, some of them a combination of almshouse and hospital.

The Royal College of Physicians established a dispensary where medical advice was given free and medicines were sold to the needy at cost. Controversies and lawsuits, however, brought an untimely end to this early clinic. Not discouraged by this experience, the Westminster Charitable Society created a similar dispensary in 1715. The same organization in 1719 founded Westminster Hospital, an infirmary built by voluntary subscription, in which the staff gave its services gratuitously. Ten years later, the Royal College of Physicians in Edinburgh opened the Royal Infirmary. London Hospital, another notable, had its origin in 1740. Admission of charity patients to the London Hospital was apparently by ticket because among its historical relics is an admission card.

Antony van Leeuwenhoek (1632 to 1723) succeeded in making some of the most important discoveries in the history of biology. Although Leeuwenhoek did not invent the first microscope, he was able to perfect it. Many of his discoveries included bacteria, free-living and parasitic microscopic protists, sperm cells, blood cells, and microscopic nematodes. His research opened up an entire world of microscopic life. Leeuwenhoek had a pronounced influence on the creation of the sciences of cytology, bacteriology, and pathology.

EARLY HOSPITALS IN THE UNITED STATES

Manhattan Island claims the first account of a hospital in the New World: a hospital that was used in 1663 for sick soldiers. Fifty years later, in Philadelphia, William Penn founded the first almshouse established in the American colonies. The Quakers supported the almshouse, which was open only to members of that faith. However, Philadelphia was rapidly growing and also in need of a public almshouse. Such an institution for the aged, the infirm, and the mentally ill was established in 1732. The institution later became the historic Old Blockley, which in turn evolved into the Philadelphia General Hospital.

Philadelphia was the site of the first incorporated hospital in America, the Pennsylvania Hospital. Dr. Thomas Bond wanted to provide a place where Philadelphia physicians might treat their private patients. With the aid of Benjamin Franklin, Bond sought a charter for the Pennsylvania Hospital, which was granted by the crown in 1751. The first staff consisted of Dr. Phineas Bond, Dr. Lloyd Zachary, and the founder, Dr. Thomas Bond, all of whom gave their services without remuneration for three years.

Dr. John Jones, an American, published a book in 1775 charging that hospitals abroad were crowded far beyond capacity, that Hotel-Dieu of Paris frequently placed three to five patients in one bed—the convalescent with the dying and fracture cases with infectious cases. He estimated that one-fifth of the 22,000 patients cared for at Hotel-Dieu died each year. Wounds were washed daily with a sponge that was carried from patient to patient. The infection rate was said to be 100%. Mortality after amputation was as high as 60%. Jones's call to action had a positive effect on American health care.

As late as 1769, New York City, with nearly 300,000 inhabitants, was without hospitals. In 1771, a small group of citizens, Dr. Jones among them, formed the Society of the New York Hospital. The society purchased a five acre site and made plans for a model hospital, which fell into the hands of British troops during the Revolution.

During postwar reconstruction, the New York Hospital broadened its services. Under the supervision of Dr. Valentine Seaman, the hospital began providing instruction in nursing, and in 1779 it introduced vaccination in the United States and established an ambulance service.

Other early American hospitals of historic interest include the first psychiatric hospital in the New World, founded at Williamsburg, Virginia, in 1773, and a branch of federal hospitals created by passage of the US Marine

Hospital Service Act in 1798. Under this act, two marine hospitals were established in 1802, one in Boston and another in Norfolk, Virginia.

The Massachusetts General Hospital, which pioneered many improvements in medicine, originated in Boston. Its first patient, admitted in 1821, was a 30-year-old sailor.

In 1832, the Boston Lying-In Hospital opened its doors to women who were unable to afford in-home medical care. It was one of the nation's first maternity hospitals, made possible because of fundraising appeals to individuals and charitable organizations.

Surgeons of the day had sufficient knowledge of anatomy to lead them to perform many ordinary operations, and as a result more surgery was probably undertaken than during any previous era. While surgeons had sought to keep wounds clean, even using wine in an attempt to accomplish this purpose, 19th-century surgeons believed suppuration (the production and discharge of pus) to be desirable and encouraged it. Hospital wards were filled with discharging wounds. Nurses of that period are said to have used snuff to make conditions tolerable. Surgeons wore their operating coats for months without washing. The same bed linens served several patients. Pain, hemorrhage, infection, and gangrene infested the wards. Mortality from surgical operations rated as high as 90% to 100%.

LATE 19TH-CENTURY RENAISSANCE

Florence Nightingale, the famous English nurse, began her career by training at Kaiserswerth on the Rhine in a hospital and deaconess home established in 1836 by Theodor Fliedner and his wife. Florence Nightingale wrote disparagingly of her training there, particularly of the hygiene practiced. Returning to England, she put her own ideas of nursing into effect and rapidly acquired a reputation for efficient work.

By 1854, during the Crimean War, the English government, disturbed by reports of conditions among the sick and wounded soldiers, selected Florence Nightingale as the one person capable of improving patient care. Upon her arrival at the military hospital in Crimea with a small band of nurses whom she had assembled, she found that the sick were lying on canvas sheets in the midst of dirt and vermin. She proceeded to establish order and cleanliness. She organized diet kitchens, a laundry service, and departments of supplies, often using her own funds to finance her projects. Ten days after her arrival, the newly established kitchens were feeding 1000 soldiers. Within three months, 10,000 soldiers were receiving clothing, food, and medicine.

As the field of nursing continued to progress, so did medicine. Crawford Long, for example, first used ether as an anesthetic in 1842 to remove a small tumor from the neck of a patient. He did not publish any accounts of his work until later, however, so the discovery is often attributed to W. T. G. Morgan, a dentist who developed sulfuric ether and arranged for the first hospital operation under anesthesia at Massachusetts General Hospital in 1846. Although not put to practical use immediately, ether soon took away some of the horror that hospitals had engendered in the public mind. Chloroform was first used as an anesthetic in 1847 for an obstetrical case in England by Sir James Simpson.

The year 1847 also brought about the founding of the American Medical Association (AMA) under the leadership of Dr. Nathan Smith Davis. The association, among its main objectives, strived to improve medical education, but most of the organization's tangible efforts in education began at the close of the century. The AMA was a strong advocate for establishing a code of ethics, promoting public health measures, and improving the status of medicine.

The culmination of Florence Nightingale's work came in 1860 after her return to England. There she founded the Nightingale School of Nursing at the St. Thomas Hospital. From this school, a group of 15 nurses graduated in 1863. They later became the pioneer heads of training schools throughout the world.

In 1886, the Royal British Nurses' Association (RBNA) was formed. The RBNA worked toward establishing a standard of technical excellence in nursing. A charter granted to the RBNA in 1893 denied nurses a register, although it did agree to maintain a list of persons who could apply to have their name entered thereon as nurses.

The first formally organized American nursing schools were established in 1872 at the New England Hospital for Women and Children in Boston (Brigham and Women's Hospital), and then in 1873 at Bellevue, New Haven, and Massachusetts General Hospital. In 1884, Alice Fisher was appointed as the first head of the nurse training at Philadelphia Hospital's (renamed as the Philadelphia General Hospital in 1902) nurses' training school. She had the distinction of being the first Nightingale-trained nurse recruited to Philadelphia upon recommendation by Florence Nightingale.

Mrs. Bedford Fenwick, a nurse leader in the English nurse registration movement, traveled to Chicago in 1893 to arrange the English nursing exhibit. As part of the Congress on Hospitals and Dispensaries, a nursing section included papers on establishing standards in hospital training schools, the establishment of a nurses' association, and nurse registration. The group formulated plans to improve nursing curriculum and hospital administration in the first concerted attempt to improve hospitals through a national organization.

Progress in Infection Control

Ignaz Philipp Semmelweis of Vienna, Austria, unknowingly laid the foundation for Pasteur's later work. In 1847, at the Vienna Lying-in Hospital, Europe's largest teaching obstetrical department, he declared that the alarming number of deaths from puerperal fever was due to infection transmitted by students who came directly from the dissecting room to take care of maternity patients. Semmelweis noted that Division 1 of the hospital was a medical student teaching service; Division 2 was utilized for midwife trainees. Maternal deaths for Division 1 averaged 10%; Division 2 averaged 3%. Medical students performed autopsies; midwives did not. As a result of these findings, an order was posted on May 15, 1847, requiring all students to scrub their hands in chlorinated lime until the cadaver smell was gone. The order was later revised to include hand washing between patients.

Semmelweis had the satisfaction of seeing the mortality rate in his obstetrical cases drop from 9.92% to 1.27% in little more than a year as a result of an aseptic technique that he devised. A few years later, Louis Pasteur demonstrated the scientific reason for Semmelweis's success when he proved that bacteria were produced by reproduction and not by spontaneous generation, as was then generally believed. From his work came the origin of modern bacteriology and clinical laboratories.

Also of great importance to hospitals and infection control was Bergmann's introduction of steam sterilization in 1886 and William Stewart Halstead's introduction of rubber gloves in 1890.

By the end of the century, Lister carried Pasteur's work a step further and showed that wound healing could be hastened by using antiseptics to destroy disease-bearing organisms and by preventing contaminated air from coming into contact with these wounds. Lister was not content with obtaining better results in his own surgical cases; he devoted his life to proving that suppuration is dangerous and that it should be prevented or reduced by use of antiseptics. Despite his successful work and eloquent pleas, his colleagues persisted in following their old methods. As time went on and antiseptics and the techniques of using them were improved, even the skeptical were impressed by the clinical results.

Discovery of Anesthesia

The discovery of anesthesia and the principle of antiseptics are to be regarded as two of the most significant influences in the development of surgical procedures and the modern hospital. Anesthesia improved pain control, and hygiene practices which helped reduce the incidence of surgical site infections.

Modern Hospital Laboratory

The study of cytology originated during the middle of the 19th century and influenced the development of the modern hospital clinical laboratory. The cell theory was first advanced in 1839 by the German anatomist Theodor Schwann and was further developed by Jacob Henle, whose writings on microscopic anatomy appeared about 1850. Rudolph Virchow was the most eminent proponent of the cell theory. His studies in cellular pathology speeded research in the etiology of disease.

Changing Hospital Structure

With nursing, anesthesia, infection control, and cytology under way, a change in hospital structure began in the last quarter of the 19th century. Buildings of the Civil War days continued with as many as 25 to 50 beds in a ward, with little provision for segregation of patients. In New York City in 1871, construction of Roosevelt Hospital, built on the lines of a one-story pavilion with small wards, set the style for a new type of architecture that came to be known as the American plan. A noteworthy feature was ventilation by means of openings in the roof, a definite improvement upon earlier hospitals that were characterized by a lack of provision for ventilation. Dr. W. G. Wylie, writing in 1877, said he favored this type of building, but he advocated that it be a temporary structure only, to be destroyed when it became infected.

Changing Hospital Function

Promoted by the wealth of bacteriological discoveries, hospitals began to care for patients with communicable diseases. During the decade 1880 to 1890, the tubercle bacillus was discovered; Pasteur vaccinated against anthrax; Koch isolated the cholera bacillus; diphtheria was first treated with antitoxin; the tetanus bacillus and the parasite of malarial fever were isolated; and inoculation for rabies was successful. Treatment of patients with some of the infections necessitated isolation, and hospitals were the logical place for observation of communicable diseases. Consequently, at the end of the century, in addition to their many surgical cases, hospitals were crowded with large numbers of patients suffering from scarlet fever, diphtheria, typhoid, and smallpox.

Discovery of the X-Ray

Wilhelm Konrad Roentgen's discovery of the X-ray in 1895 was a major scientific achievement. The first use of the X-ray symbolizes the beginning of the period that necessitated equipment so costly that the average practitioner could not afford to install it. The natural result was the founding of community hospitals in which physicians could jointly use such equipment. Nineteenth-century inventions also included the clinical thermometer, the laryngoscope, the Hermann Helmholtz ophthalmoscope, and innumerable other aids to accurate diagnosis.

20TH-CENTURY PROGRESS

The treatment of metabolic diseases, nutritional deficiencies, the importance of vitamins, and the therapy of glandular extracts played an important role in the advancement of medicine in the 20th century. As early as 1906, Gowland Hopkins began investigations of vitamins. Two years later, Carlos Finlay produced experimental rickets by means of a vitamin-deficient diet. This, in turn, was followed by Kurt Huldschinsky's discovery that rickets could be treated successfully with ultraviolet light. In quick succession came Casimir Funk's work with vitamins, Elmer McCollum's discovery of vitamins A and B, Joseph Goldberger's work in the prevention of pellagra, and Harry Steenbock's irradiation of foods and oils. Other outstanding contributions to the science of nutrition include Frederick Banting's introduction of insulin in 1922, the studies in anemia carried out by George Hoyt Whipple and Frieda Robscheit-Robbins, and the Minot and Murphy liver extract.

Einthoven's invention of the electrocardiograph in 1903 marked the beginning of an era of diagnostic and therapeutic aids. Shortly after that invention came the first basal metabolism apparatus, then the Wassermann (August Von) test in 1906, followed by tests for pancreatic function, and the invention of the fluoroscopic screen followed in 1908. Subsequently, the introduction of blood tests and examinations of numerous body secretions required well-equipped and varied laboratories. Concurrent with this progress in the field of internal medicine was the introduction of radium for the treatment of malignant growths, increasing the use of the clinical laboratory for microscopic examination of pathological tissue, and developments in antibiotics. The result of these many new aids was the conquest of diseases formerly regarded as incurable, which in turn resulted in improved public confidence in hospitals.

The 20th century is also characterized by rapid growth in nursing education. The earlier schools were maintained almost entirely for the purpose of securing nursing service at a low cost. The nurses' duties were often menial, the hours long, and classroom and laboratory study almost entirely lacking. Nurses themselves had begun to organize for educational reforms. By 1910, training increasingly emphasized theoretical studies. This movement was largely due to the work of organizations such as the American Nurses Association and the National League for Nursing, along with the organization of the Committee on the Grading of Nursing Schools. In 1943, the US Cadet Nurse Corps was organized to spur enrollment of student nurses in nursing schools to help meet the shortages due to enlistment of graduate nurses for military service. As a result, efforts increased to train practical nurses and nurses' aides to relieve the shortage of graduate nurses.

Reform in medical education began early in the century and was due almost wholly to the efforts of the Council on Medical Education and Hospitals, which was established in 1905 by the American Medical Association. Immediately after its organization, this council began inspection of medical schools. The council, by establishing standards and by grading the schools, brought about gradual elimination of most of the unethical, commercial, and unqualified institutions.

A great stimulus to the profession of hospital administration has been the work of the American Hospital Association. Organized in 1899 as the Association of Hospital Superintendents, it took its present name in 1907. Since its inception, the organization has concerned itself particularly with the problems of hospital management. As early as 1910, the association held educational programs for hospital chief executive officers and trustees.

The American College of Surgeons was founded in 1913 under the leadership of Dr. Franklin H. Martin, the first director general of the organization. One of the most dramatic of the achievements of the American College of Surgeons was the hospital standardization movement begun in 1918. The founders drew up what was known as the "minimum standard," a veritable constitution for hospitals, setting forth requirements for the proper care of the sick. An annual survey of all hospitals having 25 or more beds made the standard effective. In 1918, when the first survey was conducted, only 89 hospitals in the United States and Canada could meet the requirements.

The hospital standardization movement focused its efforts on the patient, with the goal of providing the patient with the best professional, scientific, and humanitarian care possible. The growth of this movement is remarkable, especially given that participation in the hospital standardization (now referred to as The Joint Commission) program is voluntary.

The years following 1929 will be remembered as a trying period in the history of hospitals. Due to critical economic conditions, many institutions found it difficult to keep their doors open. Lowered bed occupancy and increased charity load, coupled with steadily decreasing revenues from endowments and other sources of income, worked hardships on private institutions.

In the later half of the 20th century, competition among hospitals began to grow as for-profit hospital chains began to spring up and compete with nonprofit organizations. Advances in medical technology, such as CT, MRI, and PET scanners and robotic surgery, as well as an ever-growing list of new medications, have revolutionized the practice of medicine. Less-invasive surgical procedures and a trend toward care in outpatient settings have reduced the need for lengthy in-hospital stays.

HEALTH CARE AND HOSPITALS IN THE 21ST CENTURY

The challenges of health care are enormous and continue to test health care organizations. Some of today's health care challenges include exorbitant malpractice awards; skyrocketing insurance premiums; high expectations of society for miracle drugs and miracle cures; balancing fairly the mistakes of caregivers with the hundreds of thousands of successful events that occur each year across the nation; negative press that increases public fear; the ethical dilemmas of abortion and human cloning; the exponential growth of information and medical technology; and the ever-increasing shortage of nurses, physicians, pharmacists, physical therapists, and the like. The ability to provide affordable access to health care services to even the insured is an ongoing challenge. There are nearly 47 million uninsured Americans (16% of the population), and the numbers continue to increase. Even those with insurance are often underinsured for catastrophic occurrences. In addition, with employer-based coverage declining, many working families are left with decreasing health benefits. Unfortunately, there is little evidence that the US Congress is able to reach any consensus for effectively addressing the issue. The greatest challenge of the 21st century requires that each member of society assume a more proactive role in his or her health care.

JUST A BEGINNING

The pinnacle of hospital evolution has not been reached nor has the final page of its colorful history been written. As long as there remains a humanitarian impulse, as long as a society feels compassion, love, and sympathy for its neighbors, there will be hospitals. In the past, hospitals changed as conditions changed. In the future, they will continue to change to meet the needs of their communities. Health care leaders of the 21st century must understand their roots and the historical value of knowing the past, have the vision to preserve the good, and the passion to create an even better health care system.

2

INTRODUCTION TO LAW

This chapter introduces the reader to the development of law, the functioning of the legal system, and the roles of the different branches of government in creating, administering, and enforcing the law. It is important to understand the foundation of the US legal system before one can appreciate or comprehend the specific laws and principles relating to health care. Chief Justice Marshall, in delivering his opinion to the Court in *Marbury v. Madison*, said "The very essence of civil liberty certainly consists in the right of every individual to claim the protection of the laws, whenever he receives an injury. One of the first duties of government is to afford that protection. [The] government of the United States has been emphatically termed a government of laws, and not of men. It will certainly cease to deserve this high appellation, if the laws furnish no remedy for the violation of a vested right."[1]

Most scholars define the law as a system of principles and processes by which people in a society deal with disputes and problems, seeking to solve or settle them without resorting to force. Simply stated, laws are rules of conduct enforced by government, which imposes penalties when prescribed laws are violated.

Laws govern the relationships between private individuals and organizations and between both of these parties and government. Public law deals with relationships between individuals and government; private law deals with relationships among individuals.

One important segment of public law, for example, is criminal law, which prohibits conduct deemed injurious to public order and provides for punishment of those proven to have engaged in such conduct. In contrast, private law is concerned with the recognition and enforcement of the rights and duties of private individuals. Tort and contract actions are two basic types of private law. In a tort action, one party asserts that the wrongful conduct of another has caused harm, and the injured party seeks compensation for the harm suffered. A contract action usually involves a claim by

ting (e.g., Centers for Medicare and Medicaid Services [CMS]), and power over business practices (e.g., National Labor Relations Board [NLRB]).

Administrative agencies have legislative, judicial, and executive functions. They have the authority to formulate rules and regulations considered necessary to carry out the intent of legislative enactments. Regulatory agencies have the ability to legislate, adjudicate, and enforce their own regulations in many cases.

Rules and regulations established by an administrative agency must be administered within the scope of authority delegated to it by Congress. Although an agency must comply with its own regulations, agency regulations must be consistent with the statute under which they are promulgated. An agency's interpretation of a statute cannot supersede the language chosen by Congress. An executive regulation that defines some general statutory term in a too-restrictive or unrealistic manner is invalid. Agency regulations and administrative decisions are subject to judicial review when questions arise as to whether an agency has overstepped its bounds in its interpretation of the law.

Recourse to an administrative agency for resolution of a dispute is generally required prior to seeking judicial review. The Pennsylvania Commonwealth Court held in *Fair Rest Home v. Commonwealth, Department of Health*[5] that the department of health was required to hold a hearing before it ordered revocation of a nursing home's operating license. The department of health failed in its responsibility when "in a revocation proceeding it [did] not give careful consideration to its statutorily mandated responsibility to hear testimony."[6]

Conflict of Laws

The following case illustrates how federal and state laws can be in conflict. The plaintiff in *Dorsten v. Lapeer County General Hospital*[7] brought an action against a hospital and certain physicians on the medical board alleging wrongful denial of her application for medical staff privileges. The plaintiff asserted claims under the US Code for sex discrimination, violations of the Sherman Antitrust Act, and the like. The plaintiff filed a motion to compel discovery of peer-review reports to support her case. The US District Court held that the plaintiff was entitled to discovery of peer-review reports despite a Michigan state law purporting to establish an absolute privilege for peer-review reports conducted by hospital review boards.

GOVERNMENT ORGANIZATION

The three branches of the federal government are the legislative, executive, and judicial branches. A vital concept in the constitutional framework of government on both federal and state levels is the separation of powers. Essentially, this principle provides that no one branch of government is clearly dominant over the other two; however, in the exercise of its functions, each can affect and limit the activities, functions, and powers of the others.

Legislative Branch

On the federal level, legislative powers are vested in the Congress of the United States, which consists of the Senate and the House of Representatives. The function of the legislative branch is to enact laws that can amend or repeal existing legislation and to create new legislation. The legislature determines the nature and extent of the need for new laws and for changes in existing laws. Committees of both houses of Congress are responsible for preparing federal legislation.

Executive Branch

The primary function of the executive branch of government on the federal and state level is to administer and enforce the law. The chief executive, either the president of the United States or the governor of a state, also has a role in the creation of law through the power to approve or veto legislative proposals.

The president serves as the administrative head of the executive branch of the federal government. The executive branch includes 15 executive departments, as well as a variety of agencies, both temporary and permanent. Each department is responsible for a different area of public affairs, and each enforces the law within its area of responsibility.

On a state level, the governor serves as the chief executive officer. The responsibilities of a governor are provided for in the state's constitution. The Massachusetts State Constitution, for example, describes the responsibilities of the governor as presenting an annual budget to the state legislature, recommending new legislation, vetoing legislation, appointing and removing department heads, appointing judicial officers, and acting as Commander-in-Chief of the state's military forces (the Massachusetts National Guard).

Judicial Branch

The function of the judicial branch of government is adjudication—resolving disputes in accordance with law. As a practical matter, most disputes or controversies that are covered by legal principles or rules are resolved without resort to the courts.

The decision as to which court has jurisdiction—the legal right to hear and rule on a particular case—is determined by such matters as the locality in which each party to a lawsuit resides and the issues of a lawsuit. Each state in the United States provides its own court system, which is created by the state's constitution and statutes. Most of the nation's judicial business is reviewed and acted on in state courts. Each state maintains a level of trial courts that have original jurisdiction, meaning the authority of a court to first conduct a trial on a specific case as distinguished from a court with appellate jurisdiction, where appeals from trial judgments are held. This jurisdiction can exclude cases involving claims with damages less than a specified minimum, probate matters (i.e., wills and estates), and workers' compensation. Different states have designated different names for trial courts (e.g., superior, district, circuit, or supreme courts). Also on the trial court level are minor courts such as city, small claims, and justice of the peace courts.

Each state has at least one appellate court. Many states have an intermediate appellate court between the trial courts and the court of last resort. Where this intermediate court is present, there is a provision for appeal to it, with further review in all but select cases. Because of this format, the highest appellate tribunal is seen as the final arbiter in cases that possess importance in themselves or for the particular state's system of jurisprudence.

The trial court of the federal system is the US District Court. There are 89 district courts in the 50 states (the larger states have more than one district court) and one in the District of Columbia. The Commonwealth of Puerto Rico also has a district court with jurisdiction corresponding to that of district courts in the different states. Generally, only one judge is required to sit and decide a case, although certain cases require up to three judges. The federal district courts hear civil, criminal, admiralty, and bankruptcy cases.

The US Courts of Appeals are appellate courts for the 11 judicial circuits. Their main purpose is to review cases tried in federal district courts within their respective circuits, but they also possess jurisdiction to review orders of designated administrative agencies and to issue original writs in appropriate cases. These intermediate appellate courts were created to relieve the US Supreme Court of deciding all cases appealed from the federal trial courts.

The Supreme Court, the nation's highest court, is the only federal court created directly by the Constitution. Eight associate justices and one chief justice sit on the Supreme Court. The court has limited original jurisdiction over the lower federal courts and the highest state courts. In a few situations, an appeal will go directly from a federal or state court to the Supreme Court, but in most cases, review must be sought through the discretionary writ of certiorari, an appeal petition. In addition to the aforementioned courts, special federal courts have jurisdiction over particular subject matters. The US Court of Claims, for example, has jurisdiction over certain claims against the government. The US Court of Appeals for the Federal Circuit has appellate jurisdiction over certain customs and patent matters. The US Customs Court reviews certain administrative decisions by customs officials. Also, there is a US Tax Court and a US Court of Military Appeals.

Separation of Powers

The concept of separation of powers, a system of checks and balances, is illustrated in the relationships among the branches of government with regard to legislation. On the federal level, when a bill creating a statute is enacted by Congress and signed by the president, it becomes law. If the president vetoes a bill, it takes a two-thirds vote of each house of Congress to override the veto. The president also can prevent a bill from becoming law by avoiding any action while Congress is in session. This procedure, known as a pocket veto, can temporarily stop a bill from becoming law and can permanently prevent it from becoming law if later sessions of Congress do not act on it favorably. A bill that has become law can be declared invalid by the Supreme Court if the law violates the Constitution.

Even though a Supreme Court decision is final regarding a specific controversy, Congress and the president can generate new, constitutionally sound legislation to replace a law that has been declared unconstitutional. The procedures for amending the Constitution are complex and often time consuming, but they can serve as a way to offset or override a Supreme Court decision.

DEPARTMENT OF HEALTH AND HUMAN SERVICES

The Department of Health and Human Services (DHHS), a cabinet-level department of the executive branch of the federal government, is concerned with people and is most involved with the nation's human concerns. The DHHS is responsible for developing and implementing appropriate administrative regulations for carrying out national health and human services policy objectives. It is also the main source of regulations affecting the health care industry. The secretary of the DHHS, serving as the department's administrative head, advises the president with regard to health, welfare, and income security plans, policies, and programs.

The DHHS also is responsible for many of the programs designed to meet the needs of senior citizens, including Social Security benefits (e.g., retirement, survivors, and disability), Supplemental Security Income (which ensures a minimum monthly income to needy persons and is administered by local Social Security offices), Medicare, Medicaid, and programs under the Older Americans Act (e.g., in-home services, such as home health and home-delivered meals, and community services such as adult day care, transportation, and ombudsman services in long-term care facilities).

The Centers for Disease Control and Prevention

The Centers for Disease Control and Prevention (CDC) is recognized as the lead federal agency for protecting the health and safety of people at home and abroad, providing credible information to enhance health decisions, and promoting health. The CDC serves as the national focus for developing and applying disease prevention and control, environmental health, and health promotion and education activities.

The Centers for Medicare and Medicaid Services

The Centers for Medicare and Medicaid Services (CMS), formerly the Health Care Financing Administration, was created to combine under one administration the oversight of the Medicare program, the federal portion of the Medicaid program, the State Children's Health Insurance Program, and related quality-assurance activities.

Medicare

Medicare is a federally sponsored health insurance program for persons older than 65 and certain disabled persons. It has two complementary parts: Medicare Part A helps cover the costs of inpatient hospital care and, with qualifying preadmission criteria, skilled nursing facility care, home health care, and hospice care. Medicare Part B Medical helps pay for physicians' services and outpatient hospital services.

Medicare is funded through Social Security contributions (Federal Insurance Contributions Act payroll taxes), premiums, and general revenue. The program is administered through private contractors, referred to as intermediaries, under Part A and carriers under Part B. The financing of the Medicare program has received much attention by Congress because of its rapidly rising costs and drain on the nation's economy. However, many in Congress argue that the costs associated with the Iraq war are the real culprits draining the entire economy.

Medicaid

The Medicaid program, Title XIX of the Social Security Act Amendments of 1965, is a government program administered by the states that provides medical services (both institutional and outpatient) to the medically needy. Federal grants, in the form of matching funds, are issued to those states with qualifying Medicaid programs. In other words, Medicaid is jointly sponsored and financed by the federal government and several states. Medical care for needy persons of all ages is provided under the definition of need established by each state. Each state has set its own criteria for determining eligibility for services under its Medicaid program.

Public Health Service

The mission of the Public Health Service (PHS) is to promote the protection of the nation's physical and mental health. The PHS accomplishes its mission by coordinating with the states in setting and implementing national health policy and pursuing effective intergovernmental relations; generating and upholding cooperative international health-related agreements, policies, and programs; conducting medical and biomedical research; sponsoring and administering programs for the development of health resources, the prevention and control of diseases, and alcohol and drug abuse; providing resources and expertise to the states and other public and private institutions in the planning, direction, and delivery of physical and mental health care services; and enforcing laws to ensure drug safety and protection from impure and unsafe foods, cosmetics, medical devices, and radiation-producing objects. Within the PHS are smaller agencies that are responsible for carrying out the purpose of the division and DHHS and include the following:

- *Agency for Healthcare Research and Quality*: The Agency for Healthcare Research and Quality (AHRQ) research provides evidence-based information on health care outcomes, quality, cost, use, and access. Information from AHRQ's research helps people make more informed decisions and improve the quality of health care services.
- *Food and Drug Administration*: The Food and Drug Administration (FDA) supervises and controls the introduction of drugs, foods, cosmetics, and medical devices into the marketplace and protects society from impure and hazardous items.
- *National Institutes of Health*: The National Institutes of Health (NIH) is the principal federal biomedical research agency. It is responsible for conducting, supporting, and promoting biomedical research.

Notes

1. 5 U.S. (Cranch) 137, 163 (1803).
2. *Black's Law Dictionary* 1305 (6th ed. 1990).
3. 5 U.S.C.S. §§ 500–576 (Law. Co-op. 1989).
4. An "agency means each authority of the Government of the United States, . . . but does not include (A) the Congress; the Courts of the United States; . . ." 5 U.S.C.S. § 551(1) (Law. Co-op. 1989).
5. 401 A.2d 872 (Pa. Commw. Ct. 1979).
6. Id. at 873.
7. 88 F.R.D. 583 (E.D. Mich. 1980).

3

Tort Law

This chapter introduces the reader to the study of tort law, with an emphasis on negligence in health settings. A *tort* is a civil wrong committed against a person or property for which a court provides a remedy in the form of an action for damages. The basic objectives of tort law include: *preservation of peace* between individuals; *determining fault* for wrongdoing; *deterrence* by discouraging the wrongdoer from committing future tortous acts; and to provide *compensation* for the person/s injured.

The three basic categories of tort law are: (1) *negligent torts*; (2) *intentional torts* (e.g., assault and battery, false imprisonment, invasion of privacy, and infliction of mental distress); and (3) *strict liability*, irrespective of fault (applied where the activity, regardless of intentions or negligence, is so dangerous to others that public policy demands absolute responsibility on the part of the wrongdoer (e.g., products liability).

NEGLIGENCE

Negligence is a tort. It is the unintentional commission or omission of an act that a reasonably prudent person would or would not do under the same or similar circumstances.

Commission of an act would include, for example:

- administering the wrong medication
- administering the wrong dosage of a medication
- administering medication to the wrong patient
- performing a surgical procedure without patient consent
- performing a surgical procedure on the wrong patient
- performing the wrong surgical procedure

Omission of an act would include, for example:

- failing to conduct a thorough history and physical examination

- failing to assess and reassess a patient's nutritional needs
- failing to administer medications
- failing to order diagnostic tests
- failing to follow up on critical lab tests

Negligence is a form of conduct caused by heedlessness or carelessness that constitutes a departure from the standard of care generally imposed on reasonable members of society. It can occur when after considering the consequences of an act, a person does not exercise the best possible judgment; where one fails to guard against a risk that should be appreciated; or where one engages in behavior expected to involve unreasonable danger to others. Negligence or carelessness of a professional person (e.g., nurse practitioner, pharmacist, physician) is classified as *malpractice*.

Malpractice suits can allege various mistakes made by medical professionals, including misdiagnosis, mistreatment, delayed diagnosis, failure to diagnose, surgical errors, medical errors. It has been estimated that there are 100,000 deaths per year due to medical errors.

Not all errors in medical diagnosis and treatment are considered to be malpractice. Any medical or surgical intervention will involve some degree of risk. It is the responsibility of the treating professional to inform his or her patient as to the inherent risks, benefits, and alternatives of a proposed treatment or procedure.

Forms of Negligence

The three basic forms of negligence are:

1. *Malfeasance*: performance of an unlawful or improper act (e.g., performing an abortion in the third trimester when such is prohibited by state law)
2. *Misfeasance*: improper performance of an act, resulting in injury to another (e.g., wrong-sided surgery, such as removal of the healthy left kidney instead of the diseased right kidney; mistakenly administering a lethal dose or potentially lethal dose of a medication)
3. *Nonfeasance*: failure to act, when there is a duty to act as a reasonably prudent person would under similar circumstances (e.g., failing to administer medications, such as insulin, as ordered by the treating physician)

Degrees of Negligence

There are two generally accepted degrees of negligence:

1. *Ordinary negligence*: failure to do what a reasonably prudent person would or would not do under the circumstances of the act or omission in question
2. *Gross negligence*: the intentional or wanton omission of required care or performance of an improper act

Elements of Negligence

The elements that must be present for a plaintiff to recover damages caused by negligence are:

1. *Duty to care*
   - Obligation to conform to a recognized standard of care.
2. *Breach of duty*
   - Deviation from the recognized standard of care.
   - Failure to adhere to an obligation.
3. *Injury*
   - Actual damages must be established.
   - If there are no injuries, no damages are due the plaintiff(s).
4. *Causation*
   - The departure from the standard of care must be the cause of the plaintiff's injury.
   - The injury must be foreseeable.

All four elements of negligence must be present for a plaintiff to recover damages suffered as a result of a negligent act.

The foundation of the columns in Figure 3-1 describes examples of negligent acts (e.g., wrong site surgery). The pillars represent those elements that must be proven in order to establish that negligence has occurred. Any unproven element of negligence (e.g., injury) will defeat a lawsuit brought forward on the basis of negligence.

Duty to Care

Duty is a legal obligation of care, performance, or observance imposed on one to safeguard the rights of others. Duty can arise from a special relationship such as that between a physician and a patient. Duty to care can arise from a simple telephone conversation or out of a physician's voluntary act of assuming the care of a patient. Duty also can be established by statute or contract between the plaintiff and the defendant.

Standard of Care

A duty of care carries with it a corresponding responsibility not only to provide care, but also to provide it in an acceptable manner. The fact that an injury is suffered is not sufficient for imposing liability without proof that the defendant deviated from the standard practice of competent fellow professionals. A nurse, for example, who assumes the care of a patient has the duty to exercise that degree of skill, care, and knowledge ordinarily possessed and exercised by other nurses. The actual performance required of an individual in a given situation will be measured against what a reasonably prudent person would or would not have done. The reasonableness of conduct is judged in light of the circumstances apparent at the time of injury and by reference to different characteristics of the actor (e.g., age, sex, physical condition, education, knowledge, training, mental capacity). Deviation from the standard of care will constitute negligence if there are resulting damages.

Traditionally, in determining how a reasonably prudent person should perform in a given situation, the courts often rely on the testimony of an expert witness as to the standard of care required in the same or similar communities. Expert testimony is necessary when the jury is not trained or qualified to determine

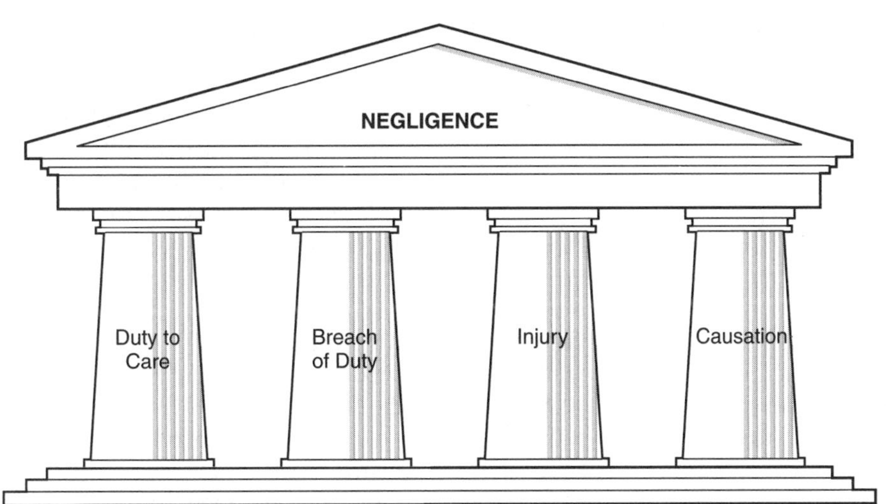

Figure 3-1 Pillars: Negligence

what the reasonably prudent professional's standard of care would be under similar circumstances. Most states hold those with special skills (e.g., physicians, nurses, and dentists) to a standard of care that is reasonable in the light of their special abilities and knowledge.

Evidence of the standard of care applicable to professional activities can be found in a variety of documents, such as regulations of government agencies (e.g., state licensure laws) and standards established by organizations, such as The Joint Commission.

Failure to Treat Emergency Patient

In *O'Neill v. Montefiore Hospital*,[1] the duty owed to a patient was clear. The plaintiff sought recovery against the hospital for failure to render necessary emergency treatment and against a physician for his failure and refusal to treat her spouse. The deceased, Mr. O'Neill, had been experiencing pain in his chest and arms. He walked with his wife to the hospital at 5:00 a.m. He claimed that he was a member of the Hospital Insurance Plan (HIP). The emergency department nurse stated that the hospital had no connection with HIP and did not take HIP patients. The nurse indicated that she would try to get a HIP physician for O'Neill. The nurse called Dr. Graig, a HIP physician, and explained the patient's symptoms to the doctor. It was suggested by Dr. Graig that Mr. O'Neill see a HIP physician at 8:00 a.m. The nurse then handed the phone to Mr. O'Neill, who said, "Well, I could be dead by 8 o'clock." Mr. O'Neill concluded his phone conversation and spoke to the nurse, indicating that he had been told to go home and come back when HIP was open. Mrs. O'Neill asked that a physician see her husband. The nurse again requested that they return at 8:00. Mr. O'Neill again commented that he could be dead by 8:00. He then left with his wife to return home, pausing occasionally to catch his breath. Shortly after arriving home, Mr. O'Neill suddenly fell to the floor and died. Dr. Graig claimed that he had offered to come to the emergency department, but that Mr. O'Neill had said he would wait and see another HIP physician at 8:00 that morning.

The New York Supreme Court, Appellate Division held that a physician who abandons a patient after undertaking examination or treatment can be held liable for malpractice. The proof of the record in this case indicated that the physician undertook to diagnose the ailments of the deceased by telephone, thus establishing at least the first element of negligence—duty to use due care.

Failure to Stabilize Patient Before Transfer

In a similar case, the surviving parents in *Hastings v. Baton Rouge Hospital*[2] brought a medical malpractice action for the wrongful death of their 19-year-old son. The action was brought against the hospital; the emergency department physician, Dr. Gerdes; and the thoracic surgeon on call, Dr. McCool. The patient had been brought to the emergency department at 11:56 p.m. because of two stab wounds and weak vital signs. Dr. Gerdes decided that a thoracotomy had to be performed. He was not qualified to perform the surgery and called Dr. McCool, who was on call that evening for thoracic surgery. Dr. Gerdes described the patient's condition, indicating he had been stabbed in a major blood vessel. At trial, Dr. McCool claimed that he did not recall Dr. Gerdes saying that a major blood vessel could be involved. Dr. McCool asked Dr. Gerdes to transfer the patient to the Earl K. Long Hospital. Dr. Gerdes said, "I can't transfer this patient." McCool replied, "No. Transfer him." Kelly, an emergency department nurse on duty, was not comfortable with the decision to transfer the patient and offered to accompany him in the ambulance. Dr. Gerdes reexamined the patient, who exhibited marginal vital signs, was restless, and was draining blood from his chest. The ambulance service was called at 1:03 a.m., and by 1:30 a.m. the patient had been placed in the ambulance for transfer. The patient began to fight wildly, the chest tube came out, and bleeding increased. The patient went into cardiac arrest. An attempt to revive him was futile and the patient died after having been moved back to the emergency department. The patient virtually bled to death.

The duty to care in this case cannot be reasonably disputed. Louisiana, by statute, imposes a duty on hospitals licensed in Louisiana to make emergency services available to all persons residing in the state regardless of insurance coverage or economic status. The hospital's own bylaws provide that patient transfer should never occur without due consideration for the patient's condition. The 19th Judicial District Court directed a verdict for the defendants, and the plaintiffs appealed. The court of appeals affirmed the district court's decision. On further appeal, the Louisiana Supreme Court held that the evidence presented to the jury could indicate the defendants were negligent in their treatment of the victim. The findings of the lower courts were reversed, and the case was remanded for trial.

Duties Created by Statute

Some duties are created by statute, which occurs when a statute specifies a particular standard that must be met. Many such standards are created by administrative agencies under the provisions of a statute. To establish liability based on a defendant's failure to follow the standard of care outlined by statute, the following elements must be present:

1. the defendant must have been within the specified class of persons outlined in the statute;
2. the plaintiff must have been injured in a way that the statute was designed to prevent; and,
3. the plaintiff must show that the injury would not have occurred if the statute had not been violated.

Duties Created by Policy

Duties can also be created by an organization through its internal policies, procedures, rules, and regulations. The courts hold that such internal rules are indicative of the organization's knowledge of the proper procedure to follow and, hence, create a duty. Thus, if an employee fails to follow an operating rule of an organization and, as a result, a patient is injured, then the employee who violated the rule would be considered negligent for causing the injury.

Duty to Hire Competent Employees

Texas courts recognize that an employer has a duty to hire competent employees, especially if they are engaged in an occupation that could be hazardous to life and limb and requires skilled or experienced persons. For example, the appellant in *Deerings West Nursing Center v. Scott*[3] was found to have negligently hired an incompetent employee that it knew or should have known was incompetent, thereby causing unreasonable risk of harm to others. In this case, an 80-year-old visitor had gone to Deerings to visit her infirm older brother. During one visit, Nurse Hopper, a 6-foot-4-inch male employee of Deerings, confronted the visitor to prevent her from visiting. The visitor recalled that he was angry and just stared. She stated that upon his approach she had thrown up her hands to protect her face, but he hit her on the chin, slapped her down onto the concrete floor, and got on top of her, pinning her to the floor.

Hopper testified that he was hired sight unseen over the telephone by Deerings's director of nursing. Even though the following day, Hopper completed an application at the nursing facility, he still maintained that he was hired over the phone. In his application, he falsely stated that he was a Texas licensed vocational nurse (LVN). Additionally, he claimed that he had never been convicted of a crime. In reality, he had been previously employed by a bar, was not a LVN, had committed more than 56 criminal offenses of theft, and was on probation at the time of his testimony.

Deerings showed a clear duty to care. The appellant violated the very purpose of Texas licensing statutes by failing to verify whether

Hopper held a current LVN license. The appellant then placed him in a position of authority by allowing him to dispense drugs and by making him a shift supervisor. This negligence eventually resulted in the assault on an elderly woman. The employee's failure to obtain a nursing license was the proximate cause of the visitor's damages. Deerings's hiring of Hopper showed a heedless and reckless disregard of the rights of others.

It is common knowledge that the bleakness and rigors of old age, drugs, and the diseases of senility can cause people to become confused . . . and cantankerous. It is predictable that elderly patients will be visited by elderly friends and family. It is reasonable to anticipate that a man of proven moral baseness would be more likely to commit a morally base act on an 80-year-old woman. Fifty-six convictions for theft is some evidence of mental aberration. Hopper was employed not only to administer medicine but also to contend with the sometimes erratic behavior of the decrepit. The investigative process necessary to the procurement of a Texas nursing license would have precluded the licensing of Hopper. In the hiring of an unlicensed and potentially mentally and morally unfit nurse, it is reasonable to anticipate that an injury would result as a natural and probable consequence of that negligent hiring.[4]

Breach of Duty

When a duty to care has been established, the plaintiff must demonstrate that the defendant breached that duty by failing to comply with the accepted standard of care. Breach of duty is the failure to conform to or the departure from a required duty of care owed to a person. The obligation to perform according to a standard of care can encompass either doing or refraining from doing a particular act.

The court in *Hastings v. Baton Rouge Hospital*,[5] discussed earlier, found a severe breach of duty when a patient did not receive adequate care. Hospital regulations provided that when a physician cannot be reached or refuses a call, the chief of service must be notified so that another physician can be obtained. This was not done. A plaintiff need not prove that a patient would have survived if proper treatment had been administered but only that the patient would have had a chance of survival. As a result of Dr. Gerdes's failure to make arrangements for another physician and Dr. McCool's failure to perform the necessary surgery, the patient had no chance of survival. The duty to provide for appropriate care under the circumstances was breached.

Injury/Actual Damages

Without harm or injury, there is no liability. Injury includes physical harm, pain, suffering, and loss of income or reputation. The mere occurrence of an injury does not establish negligence for which the law imposes liability because the injury might be the result of an unavoidable accident or an act of God.

Failure to Render Care

Injury was obvious in *Lucas v. HCMF Corp.*,[6] where the patient had been transferred to a nursing facility following hospitalization for several ailments, including early decubitus ulcers. The resident was returned to the hospital 24 days later. An ulcer on her buttocks had grown from one inch in diameter to eight inches in diameter and extended to the bone. The standard of care required in preventing and treating decubitus ulcers required that the resident be mobilized and turned every two hours to prevent deterioration of tissue. Treatment records reflected that the resident was not turned from September 22 through October 1, nor was she turned on October 4, 7, or 12. Failure to periodically turn the resident and move her to a chair had caused the deterioration in her condition.

Causation

The element of *causation* requires that there be a reasonable, close, and causal connection or relationship between the defendant's negligent conduct and the resulting damages. In other words, the defendant's negligence must be a substantial factor causing the injury. *Proximate cause* is a term that refers to the relationship between a breach of duty and the resulting injury. The breach of duty must be the proximate cause of the resulting injury. The mere departure from a proper and recognized procedure is not sufficient to enable a patient to recover damages unless the plaintiff can show that the departure was unreasonable and the proximate cause of the patient's injuries. Causation in the *Hastings v. Baton Rouge Hospital*[7] case was well established. In the ordinary course of events, Hastings would not have bled to death in a hospital emergency department over a two-hour period if surgical intervention had been introduced in a timely manner to save his life.

Negligent Misreading of CT Scan

The patient–plaintiff in *Dic v. Brooklyn Hospital Center*[8] was admitted into the hospital complaining of a severe headache, an inability to open her eyes, and the absence of feeling in her legs. A CT scan was taken and read by a staff physician as normal. After discharging the plaintiff, the hospital's radiologist reviewed the CT scan and concluded it was "not" normal. The defendant did not contact the plaintiff to alert her about the revised finding. The hospital conceded that its employee's initial misreading of the CT scan and its failure to alert the plaintiff to the misreading were departures from accepted medical practice. The jury found that those departures were the proximate causes of the plaintiff's injury.

Delay in Diagnosing Breast Cancer

The plaintiff, while in the custody of a penal institution, alleged that because the institution's employees failed to timely diagnose her breast cancer, her right breast had to be removed. Pursuant to the institution's policy of medically evaluating all new inmates, on May 26, 1989, Dr. Evans gave the plaintiff a medical examination. He testified that his physical evaluation of the plaintiff's breasts was cursory.

The day following her examination, the plaintiff examined her own breasts. At that time she discovered a lump in her right breast, which she characterized as being about the size of a pea. The plaintiff then sought an additional medical evaluation at the defendant's medical clinic. Testimony indicated that fewer than half of the inmates who sign the clinic list are actually seen by medical personnel the next day. Also, those not examined on the day for which the list is signed are given no preference in being examined on the following day. The evidence indicated that after May 27, the plaintiff constantly signed the clinic list and provided the reason she was requesting medical care. A nurse examined the plaintiff on June 21. The nurse noted in her nursing notes that the plaintiff had a "moderate large mass in right breast." The nurse failed to measure the mass. She testified that no measuring device was available. The missing measuring device was a simple ruler. The nurse concluded that Dr. Evans should again examine the plaintiff.

On June 28, Dr. Evans again examined the plaintiff. He recorded in the progress notes that the plaintiff had "a mass on her right wrist. Will send her to hospital and give her Benadryl for allergy she has." Dr. Evans meant to write "breast" not "wrist." He again failed to measure the size of the mass on the plaintiff's breast.

The plaintiff was transferred to the Franklin County Prerelease Center (FCPR) on September 28. On September 30, a nurse at FCPR examined the plaintiff; the nurse recorded that the plaintiff had a "golf-ball"-sized lump in her right breast. The plaintiff was transported to the hospital on October 27, where Dr. Walker treated her. The plaintiff received a mammogram examination, which indicated that the tumor was probably malignant. This diagnosis was confirmed by a biopsy performed on November 9. The plaintiff was released from confinement on November 13.

On November 16, a surgeon examined the plaintiff. He noted the existence of the lump in the plaintiff's breast and determined that the size of the mass was approximately 4 to 5 centimeters and somewhat fixed. He performed a modified radical mastectomy upon the plaintiff's right breast.

The Ohio Court of Appeals was appalled that the physician had characterized his evaluation as a medical examination or had implied that what he described as a "cursory breast examination" should be considered to be a medically sufficient breast examination. It was probable that an earlier procedure would have safely and reliably conserved a large part of the plaintiff's right breast. Through inexcusable delays, the plaintiff lost this option. The court concluded that the defendant's negligence was the sole and proximate cause of the plaintiff's losses.[9]

Failure to Administer Proper Nourishment

Under the Illinois Nursing Home Care Reform Act, the owner and licensee of a nursing home are liable to a resident for any intentional or negligent act or omission of their agents or employees that injures a resident. The act defines *neglect* as a failure in a facility to provide adequate medical or personal care or maintenance, when failure results in physical or mental injury to a resident or in the deterioration of the resident's condition. Personal care and maintenance include providing food, water, and assistance with meals necessary to sustain a healthy life.

The nursing facility in this case maintained no records of the resident's fluid intake and output. A nurse testified that such a record was a required nursing facility procedure that should have been followed for a person in the resident's condition but was not. The resident's condition deteriorated after staying six and a half days at the facility. Upon entering a hospital, the resident was diagnosed as suffering from severe dehydration. The nursing facility offered no alternative explanation for the resident's dehydrated condition. As a result of the facility's failure to maintain adequate records, the resident suffered severe dehydration that required hospital treatment. The evidence demonstrated that the proximate cause of the resident's dehydration was the nursing facility's failure to administer proper nourishment.[10]

Foreseeability

Foreseeability is the reasonable anticipation that harm or injury is likely to result from an act or an omission to act. The test for foreseeability is whether a reasonable person should have anticipated the danger to others caused by a negligent act. The test is not what the wrongdoer believed would occur; it is whether he or she ought reasonably to have foreseen that the event in question would occur.

When a defendant's actions fail to meet the standard of care, negligence has occurred, and the jury must make two determinations. First, was it foreseeable that harm would occur from the failure to meet the standard of care? Second, was the carelessness or negligence the proximate or immediate cause of the harm or injury to the plaintiff?

Patient Fails to Provide Known Allergies

There is no expectation that a person can guard against events that cannot reasonably be foreseen or that are so unlikely to occur that they would be disregarded. For example, in *Haynes v. Hoffman*,[11] the plaintiff brought a medical malpractice action against the defendant physician for his alleged negligence in prescribing a medication to which the plaintiff suffered an allergic reaction. The trial court returned a verdict in favor of the defendant, and the plaintiff appealed. The evidence at trial revealed that the plaintiff had not disclosed her history of allergies to the physician. The physician testified that, at the time of the physical examination of the plaintiff, she denied having any allergies. The physician testified that he would not have prescribed the drug had he known the plaintiff's complete history. By failing to disclose her allergies to the physician, the plaintiff through her negligence contributed to her own injury. Foreseeability involves guarding against that which is probable and likely to happen, not against that which is only remotely and slightly possible. Generally, the issue of foreseeability is for the trial court to decide. A duty to prevent a wrongful act by a third party will be imposed only where those wrongful acts can be reasonably anticipated.

SUMMARY CASE

All the elements necessary to establish negligence were well established in *Niles v. City of San Rafael*.[12] On June 26, 1973, at approximately 3:30 p.m., Kelly Niles, a young boy, got into an argument with another boy on a ball field, and he was hit on the right side of his head. He rode home on his bicycle and waited for his father, who was to pick him up for the weekend. At approximately 5:00 p.m., his father arrived to pick him up. By the time they arrived in San Francisco, Kelly appeared to be in a great deal of pain. His father then decided to take him to Mount Zion Hospital, which was a short distance away. He arrived at the hospital emergency department at approximately 5:45 p.m. On admission to the emergency department, Kelly was taken to a treatment room by a registered nurse. The nurse obtained a history of the injury and took Kelly's pulse and blood pressure. During his stay in the emergency department, he was irritable, vomited several times, and complained that his head hurt. An intern who had seen Kelly wrote, "pale, diaphoretic, and groggy," on the patient's chart. Skull X-rays were ordered and found to be negative except for soft tissue swelling that was not noted until later. The intern then decided to admit the patient. A second-year resident was called, and he agreed with the intern's decision. An admitting clerk called the intern and indicated that the patient had to be admitted by an attending physician. The resident went as far as to write "admit" on the chart and later crossed it out. A pediatrician who was in the emergency department at the time was asked to look at Kelly. The pediatrician was also the paid director of the Mount Zion Pediatric Out-Patient Clinic. The pediatrician asked Kelly a few questions and then decided to send him home. The physician could not recall what instructions he gave the patient's father, but he did give the father his business card.

The pediatrician could not recall giving the father a copy of the emergency department's head injury instructions, an information sheet that had been prepared for distribution to patients with head injuries. The sheet explained that an individual should be returned to the emergency department should any of the following signs appear: a large, soft lump on the head; unusual drowsiness (cannot be awakened); forceful or repeated vomiting; a fit or convulsion (jerking or spells); clumsy walking; bad headache; and/or one pupil larger than the other.

Kelly was taken back to his father's apartment at about 7:00 p.m. A psychiatrist friend stopped by at approximately 8:45 p.m. He examined Kelly and noted that one pupil was larger than the other. Because the pediatrician could not be reached, the patient was taken back to the emergency department. A physician on duty noted an epidural hematoma during his examination and ordered that a neurosurgeon be called.

Today, Kelly can move only his eyes and neck. A lawsuit against Mount Zion and the pediatrician for $5 million was instituted. Expert testimony by two neurosurgeons during the trial indicated that the patient's chances of recovery would have been very good if he had been admitted promptly. This testimony placed the proximate cause of the injury with the hospital. The final judgment was $4 million against the medical defendants, $2.5 million for compensatory damages, and another $1.5 million for pain and suffering.

Case Lessons

Each case presented in this book illustrates actual experiences of plaintiffs and defendants, enabling the reader to apply the lessons learned to real-life situations. The many lessons in *Niles v. City of San Rafael* include the following:

- An organization can improve the quality of patient care rendered in the facility by establishing and adhering to policies, procedures, and protocols that facilitate the delivery of quality care across all disciplines.
  - The provision of quality health care requires collaboration across disciplines.
  - A physician must conduct a thorough and responsible examination and order the appropriate tests for each patient, evaluating the results of those tests, and providing appropriate treatment prior to discharging the patient.
  - A patient's vital signs must be monitored closely and documented in the medical record.
  - Corrective measures must be taken when a patient's medical condition signals a medical problem.
  - A complete review of a patient's medical record must be accomplished before discharging a patient. Review of the record must include review of test results, nurses' notes, residents' and interns' notes, and the notes of any other physician or consultant who might have attended the patient.
  - An erroneous diagnosis leading to the premature dismissal of a case can result in liability for both the organization and physician.

INTENTIONAL TORTS

There are two main differences between intentional and negligent wrongs. The first is intent, which is present in intentional but not in negligent wrongs. For a tort to be considered intentional, the act must be committed intentionally, and the wrongdoer must realize to a substantial certainty that harm would result. The second difference is less obvious. While a negligent wrong can simply be the failure to act when there is a legal duty to act, an intentional wrong always involves a willful act that violates another's interests. Intentional wrongs include such acts as assault, battery, false imprisonment, defamation of character, fraud, invasion of privacy, and infliction of emotional distress.

Assault and Battery

It has long been recognized by law that a person possesses a right to be free from aggression and the threat of actual aggression against one's person. The right to expect others to respect the integrity of one's body has roots in both common and statutory law. The distinguishing feature between assault and battery is that assault effectuates an infringement on the mental security or tranquility of another whereas battery constitutes a violation of another's physical integrity.

Assault

An assault is defined as the deliberate threat, coupled with the apparent present ability, to do physical harm to another. No actual contact is necessary. To commit the tort of assault, two conditions must exist: First, the person attempting to touch another unlawfully must possess the apparent present ability to commit the battery; second, the person threatened must be aware of or have actual knowledge of and fear of an immediate threat of a battery.

Battery

Battery is the intentional touching of another's person in a socially impermissible manner, without that person's consent. The law provides a remedy if consent to a touching has not been obtained or if the act goes beyond the consent given. Therefore, the injured person can initiate a lawsuit against the wrongdoer for damages suffered.

In the health care context, the principle of law concerning battery and the requirement of consent to medical and surgical procedures is critically important. Liability of organizations and health care professionals for acts of battery is most common in situations involving lack of patient consent to medical and surgical procedures.

It is of no legal importance that a procedure constituting a battery has improved a patient's health. If the patient did not consent to the touching, the patient might be entitled to such damages as can be proved to have resulted from commission of the battery. In *Perna v. Pirozzi*,[13] the New Jersey Supreme Court held that a patient who consents to surgery by one surgeon and is actually operated on by another has an action for medical malpractice or battery. Proof of unauthorized invasion of the plaintiff's person, even if harmless, can entitle one to nominal damages.

False Imprisonment

False imprisonment is the unlawful restraint of an individual's personal liberty or the unlawful restraint or confinement of an individual. The personal right to move freely and without hindrance is basic to the legal system. Any intentional infringement on this right can constitute false imprisonment. Actual physical force is not necessary to constitute false imprisonment; false imprisonment can occur when an individual who is physically confined to a given area reasonably fears detainment or intimidation without legal justification. Both intimidation and forced detainment can be implied by words, threats, or gestures. Excessive force used to restrain a patient can produce liability for both false imprisonment and battery.

To recover for damages for false imprisonment, a plaintiff must be aware of the confinement and have "no" reasonable means of escape. Availability of a reasonable means of escape can bar recovery. To lock a door when another is reasonably available to pass through is not imprisonment. However, if the only other door provides a way of escape that is dangerous, the law might consider it an unreasonable way of escape and, therefore, false imprisonment can be a cause of action.

Some occasions and circumstances allow for a person's confinement, such as when a person presents a self-danger or a danger to others. Criminals are incarcerated, as are sometimes the mentally ill who can present a danger to themselves or others. Patients are sometimes restrained to prevent falls. Children are retained after school for disciplinary reasons. In these examples, the right to move about freely has been violated, but the infringement occurs for reasons that are justifiable under the law.

Physically Violent Persons

In *Celestine v. United States*,[14] the right to move about freely had been violated; however, the infringement was permissible for reasons justifiable under the law. In this case, the plaintiff had brought an action alleging battery and false imprisonment because security guards had placed him in restraints. The plaintiff–appellant sought psychiatric care at a veterans administration (VA) hospital. He became physically violent while waiting to be seen by a physician. The VA security guards placed him in restraints until a psychiatrist could examine him. The US Court of Appeals for the Eighth Circuit held that the record supported a finding that the hospital was justified in placing the patient under restraint. Under Missouri law, no false imprisonment or battery occurred in view of the common-law principle that a person believed to be mentally ill could be restrained lawfully if such was considered necessary to prevent immediate injury to that person or others.

Contagious Diseases

Protocols should be instituted for handling patients diagnosed as having contracted a highly contagious disease. Detaining such patients, without statutory protection, constitutes false imprisonment. State health codes generally provide guidelines for caring for such patients.

Behavioral Health Patients

Statutes in many states allow mentally ill and intoxicated individuals to be detained if they are found to be dangerous to themselves or others. Those who are mentally ill, however, can be restrained only to the degree necessary to prevent them from harming themselves or others. If a mentally ill patient cannot be released, procedures should be followed to provide commitment to an appropriate institution for the patient's care.

Restraints

Restraints generally are used to control behavior when patients are disoriented or can cause harm to themselves (e.g., from falling, contaminating wounds, or pulling out intravenous lines) or to others. The use of restraints raises many questions of a patient's rights in the areas of autonomy, freedom of movement, and the accompanying health problems that can result from continued immobility. In general, a patient has a right to be free from any physical restraints imposed or psychoactive drugs administered for purposes of discipline or convenience and that are not required to treat a patient's medical symptoms.

Although the motivations for using restraints appear to be sound, there has been a tendency toward overuse. The fear of litigation over injuries sustained because of the failure to apply restraints further compounds the problem of overuse. As a result, regulations governing the use of restraints under the Omnibus Budget Reconciliation Act of 1987 make it clear that restraints are to be applied as a last resort rather than as a first option in the control of a resident's behavior. Because prescription drugs are sometimes used to restrain behavior, the regulations represent the first time that prescription drugs must by law "be justified by indications documented in the medical chart."[15]

To avoid legal problems, health care organizations should implement policies aimed at eliminating or reducing the use of restraints. Programs for the effective use of restraints should include the following:

- written policies that conform to federal and state guidelines (e.g., a policy prescribing that the least-restrictive device will be utilized to maintain the safety of the patient, a policy requiring the periodic review of patients under restraint, and a policy requiring physician orders for restraints)
- procedures for implementing organizational policies (e.g., alternatives to follow before restraining a patient can include family counseling to encourage increased visitations, environmental change, activity therapies, and patient counseling)
- periodic review of policies and procedures, with revision as necessary
- education and orientation programs for the staff to be conducted inside and outside the organization
- education programs for patients and their families
- a sound appraisal of each patient's needs
- informed consent from the patient or legal guardian
- the application of the least-restrictive restraints
- constant monitoring of the patient to determine the continuing need for restraints, injury to the patient, and complaints by the patient
- documentation that includes:
  - the need for restraints
  - time-limited orders ("as needed" PRN orders are not acceptable)
  - consents for the application of restraints
  - patient monitoring
  - reappraisal of the continuing need for restraints

Discharge Against Medical Advice

Patients who decide to leave a facility against medical advice should be requested to sign a discharge against advice form. Should a patient refuse to sign such a form, such refusal should be noted in the patient's record.

Defamation of Character

Another type of intentional tort comes in the form of defamation of character. *Defamation of character* is a communication to someone about another person that tends to hold that person's reputation up to scorn and ridicule. To be an actionable wrong, defamation must be communicated to a third person; defamatory statements communicated only to the injured party are not grounds for an action. *Libel* is the written form of defamation and can be presented in such forms as signs, photographs, letters, and cartoons. *Slander* is the verbal form of defamation and tends to form prejudices against a person in the eyes of third persons.

Slander

Slander lawsuits are rare because of the difficulty in proving defamation, the small awards, and high legal fees. With slander, the person who brings suit generally must prove special damages; however, when any allegedly defamatory words refer to a person in a professional capacity, the professional need not show that the words caused damage. It is presumed that any slanderous reference to someone's professional capacity is damaging.

Professionals who are called incompetent in front of others have a right to sue to defend their reputation. However, it is difficult to prove that an individual comment was injurious. If the person making an injurious comment cannot prove that the comment is true, then that person can be held liable for damages.

Libel

In a libel or slander per se (on its face) action, a court will presume that certain words and accusations cause injury to a person's reputation without proof of damages. Words or accusations that require no proof of actual harm to one's reputation are: (1) accusing someone of a crime, (2) accusing someone of having a loathsome disease, (3) using words that affect a person's profession or business, and (4) calling a woman unchaste. Health care professionals are, however, legally protected against libel when complying with a law that requires the reporting of venereal or other diseases. Damages typically consist of economic losses, such as loss of business or employment.

Defenses to a Defamation Action

Essentially, the two defenses to a defamation action are truth and privilege. When a person has said something that is damaging to another person's reputation, the person making the statement will not be liable for defamation if it can be shown that the statement is true. A privileged communication differs from a defamatory statement in that the person making the communication has a responsibility to do so. For example, many states have statutes providing immunity to physicians and health care institutions in connection with peer review activities. The person making the communication must do so in good faith, on the proper occasion, in the proper manner, and to persons who have a legitimate reason to receive the information.

An administrator's statements made to a physician's supervisor regarding the physician's alleged professional misconduct are not grounds for a defamation action as long as the statements are made in good faith. A hospital administrator has a duty to report complaints about alleged professional misconduct of physicians working in the hospital. The administrator has qualified privilege to report such complaints to the physician's supervisor and other hospital officials as necessary.[16]

It is important to note that public figures have more difficulty in pursuing defamation litigation than the average individual. Legal action against a public figure generally will be denied in the absence of any showing of actual malice in connection with alleged defamatory references to a plaintiff. Actual malice applies only in cases involving public figures and encompasses knowledge of falsity or recklessness as to truth.

Performance Appraisals Not for General Publication

A statement in a hospital newsletter regarding the discharge of a nursing supervisor constituted libel per se in *Kraus v. Brandsletter*.[17] The newsletter indicated that the hospital's medical board had discharged the nursing supervisor after a unanimous vote of no confidence. Couching the board's determination in terms of a vote gave the impression that the board's determination had been based on facts that justified the board's opinion. The statement tended to injure the nurse's reputation as a professional because it did not refer to specifics of her performance but rather to her abilities as a professional in general. The reasonable interpretation of the statement in the newsletter was that the supervisor was incompetent in her professional capacity, thus giving rise to a cause of action for libel per se.

On the flip side in the same case, an alleged statement that a physician said, "You nurses will receive your Christmas bonus early, your boss is going to get fired," was not slander per se in that it did not injure the nurse in her professional capacity.[18] In addition, the statement that she was going to be fired was true.

Performance Appraisal Statements Not Libelous

In *Schauer v. Memorial Care System*,[19] the plaintiff applied for and was given a supervisory position at Memorial Hospital's new cateterization laboratory. In March 1989, she received an employment appraisal for the period June 1988 through December 1988. At that time, Schauer's supervisor rated her performance as "commendable" in two categories and "fair" in eight categories, with an overall rating of "fair." Although Schauer did not lose her job as a result of the appraisal, she brought an action against the hospital and her former supervisor for libel and emotional distress as a result of the appraisal. The hospital moved for summary judgment on the grounds that the employment appraisal was not defamatory as a matter of law, the hospital had qualified privilege to write the performance appraisal, and the claim for emotional distress did not reach the level of severity required for a claim for intentional infliction of emotional distress. The trial court granted the hospital's motion for summary judgment, and Schauer appealed.

The Texas Court of Appeals held that the statements contained in the performance appraisal were not libelous and that the appraisal was subject to qualified privilege. Moreover, the hospital's conduct and the statements contained in the appraisal did not support the claim for intentional infliction of emotional distress.

To sustain her claim of defamation, Schauer had to show that the hospital published her appraisal in a defamatory manner that injured her reputation in some way. A statement can be unpleasant and objectionable to the plaintiff without being defamatory. The hospital argued that the statements contained in the appraisal were truthful, permissible expressions of opinion and not capable of a defamatory meaning. Schauer's supervisor prepared the appraisal as part of her supervisory duties. The appraisal was not published outside the hospital and was prepared in compliance with the hospital policy for all employees. Schauer disputed her overall rating of "fair" as being libelous. "Clearly, this is a statement of her supervisor's opinion and is not defamatory as a matter of law."[20]

In her performance appraisal, Schauer objected to the statement, "Ms. Schauer was not sensitive to employee relations."[21] Schauer conceded in her deposition that there were a number of interpersonal problems in the catheterization laboratory and that she did not get along with everyone. The court found that given these admissions, the statement was not defamatory.

Newspaper Articles

A libel suit was brought against the Miami Herald Publishing Company more than two years after its publication of an editorial cartoon depicting a nursing facility in a distasteful manner.[22] The cartoon was described in the following manner:

> On October 29, 1980, *The Herald* published an editorial cartoon which depicted three men in a dilapidated room. On the back wall was written

> "Krest View Nursing Home," and on the side wall there was a board which read "Closed by Order of the State of Florida." The room itself was in a state of total disrepair. There were holes in the floor and ceiling, leaking water pipes, and exposed wiring. The men in the room were dressed in outfits resembling those commonly appearing in caricatures of gangsters. Each man carried a sack with a dollar sign on it. One of the men was larger than the other two and was more in the forefront of the picture. One of the others addressed him. The caption read: "Don't Worry, Boss, We Can Always Reopen It As a Haunted House for the Kiddies."[23]

The court held that the newspaper's editorial cartoon depicting persons resembling gangsters in a dilapidated building, identified as a particular nursing facility that had been closed by state order, was an expression of pure opinion and was protected by the First Amendment against the libel suit alleging that the cartoon defamed the owner of the facility.

Fraud

Fraud is defined as willful and intentional misrepresentation that could cause harm or loss to a person or property. Fraud includes any cunning, deception, or artifice used, in violation of legal or equitable duty, to circumvent, cheat, or deceive another. The forms it can assume and the means by which it can be practiced are as multifarious as human ingenuity can devise, and the courts consider it unwise or impossible to formulate an exact, definite, and all-inclusive definition of the action.

To prove fraud, the following facts must be shown:

- an untrue statement known to be untrue by the party making it and made with the intent to deceive
- justifiable reliance by the victim on the truth of the statement
- damages as a result of that reliance

Concealment of Information from Patient

The plaintiff in *Robinson v. Shah*[24] was a long-time patient of defendant, Dr. Shah, from 1975 to 1986. During that period of time, the defendant treated the plaintiff for various gynecological disorders. On November 9, 1983, the defendant performed a total abdominal hysterectomy and bilateral salpingo-oophorectomy on the plaintiff. Approximately one week following surgery, the plaintiff was discharged from the hospital and was assured that there were no complications or potential problems that might arise as a result of the surgery. On the day after the plaintiff was discharged from the hospital, she began to experience abdominal distress. She consulted the defendant about these symptoms, and the defendant ordered X-rays to be taken of the plaintiff's kidneys, ureter, and bladder in an effort to explain her discomfort.

The X-rays were taken at a hospital and were read and interpreted by Dr. Cavanaugh, presumably a radiologist associated with that facility. After reading the X-rays, Cavanaugh called the defendant and reported that the slides showed the presence of surgical sponges that had been left in the plaintiff's abdomen after surgery. Cavanaugh also sent the defendant a copy of a written report that reflected the findings.

The defendant fraudulently concealed from the plaintiff the findings of the X-rays. The defendant told the plaintiff that the X-rays were negative and that there were no apparent or unusual complications from the recent abdominal surgery, and she assured the plaintiff that she did not require further treatment. At no time did the defendant reveal to the plaintiff the fact that she had left surgical sponges in the plaintiff's abdomen.

Over the next several years, the plaintiff continued to see the defendant for gynecological checkups. She continued to experience abdominal pain and discomfort. The defendant, however, continued to conceal from the plaintiff the existence of the surgical sponges left in the plaintiff's abdomen. The plaintiff ceased seeing the defendant as her physician in 1986. However, she consulted other physicians and continued to experience frequent pain and discomfort in her abdomen as well as intestinal, urological, and gynecological problems. Although the plaintiff brought her complaints to the attention of other physicians, no one was able to diagnose the source of her problems.

In 1993, one of the physicians attending to the plaintiff's problems diagnosed a pelvic mass, which he felt could be causing some discomfort. The plaintiff underwent pelvic sonograms and X-rays, which revealed the existence of retained surgical sponges. The plaintiff contended that the defendant, from and after November 18, 1983, had knowledge of the presence of retained surgical sponges in her abdomen and knew the potential of future complications that could arise from this condition. Despite this knowledge, the plaintiff contended, the defendant fraudulently concealed the existence of this condition from the plaintiff.

The appeals court held that although the action in this case was filed more than 10 years after the fraud was perpetrated, the statute of limitations was not tolled because of the defendant's fraudulent concealment of information from the patient. The court decided that a physician may not blunt a malpractice cause of action by misrepresenting facts to a patient.

Invasion of Privacy

The right to privacy is implied in the Constitution. It is recognized by the law as the right to be left alone—the right to be free from unwarranted publicity and exposure to public view, as well as the right to live one's life without having one's name, picture, or private affairs made public against one's will. Health care organizations and professionals can become liable for invasion of privacy if, for example, they divulge information from a patient's medical record to improper sources or if they commit unwarranted intrusions into a patient's personal affairs.

Patients have a right to personal privacy and a right to the confidentiality of their personal and clinical records. The information in a patient's medical record is confidential and should not be disclosed without the patient's permission, with the exception of occasions when there is a legal obligation or duty to disclose the information (i.e., reporting of communicable diseases, gunshot wounds, and child abuse). Those who come into possession of the most intimate personal information about patients have both a legal and an ethical duty not to reveal confidential communications.

Intentional Infliction of Mental Distress

The intentional or reckless infliction of mental distress is characterized by conduct that is so outrageous that it goes beyond the bounds tolerated by a decent society. Mental distress includes mental suffering resulting from painful emotions such as grief, public humiliation, despair, shame, and wounded pride. Liability for the wrongful infliction of mental distress can be based on either intentional or negligent misconduct. A plaintiff may recover damages if he or she can show that the defendant intended to inflict mental distress and knew or should have known that his or her actions would give rise to it.

Mother Shown Her Premature Infant

The mother of a premature infant who died shortly after birth went to her physician for a six week checkup. She noticed a report in her medical chart that stated that the child was past the fifth month in development and that hospital rules and state law prohibited disposal of the infant as a surgical specimen. The mother questioned her physician regarding the infant. The physician requested that his nurse take the mother to the hospital. An employee at the hospital took the mother to a freezer. The freezer was opened and the mother was handed a jar containing her premature infant. The circuit court found that the hospital, through its employees, committed intentional infliction of emotional distress. On appeal, the court of appeals held that the jury could find that the hospital's conduct in displaying the infant was outrageous conduct.[25]

Verbal Abuse of a Patient

In another mental distress case, an action in *Greer v. Medders*[26] was brought by a patient and his wife against a physician. The defendant physician had been covering for the attending physician who was on vacation. When the hospitalized plaintiff had not seen the covering physician for several days, he called the physician's office to complain. The physician later entered the patient's room in an agitated manner and became verbally abusive in the presence of the patient's wife and a nurse. He said to the patient, "Let me tell you one damn thing, don't nobody call over to my office raising hell with my secretary. . . . I don't have to be here every damn day checking on you because I check with physical therapy. . . . I don't have to be your damn doctor."[27] When the physician left the room, the plaintiff's wife began to cry, and the plaintiff experienced episodes of uncontrollable shaking for which he received psychiatric treatment. The Georgia Court of Appeals held that the physician's abusive language willfully caused emotional upset and precluded summary judgment for the defendant.

STRICT LIABILITY

Strict liability is a legal doctrine that makes some persons or entities responsible for damages their actions or products cause, regardless of "fault" on their part. Strict liability often applies when people engage in inherently hazardous activities, such as blasting in a city. If the blasting injures a person, no matter how careful the blasting company was, it can be liable for any injuries suffered. Strict liability also applies in the case of manufactured products such as drugs. This section focuses on products liability.

Products liability is the accountability of a manufacturer, seller, or supplier of chattels to a buyer or other third party for injuries sustained because of a defect in a product. An injured party may proceed with a lawsuit against a seller, manufacturer, or supplier on three legal theories: (1) negligence, (2) breach of warranty (express or implied), and (3) strict liability. Three types of product defects that incur liability are design defects, manufacturing defects, and defects in marketing (e.g., providing improper instructions for the product's use).

Negligence

Negligence, as applied to products liability, requires the plaintiff to establish duty, breach, injury, and causation. The manufacturer of a product is not liable for injuries suffered by a patient if they are the result of negligent use by the user. Product users must conform to the safety standards provided by the manufacturers of supplies and equipment. Failure to follow proper safety instructions can prevent recovery in a negligence suit if injury results from improper use.

Because manufacturers are liable for injuries that result from unsafe product design, they generally provide detailed safety instructions to the users of their products. Failure to provide such instructions could be considered negligence on the part of the manufacturer.

An action in *Airco v. Simmons National Bank, Guardian, et al.*[28] was brought against a physician partnership that provided anesthesia services to the hospital and Airco, Inc., the manufacturer of an artificial breathing machine used in the administration of anesthesia. It was alleged that the patient suffered irreversible brain damage because of the negligent use of the equipment and its unsafe design. The machine had been marketed despite prior reports of a foreseeable danger of human error brought about by the presence of several identical black hoses and the necessity of connecting them correctly to three ports of identical size placed closely together. The machine lacked adequate labels and warnings, according to the reports. The jury awarded $1,070,000 in compensatory damages against the physician partnership and Airco, Inc. Punitive damages in the amount of $3 million were awarded against Airco, Inc. On appeal of the punitive damages award, the Arkansas Supreme Court held that the evidence for punitive damages was sufficient for the jury. The manufacturer acted in a persistent reckless disregard of the foreseeable dangers in the machine by continuing to sell it with the known hazardous design.

Negligence, as well as breach of warranty and strict liability, was not established in the well-publicized case of the 1980s involving a woman who died after ingesting Tylenol capsules tainted with potassium cyanide. The decedent's estate in *Elsroth v. Johnson & Johnson*[29] sued the manufacturer and the retail grocery store that sold the over-the-counter drug. The defendants moved for a summary judgment. The US district court held that the retailer did not have a duty to protect the decedent from acts of tampering by an unknown third party. The manufacturer was not liable under an inadequate warning theory. Manufacturers are under a duty to warn of the dangers that might be associated with the normal and lawful use of their products, but they need not warn that their products might be susceptible to criminal misuse.

Failure to Warn

Merck pulled its painkiller Vioxx off pharmacy shelves, a drug it manufactures for the treatment of arthritis, after participants in a study experienced adverse cardiovascular events compared to those taking a placebo. Following a 3-year battle, Merck announced in November 2007 that it would pay $4.85 billion to settle claims of 47,000 plaintiffs over injuries linked to Vioxx. The company paid the money into a fund, and people who claim they were hurt by Vioxx can petition for money. The deal was not a class action settlement, and individual cases will be examined before payments are made.

Breach of Warranty

A *warranty* is a particular type of guarantee (a pledge or assurance of something) concerning goods or services provided by a seller to a buyer. Nearly everything purchased is covered by a warranty. To recover under a cause of action based on a breach of warranty theory, the plaintiff must establish whether there was an express or implied warranty.

Express Warranty

An *express warranty* includes specific promises or affirmations made by the seller to the buyer, such as "X" drug is not subject to addiction. If the product fails to perform as advertised, it is a breach of express warranty. For example, in *Crocker v. Winthrop Laboratories*,[30] the patient, Mr. Crocker, was admitted to the hospital for a hernia operation. His physician prescribed both Demerol and Talwin for pain. After discharge from the hospital, Crocker developed an addiction to Talwin and was able to obtain prescriptions from several physicians to support a habit he developed. He was eventually admitted to the hospital for detoxification. After six days, Crocker walked out of the hospital and went home. He became agitated and abusive, threatening his wife, and she eventually called a physician at his request. The physician arrived and gave Crocker an injection of Demerol. Crocker then retired to bed and subsequently died. Action was brought against the drug company for the suffering and subsequent wrongful death that occurred as the proximate result of the decedent's addiction to Talwin.

The district court rendered a judgment for the plaintiff, and the court of appeals reversed. On further appeal, the Texas Supreme Court held that when a drug company positively and specifically represents its product to be free and safe from all dangers of addiction and when the treating physician relies on such representation, the drug company is liable when the representation proves to be false and injury results.

Implied Warranty

An *implied warranty* is a guarantee of a product's quality that is not expressed in a purchase contract. An implied warranty assumes that the item sold can perform the function for which it is designed. Implied warranties are in effect when the law implies that one exists by operation of law as a matter of public policy for the protection of the public.

Strict Liability

Strict liability refers to responsibility without fault and makes possible an award of damages without any proof of manufacturer negligence. The plaintiff needs only to show that he or she suffered injury while using the manufacturer's product in the prescribed way.

The following elements must be present for a plaintiff to proceed with a case on the basis of strict liability:

- The product must have been manufactured by the defendant.
- The product must have been defective at the time it left the hands of the manufacturer or seller. The defect in the product normally consists of a manufacturing defect, a design defect in the product, or an absence or inadequacy of warnings for the use of the product.
- The plaintiff must have been injured by the specific product.
- The defective product must have been the proximate cause of injury to the plaintiff.

Negligent blood handling held a blood bank strictly liable in *Weber v. Charity Hospital of Louisiana at New Orleans*[31] when a hospital patient developed hepatitis from a transfusion of defective blood during surgery. Evidence established that the blood bank collected, processed, and sold the blood to the hospital. Although the hospital administered the blood, absent any negligence in its handling or administration, it was not liable for the patient's injury. Many states have enacted statutes to exempt blood from the product category and thus remove blood products from the theory of strict liability.

Res Ipsa Loquitur

Liability also can be based on the concept of *res ipsa loquitur* (the thing speaks for itself) by showing all of the following:

- The product did not perform in the way intended.
- The product was not tampered with by the buyer or third party. The defect existed at the time it left the defendant manufacturer. For example, a manufacturer mislabeled a box of Duragesic patches, a strong prescription medication for moderate to severe chronic pain, marking the box as containing 25 mcg patches. In actuality, the box contained 100 mcg patches. The patient placed a patch on her back to provide relief of severe back pain. Instead of receiving the 25 mcg dosage recommended by her physician, she received 100 mcg, four times the recommended dosage. The patient went into a coma and eventually died.

Products Liability Defenses

Defenses against recovery in a products liability case include:

- assumption of a risk (e.g., voluntary exposure to such risks as radiation treatments and chemotherapy treatments)
- intervening cause (e.g., an intravenous solution contaminated by the negligence of the product user, rather than that of the manufacturer)
- contributory negligence (e.g., use of a product in a way that it was not intended to be used)

- comparative fault (e.g., injury is the result of the concurrent negligence of both the manufacturer and the plaintiff)
- disclaimers (e.g., manufacturers' inserts and warnings regarding usage and contraindications of their products)

Notes

1. 11 A.2d 132 (N.Y. App. Div. 1960).
2. 498 So. 2d 713 (La. Ct. App. 1986).
3. 787 S.W.2d 494 (Tex. Ct. App. 1990).
4. Id. at 496.
5. 498 So. 2d 713 (La. Ct. App. 1986).
6. 384 S.E.2d 92 (Va. 1989).
7. 498 So. 2d 713 (La. Ct. App. 1986).
8. No. 2003-01976 (N.Y. App. Div. 2004).
9. *Tomcik v. Ohio Dep't of Rehabilitation & Correction*, 598 N.E.2d 900 (Ohio Ct. App. 1991).
10. *Caruso v. Pine Manor Nursing Ctr.*, 538 N.E.2d 722 (Ill. App. Ct. 1989).
11. 296 S.E.2d 216 (Ga. Ct. App. 1982).
12. 116 Cal. Rptr. 733 (Cal. Ct. App. 1974).
13. 457 A.2d 431 (N.J. 1983).
14. 841 F.2d 851 (8th Cir. 1988).
15. Garrard, Evaluation of Neuroleptic Drug Use by Nursing Home Elderly under Proposed Medicare and Medicaid Regulations, 265(4) JAMA 463 (1991).
16. *Miller-Douglas v. Keller*, 579 So. 2d 491 (La. Ct. App. 1991).
17. 562 N.Y.2d 127 (N.Y. App. Div. 1990).
18. *Id.* at 129.
19. 856 S.W.2d 437 (Tex. Ct. App. 1993).
20. *Id.* at 447.
21. *Id.*
22. *Keller v. Miami Herald Publishing Company*, 778 F.2d 711 (11th Cir. 1985).
23. *Id.* at 713.
24. 936 P.2d 784 (Kans. App. 1997).
25. 527 S.W.2d 133 (Tenn. Ct. App. 1975).
26. 336 S.E.2d 329 (Ga. App. 1985).
27. *Id.*
28. 638 S.W.2d 660 (Ark. 1982).
29. 700 F. Supp. 151 (S.D.N.Y. 1988).
30. 514 S.W.2d 429 (Tex. 1974).
31. 487 So. 2d 148 (La. Ct. App. 1986).

4

Criminal Aspects of Health Care

Criminal law (also known as penal law) is the body of statutory and common law that deals with crime and the legal punishment of criminal offenses. Criminal law represents society's expression of the limits of acceptable human behavior. A crime is any social harm defined and made punishable by law.

Crimes are classified as misdemeanors or felonies, dependent upon the severity of the crime. A *misdemeanor* is an offense generally punishable by less than one year in jail and/or a fine (e.g., petty larceny). A *felony* is a much more serious crime (e.g., rape or murder) and is punishable by imprisonment in a state or federal penitentiary for more than one year.

Criminal law distinguishes crimes from civil wrongs such as tort or breach of contract. Criminal law has been seen as a system of regulating the behavior of individuals and groups in relation to societal norms at large whereas civil law is aimed primarily at the relationship between private individuals and their rights and obligations under the law.

The objectives of criminal law are to maintain public order and safety, to protect the individual, to use punishment as a deterrent to crime, and to rehabilitate the criminal for return to society.

Particular to health care organizations is the fact that patients are often helpless and at the mercy of others. Health care facilities are far too often places where the morally weak and mentally deficient prey on the physically and sometimes mentally helpless. The very institutions designed to make the public well and feel safe can sometimes provide the setting for criminal conduct. The US Department of Justice and state prosecutors vigorously pursue and prosecute health care organizations and individuals for criminal conduct. Health care fraud, murder, patient abuse, and other such crimes have caused law enforcement agencies to assume a zero-tolerance policy for such acts.

CRIMINAL PROCEDURE

Criminal procedure regulates the process for addressing violations of criminal law. The process begins with an alleged crime. A complainant makes an accusation, which is investigated by the police who act as agents of the government. When necessary, detectives can be assigned to a case to gather evidence, interview crime suspects and witnesses, and assist in preparing a case for possible trial. When a misdemeanor or felony has been committed, evidence has been gathered, and a target defendant has been identified, an arrest by a police officer is made. Upon arrest, the defendant is taken to the appropriate law enforcement agency for processing, which includes paperwork and fingerprinting. The police prepare and file accusatory statements, such as misdemeanor or felony complaints with a court in the appropriate jurisdiction. After processing has been completed, the defendant is either detained or released on bond. If the alleged offense is classified as a felony, the US Constitution requires that the case be referred to a grand jury for an indictment. An indictment is the official charging instrument accusing the defendant of criminal conduct.

A prosecuting attorney represents the interests of the state, while the interests of the defendant are represented by his or her defense attorney. Although the specific process varies according to local law, in virtually every jurisdiction the process culminates with a trial, followed by appeals to higher courts.

Criminal statutes spell out the exact circumstances that constitute a crime. These circumstances are known as the elements of the offense. Unless all the elements are proven by the prosecuting authority, the defendant is not guilty of the offense. There are three kinds of elements: the act itself (the actus reus or guilty act); the requisite mental state (the mens rea or guilty mind); and the attendant circumstances.

Criminal cases are presented to a grand jury by a prosecutor. When the grand jury is presented with the prosecution's evidence, it may indict the target if jurors find in the evidence reasonable cause to believe that all the elements of a particular crime are present. Before indictment, the grand jury may request that witnesses be subpoenaed to testify. Finally, actions of a grand jury are handed to a judge, after which the defendant will be notified to appear to be arraigned for the crimes charged in the indictment.

Arraignment

The arraignment is a formal reading of the accusatory instrument (a generic term that describes a variety of documents, each of which accuses a defendant of an offense) and includes the setting of bail. After the charges are read, the defendant pleads guilty or not guilty. On a plea of not guilty, the defense attorney and prosecutor make arguments regarding bail. After the defendant's arraignment, the judge sets a date for the defendant to return to court. Between the time of arraignment and the next court date, the defense attorney and the prosecutor confer about the charges and evidence in the possession of the prosecutor. At that time, the defense will offer any mitigating circumstances it believes will convince the prosecutor to lessen or drop the charges.

Conference

If the defendant does not plead guilty, both felony and misdemeanor cases are taken to conference, and plea bargaining commences with the goal of an agreed-upon disposition. If no disposition can be reached, the case is adjourned, motions are made, and the case is set for trial.

Criminal Trial

Most of the processes of a criminal trial are similar to those of a civil trial and include jury selection, opening statements, presentation of witnesses and other evidence, summations, instructions to the jury by the judge, jury deliberations, verdict, and opportunity for appeal to a higher court. In a criminal trial, the jury verdict must be unanimous, and the standard of proof must be beyond a reasonable doubt. Criminal trials involving health care professionals and organizations often involve health care fraud, falsification of records, misuse and theft of drugs, patient abuse, and murder. A variety of such cases are reviewed here.

FALSE CLAIMS

The False Claims Act of 1986 prohibits: knowingly presenting, or causing to be presented, to the government a false claim for payment; knowingly making, using, or causing to be made or used a false record or statement to get a false claim paid or approved by the government; conspiring to defraud the government by getting a false claim allowed or paid; and knowingly making, using, or causing to be made or used a false record to avoid or decrease an obligation to pay or transmit property to the government.

As part of the effort to reduce fraud and abuse in federal health care programs, the Office of Inspector General (OIG) can impose monetary penalties as well as exclude providers that violate the False Claims Act from participation in Medicare and other federal health care programs. Where the best interests of the programs are served by allowing continued participation by the provider, the OIG will often require that the provider adopt specific measures to better ensure its integrity. These measures are set forth in a corporate, institutional, or individual integrity agreement (collectively referred to as a corporate integrity agreement or CIA).

KICKBACKS

The Medicare and Medicaid Patient Protection Act of 1987, as amended, 42 U.S.C. §1320a-7b (the "Anti-Kickback Statute"), provides for criminal penalties for certain acts impacting Medicare and state health care (e.g., Medicaid) reimbursable services. The Anti-Kickback Statute, as amended, prohibits certain solicitations or receipt of remuneration. The statute penalizes anyone who knowingly and willfully solicits, receives, offers, or pays anything of value as an inducement in return for: referring an individual to a person for the furnishing or arranging for the furnishing of any item or service payable under the Medicare or Medicaid programs; and purchasing, leasing, or ordering or arranging for or recommending purchasing, leasing, or ordering any good, facility, service, or item payable under the Medicare or Medicaid programs.

The OIG investigates violations of the Medicare and Medicaid Anti-Kickback Statute. Violators are subject to criminal penalties or exclusion from participation in the Medicare and Medicaid programs. The OIG specifically targets four billing practices: claims for services not provided, claims for beneficiaries not homebound, claims for visits not made, and claims for visits not authorized by a physician.

Laboratory Kickback

In the case of *United States v. Katz*,[1] the owner of a diagnostic medical lab agreed to kick back 50% of Medicare payments received by the lab for referrals from Total Health Care, a medical service company. Under the scheme, Total Health Care collected blood and urine samples from medical offices and clinics in southern California and sent them to the medical lab for testing. The lab billed Total Health, which in turn billed the private insurance carrier or the government-funded insurance programs Medi-Cal and Medicare for reimbursement. The lab then kicked back half of its receipts to Total Health. The owners of the lab and Total Health arranged an identical scheme with a community medical clinic; Katz, the appellant, subsequently purchased a 25% interest in the clinic and began collecting payments under the scheme. Katz was convicted of conspiracy to commit Medicare fraud and of receipt of kickbacks in exchange for referral of Medicare patients. He appealed the decision. The court of appeals, however, affirmed the charges against him.

Architectural Contract Kickback

In *United States v. Thompson*,[2] three members of a county council, which served as the governing body of a county hospital, were convicted by a jury for soliciting and receiving kickbacks from architects. The architects testified that the appellants and others sought a 1% kickback on a hospital project, financed by federal funds, in return for being awarded the architectural contract. Mr. Galloway, of the architectural firm of Galloway and Guthrey, had delivered $6,000 to appellant Campbell at the Knoxville airport. The architects had informed the FBI, and an investigation was conducted. After the investigation, indictments, and trial by jury, the defendants were each sentenced to 1 year in prison. On appeal, the US Court of Appeals for the Sixth Circuit held that the receipt of a kickback constituted an overt act in furtherance of a conspiracy to obstruct lawful government function and was a violation of the general conspiracy statute and a crime against the United States. It had been previously observed that "to conspire to defraud the United States means primarily to cheat the government out of property or money, but it also means to interfere with or obstruct one of its lawful governmental functions by deceit, craft or trickery, or at least by means that are dishonest."[3] Proof that part of the architects' fee was reimbursed with federal funds was not necessary for a conviction. The criminal convictions were affirmed.

HEALTH CARE FRAUD

In 1989, the Ethics in Patient Referral Act prohibits physicians who have ownership interest or compensation arrangements with a clinical laboratory from referring Medicare patients to that laboratory. The law also requires all Medicare providers to report the names and provider numbers of all physicians or their immediate relatives with ownership interests in a provider entity.

HIPAA

The Health Insurance Portability and Accountability Act of 1996 (HIPAA) provides new criminal and civil enforcement tools and funding dedicated to the fight against health care fraud. In addition, HIPAA requires the US Attorney General and the US Secretary of the Department of Health and Human Services (DHHS), acting through the Office of Inspector General (OIG), to established a national health care fraud and abuse control program. The program provides a coordinated national framework for federal, state, and local law enforcement agencies; the private sector; and the public to fight health care fraud. To combat fraud in home care settings, the DHHS announced Operation Restore Trust, an antifraud enforcement initiative targeted at home care agencies, nursing homes, and durable equipment suppliers. DHHS provided a toll-free telephone number (800-HHS-TIPS) to gather allegations of health care fraud from the public as well as from organizational whistle-blowers.

Scheme to Defraud Medicare and Medicaid

The defendant physician in *United States v. Raithath*[4] owned and operated two clinics. The defendant was convicted by a jury of making false statements and scheming to defraud. The defendant, sentenced to 27 months of imprisonment, appealed his conviction and sentence.

The indictment filed against the defendant included charges for instructing billing staff to raise the current procedural terminology (CPT) codes on invoices when the physician reported a lower level of service; submit invoices to insurance companies for services performed by other physicians as if the defendant had performed them; submit claims with a diagnosis listing an illness, when the patient did not have an illness; and causing patients to present themselves for medically unnecessary visits by refusing to authorize refills on prescriptions and preventing employees from authorizing refills of prescriptions.

Charges also included making unannounced home visits to patients; approaching people on the street and ushering them into the clinic for unscheduled examinations; examining people who had come into the clinic for nonmedical reasons, such as to pay debts owed to the defendant; ordering medical tests not related to patients' conditions; falsely representing that other physician employees had specialties so that patients would be examined an additional time by a "specialist"; and refusing to give test results until an additional appointment was kept.

The defendant was also charged with defrauding Medicare/ Medicaid by submitting a cost report for 1997 that included personal expenses unrelated to patient care. Included in those expenses was money that was actually spent to furnish and complete the defendant's home.

The defendant, on appeal, argued that there was insufficient evidence to sustain his conviction for defrauding or attempting to defraud. The defendant's staff members testified that the defendant instructed them to bill office visits covered by private insurance under CPT codes 99213 or 99203, regardless of the CPT code entered by the attending physician on the encounter form. Staff members were aware that this "up-coding" scheme resulted in higher reimbursement from private insurance companies.

In addition, staff members testified that the defendant routinely ordered tests unrelated to his patients' conditions and supported the tests with false diagnoses. Zeren, a nurse practitioner working at the McKee clinic, testified that after she performed sports physicals on children at local schools and found no indication of upper-respiratory infections, the defendant, who had not been present at the examinations, falsely diagnosed them as having upper respiratory infections.

A reasonable juror could have reasonably found the defendant–physician guilty of defrauding or attempting to defraud Medicare/ Medicaid. The conviction and sentence of the district court was affirmed.

False Medicaid Claims by Physician and Office Manager

In *United States v. Larm*,[5] a physician and his office manager were convicted on charges that they violated 42 U.S.C. § 139h(a)1 by submitting false Medicaid claims for medical services they never rendered to patients. Claims sometimes were submitted even when patients administered allergy injections themselves. In addition, sometimes more expensive serums were billed rather than those that were actually administered.

Pharmacist Submits False Drug Claims

The pharmacist in *State v. Heath*[6] submitted claims for reimbursement on brand-name medications rather than on the less-expensive generic drugs that were actually dispensed. A licensed pharmacist and former employee of the defendant contacted the Medicaid Fraud Unit of the Louisiana Attorney General's office and reported the defendant's conduct in substituting generic drugs for brand-name drugs. As a result of the complaint, the Medicaid Fraud Unit conducted a call out, in which the unit sent letters to Medicaid recipients in the pharmacy's surrounding area.

> In a recipient call out, the Medicaid Fraud Unit sends letters to Medicaid recipients in the general area of the pharmacy involved and asks them to bring all their prescription drugs to the welfare office on a specific date. The call out revealed that some of the prescription vials issued by the aforesaid pharmacies contained generic

drugs while the labels indicated that they should contain brand name drugs.

The pharmacist was convicted on three counts of Medicaid fraud.[7]

Inflating Insurance Claims

The North Carolina Court of Appeals held that a chiropractor's license was properly suspended for 6 months in *Farlow v. North Carolina State Board of Chiropractic Examiners*[8] for inflating the insurance claims of victims of an automobile accident. Dr. Farlow prescribed a course of treatment for several patients that was not justified by the injuries they received. Instead, the treatment was prescribed to inflate insurance claims.

Fraud and Ethics

Behind every act of health care fraud lies a lapse in ethics. One particular type of fraud occurs when physicians refer their patients to hospitals and ancillary health care providers where the physician owns a financial interest in the provider to which the patient has been referred. The ethical risks inherent in physician self-referral were first noted in a 1986 Institute of Medicine study, and then again in a 1989 Health and Human Services inspector general study. The 1989 study concluded that physicians who owned or invested in independent clinical laboratories referred Medicare patients for 45% more laboratory services than did physicians without financial interests. It was in 1989 that the Ethics in Patient Referral Act was enacted, prohibiting unethical referrals, which were further defined in 1991, when the American Medical Association (AMA) Council on Ethical and Judicial Affairs concluded that physicians should not refer patients to a health care facility in which they have a financial interest and they do not directly provide services. In the following year, the AMA House of Delegates voted to declare self-referral to be unethical in most instances.

The Omnibus Budget Reconciliation Act of 1989 (which took effect January 1, 1992) backed the AMA's position on self-referral, barring the referral of Medicare patients to clinical laboratories by physicians who have, or whose family members have, a financial interest in those laboratories. The scope of the ban on self-referral was expanded with the enactment of the Omnibus Reconciliation Act of 1993 (effective January 1, 1995), which added 10 additional designated health services, including physical therapy; occupational therapy; radiology services; radiation therapy services and supplies; durable medical equipment and supplies; parenteral and enteral nutrients, equipment, and supplies; orthotics, prosthetics, and prosthetic devices and supplies; home health services; outpatient prescription drugs; and inpatient and outpatient hospital services. The 1993 law also expanded and clarified exceptions and applied the referral limits to Medicaid.

Falsification of Records

As with health care fraud, falsification of medical and business records is grounds for criminal prosecution. Anyone who suffers damage as a result of falsification of records can claim civil liability, which could result in the provider's loss of Medicare and Medicaid funding.

Misuse and Theft of Drugs

Perhaps one of the most tempting and accessible crimes for a health care professional involves the misuse or theft of drugs. Drugs can offer significant financial gain when they fall into the hands of the wrong people. Such was the case in *United States v. Nelson*,[9] where a doctor cooperated in an Internet pharmacy and had the proceeds transferred to an offshore account for himself. Fuchs, an unindicted coconspirator, operated an Internet pharmacy called NationPharmacy.com, where customers could obtain prescription and nonprescription drugs. In accord with federal law, all requests for prescription drugs were first reviewed by a physician, defendant Nelson, who either approved or denied the request. Nelson, however, approved 90% to 95% of all prescription drug requests and did so without ever examining his purported patient. Customers who used Fuchs's Internet pharmacy would have their orders routed through a brick-and-mortar pharmacy called Main Street Pharmacy. Nelson would physically visit Main Street Pharmacy to sign the prescription requests, and customers would receive prescriptions by mail and pay Fuchs directly. Nelson, the prescribing physician, was never paid by any customer. Instead, Nelson received a total of $175,000, which was wired directly from Fuchs into an offshore account.

Nelson was charged and convicted of both conspiracy to distribute controlled prescription drugs outside the usual course of professional practice, in violation of 21 U.S.C. § 846, and conspiracy to launder money, in violation of 18 U.S.C. § 1956(h). Nelson appealed his conviction, arguing that there was insufficient evidence to support a conviction because there was no evidence of a conspiracy.

The most significant evidence came from testimonies by Weeks, the person who set up the Web site; Shadid, the resident pharmacist at Main Street Pharmacy; Thompson, another pharmacist at Main Street Pharmacy; and Dupes, the office manager for Fuchs. Weeks's testimony described the general workings of the Fuchs Web site. He testified he established this Web site at Fuchs's behest as a means of providing prescription and nonprescription drugs over the Internet. Weeks testified that only those orders for prescription drugs that were specifically approved by Nelson were processed. He testified that he provided Nelson the means to review and approve prescription drug requests with a unique user name and password that enabled Nelson to access the medical history questionnaires required to be filled out by all customers who requested prescription drugs.

Shadid and Thompson testified at trial as to Nelson's personal participation in this scheme. Both men were pharmacists at Main Street Pharmacy, which processed all orders taken through NationPharmacy.com. Both testified that on numerous occasions, Nelson would personally come to Main Street Pharmacy to sign prescriptions and that Nelson signed "thousands" of prescriptions for Nation Pharmacy.com. Finally, Dupes testified that she transferred money, a total of $175,000, from an account controlled by Fuchs to an offshore account controlled by Nelson.

The evidence described a scheme that depended upon the participation of Nelson. Without his approval, requests for controlled prescription drugs taken on the Web site would not have been filled. Given the concert of action between Nelson and Fuchs in the common purpose of operating a Web site pharmacy, a reasonable jury could infer the existence of an agreement constituting a conspiracy to distribute prescription drugs outside the usual course of professional practice and to launder the proceeds of that distribution.

Physicians Can Be Victims of Fraud

Physicians are not immune from being the victims of fraud. The detection, investigation, and prosecution of financial crimes against physicians are not uncommon occurrences. They involve such areas as computer billing crime, bookkeeper/office manager theft, insurance fraud, cash larceny, checkbook scams, and patient record tampering.

Physicians should be aware of how to analyze larcenous transactions, identify embezzled funds, and recognize the criminal employee. Physicians should be wary of bookkeepers who make themselves indispensable because of their perceived ability to operate the office computer system. To avoid being victimized by employee fraud, physicians should:

- Familiarize themselves with patient billing and record keeping practices.
- Avoid having one individual in charge of billing and collection procedures.
- Arrange for an annual audit of office procedures and records by an outside auditor.

PATIENT ABUSE

> Gale . . . wasn't prepared for the rough treatment and cruel taunts she says her ailing mother suffered at the nursing home. She cried as a nurse's aide upbraided her mother for failing to straighten her arthritis-stricken legs. And she watched in disbelief as an assistant jerked her mother off her rubber bed pad and pushed her into the bed's metal rails.
>
> All of these images were caught . . . by a "granny cam"—a camera hidden in her mother's room.
>
> *USA Today*, September 14, 1999

Patient abuse is the mistreatment or neglect of individuals who are under the care of a health care organization. Abuse is not limited to an institutional setting and can occur in an individual's home as well as in an institution. Abuse can take many forms: physical, psychological, medical, and financial. To compound the issue, abuse is not always easy to identify because injuries often can be attributed to other causes, especially in elderly patients with their advanced age and failing health. In the hospital setting, patients are not generally as dependent upon the facility operator in the same manner as a resident in a nursing facility is. Persons are usually hospitalized for only brief periods of time, whereas nursing facility residents might be dependent upon the facility operator for a period of years. Thus, the potential for long-term abuse and neglect is far greater for nursing facility residents than hospital patients.

The abuse of the elderly is not a localized or isolated problem. Unfortunately, it permeates society. *Behind Closed Doors*, a landmark book on family violence, stated that the first national study of violence in American homes estimated that one in two homes is the scene of family violence at least once per year.[10]

The plaintiffs in *In re Estate of Smith v. O'Halloran*[11] instituted a lawsuit in an effort to improve deplorable conditions at many nursing homes. The court concluded that:

> The evidentiary record . . . supports a general finding that all is not well in the nation's nursing homes and that the enormous expenditures of public funds and the earnest efforts of public officials and public employees have not produced an equivalent return in benefits. That failure of expectations has produced frustration and anger among those who are aware of the realities of life in some nursing homes which provide so little service that they could be characterized as orphanages for the aged.[12]

Abuse of nursing facility residents gave impetus to the strengthening of resident rights under the Omnibus Budget Reconciliation Act of 1989. The act provides that a "resident has the right to be free from verbal, sexual, physical, or mental abuse, corporal punishment, and involuntary seclusion."[13] Although resident rights have been significantly strengthened, resident abuse is often in the headlines. For example, the headline "Nurse's Aide Jailed for Punching Patient" topped a story about a nurse's aide who was jailed for punching a 91-year-old senile man in the nose.[14] The aide had been previously convicted of resident abuse.

Criminal Negligence

Criminal negligence is the reckless disregard for the safety of others. It is the willful indifference to an injury that could follow an act. The defendants in *State v. Brenner*[15] were charged with cruelty to the infirm. The state alleged that the administrator of the nursing facility neglected and mistreated residents by failing to ensure: the facility was maintained in a sanitary manner, necessary health services were performed; staff were properly trained; there were adequate medical supplies and sufficient staff; records were maintained properly; and the residents were adequately fed and cared for. In addition to allegations of neglect and mistreatment of residents, other allegations charged the director with failing to properly train the staff at the facility in correct nursing procedures. The controller was alleged to have failed to purchase adequate medical supplies for proper treatment. The admissions director allegedly failed to exercise proper judgment regarding admissions procedures, and the physical therapist allegedly failed to provide adequate physical therapy services. The defendants asserted that the term "neglect" was unconstitutionally vague. The Louisiana Supreme Court, on appeal by the defendants from two lower courts, held that the phrases "intentional or criminally negligent mistreatment or neglect" and "unjustifiable pain and suffering" were not vague and that they were sufficiently clear in meaning to afford a person of ordinary understanding fair notice of the conduct that was prohibited.[16]

Neglect of Residents

The defendant in *State v. Cunningham*[17] was the owner and administrator of a residential care facility that housed 30 to 37 mentally ill, mentally retarded, and elderly residents. The Iowa Department of Inspections and Appeals conducted surveys at the defendant's facility. A grand jury charged the defendant with several counts of resident neglect in violation of Iowa Code section 726.7 (1989).

The district court held that the defendant had knowledge of the dangerous conditions that existed in the health care facility but willfully and consciously refused to provide or exercise adequate supervision to remedy or attempt to remedy the dangerous conditions. The residents were exposed to physical dangers, unhealthy and unsanitary physical conditions, and were grossly deprived of much-needed medical care and personal attention. The conditions were likely to and did cause injury to the physical and mental well-being of the facility's residents. The defendant was found guilty on five counts of neglect. The district court sentenced the defendant to one year in jail for each of the five counts, to run concurrently. The district court suspended all but two days of the defendant's sentence and ordered him to pay $200 for each count, plus a surcharge and costs, and to perform community service. A motion for a new trial was denied, and the defendant appealed.

The Iowa Court of Appeals held that there was substantial evidence to support a finding that the defendant was responsible for not properly maintaining the facility, which led to prosecution for wanton neglect of the facility's residents. The defendant was found guilty of knowingly acting in a manner likely to be injurious to the physical or mental welfare of the facility's residents by creating, directing, or maintaining the following five hazardous conditions and unsafe practices:

1. There were fire hazards and circumstances that impeded safety from fire. For example, cigarette stubs were found in a cardboard box, and burn holes were found in patient clothing, on furniture, and in nonsmoking areas. Also, exposed electrical wiring was found, along with a bent and rusted fire door that could not close or latch.
2. The facility was not properly maintained and demonstrated many health and safety violations, including broken glass in patients' rooms, excessively hot water in faucets, dried feces on public bathroom walls and grab bars, no soap in the kitchen, insufficient towels and linens, dead and live cockroaches and worms in the food preparation area, and debris, bugs, and grease throughout the facility.
3. Dietary facilities were unsanitary and inadequate to meet the dietary needs of the residents. In one particular case, an ordered "no concentrated sweets" diet for a diabetic patient was not followed, subjecting the patient to life-threatening blood sugar levels.
4. There were inadequate staffing patterns and supervision in the facility. No funds were spent on employee training, and the defendant did not spend the minimum

amount of time at the facility, as required by administrative standards.

5. Improper dosages of medications were administered to the residents. For example, physicians distributed an ongoing overdose of heart medication to one resident while failing to administer medication to another (which resulted in a seizure).[18]

The defendant argued that he did not create the unsafe conditions at the facility. The court of appeals disagreed. The statute does not require that the defendant create the conditions at the facility to sustain a conviction. The defendant was the administrator of the facility and responsible for the conditions that existed.

Abuse and Revocation of License

The operator of a nursing facility appealed an order by the department of public welfare revoking his license because of resident abuse in *Nepa v. Commonwealth Department of Public Welfare*.[19] Substantial evidence supported the department's finding. Three former employees testified that the nursing facility operator had abused residents in the following incidents: he unbuckled the belt of one of the residents, causing his pants to drop, and then grabbed a second resident, forcing the two to kiss (the petitioner's excuse for this behavior was to shame the resident because of his masturbating in public); on two occasions he forced a resident to remove toilet paper from a commode after she had urinated and defecated in it (denying that there was fecal matter in the commode, the petitioner's excuse was that this was his way of trying to stop the resident from filling the commode with toilet paper); and he verbally abused a resident who was experiencing difficulty in breathing and accused him of being a fake as he attempted to feed him liquids.[20]

The nursing facility operator claimed that the findings of fact were not based on substantial evidence and that even if they were, the incidents did not amount to abuse under the code. The court held that there was substantial evidence supporting the department's decision and that the activities committed by the operator were sufficient to support revocation of his license.

> We believe Petitioner's treatment of these residents as found by the hearing examiner to be truly disturbing. These residents were elderly and/or mentally incapacitated and wholly dependent on Petitioner while residing in his home. As residents, they are entitled to maintain their dignity and be cared for with respect, concern, and passion.[21]

Abusive Search

A nurse in *People v. Coe*[22] was charged with a willful violation of the public health law in connection with an allegedly abusive search of an 86-year-old resident at a geriatric center and with the falsification of business records in the first degree. The resident, Mr. Gersh, had heart disease and difficulty in expressing himself verbally. Another resident claimed that two $5 bills were missing. Nurse Coe assumed that Gersh had taken them because he had been known to take things in the past. The nurse proceeded to search Gersh, who resisted. A security guard was summoned, and another search was undertaken. When Gersh again resisted, the security guard slammed a chair down in front of him and pinned his arms while the defendant nurse searched his pockets, failing to retrieve the two $5 bills. Five minutes later, Gersh collapsed, gasping for air, in a chair. Coe administered cardiopulmonary resuscitation but was unsuccessful, and Gersh died.

Coe was charged with violation of Section 175.10 of the New York Penal Law for falsifying records because of the defendant's "omission" of the facts relating to the search of

Gersh. These facts were considered to be relevant and should have been included in the nurse's notes regarding this incident. "The first sentence states, 'Observed resident was extremely confused and talks incoherently. Suddenly became unresponsive . . . .' This statement is simply false. It could only be true if some reference to the search and the loud noise was included."[23] A motion was made to dismiss the indictment at the end of the trial.

The court held that the search became an act of physical abuse and mistreatment, the evidence was sufficient to warrant a finding of guilt on both charges, and the fact that searches took place frequently did not excuse an otherwise illegal procedure.

It may well be that this incident reached the attention of the criminal justice system only because, in the end, a man had died. In those instances that are equally violative of residents' rights and equally contrary to standards of common decency but that do not result in visible harm to a patient, the acts are nevertheless illegal and subject to prosecution. A criminal act is not legitimized by the fact that others have, with impunity, engaged in that act.[24]

Physical Abuse

The revocation of a personal care home license was found to be proper in *Miller Home, Inc. v. Commonwealth, Department of Public Welfare*[25] because of repeated medication violations and resident abuse. Evidence was presented that the son of the personal care home's manager was hired as a staff member after having acted as a substitute, even though he had physical altercations with residents of the home. On one occasion, the manager's son punched a female resident, resulting in her hospitalization for broken bones around the eye, and on two prior occasions he had been involved in less-physical altercations that required police intervention.

The nursing facility resident in *Stiffelman v. Abrams*[26] died from:

> ". . . blows, kicks, kneeings, or bodily throwings intentionally, viciously, and murderously dealt him from among the facility's staff over a period of approximately two to three weeks prior to his death"; that the "beatings were repeated and were received by the decedent at ninety years of age and in a frail, defenseless, and dependent condition"; that the beatings so administered to the decedent were "physically and mentally tortuous"; that he was caused by them to live out his final days in agony and terror; and that his physical injuries included thirteen fractures to his ribs, subpleural hemorrhaging, and marked lesions to his chest, flanks, abdomen, legs, arms, and hands; that during and following the period of the beatings the decedent lay at the facility for days unattended and unaided as to the deterioration and grave suffering he was undergoing.[27]

The executors of the estate had brought suit against the operator and individual and corporate owners of the facility for damages for personal injuries resulting in the death of the resident. The executors were requesting under Count I, $1.5 million in survival damages because of the physical and mental pain and suffering of the decedent, as well as $3 million for punitive damages, and under Count II, $1,504,084 in contractual breaches of the resident's admission contract with the facility. The executors claimed that certain standards of care and personal rights contained in the contract were violated. The trial court sustained the nursing facility's motion for dismissal of the case on the grounds that the plaintiffs failed to state a claim on which relief could be granted. On appeal, the judgment of the trial court was reversed with respect to Count I, and the dismissal of Count II was sustained. The case was remanded, requiring the executors to proceed under appropriate statutory authority and not under contract.

MURDER

The tragedy of murder in institutions that are dedicated to the healing of the sick has been an all-too-frequent occurrence. As was the case in *People v. Diaz*,[28] where the defendant, a registered nurse working nights at a community hospital, had an unusual number of deaths on her shift. During a three-and-a-half-week period, 13 patients on the night shift had seizures, cardiac arrest, and respiratory arrest; nine died. The unit closed and the defendant went to work at another hospital. Within three days, a patient died after exhibiting the same symptoms as those in the previous hospital while the defendant was on duty. The defendant was arrested and tried for 12 counts of murder.

The testimony revealed that the defendant injected the patients with massive doses of Lidocaine (a rhythm-controlling drug). Evidence showed that the defendant assisted the patients before they exhibited seizures, providing opportunity for the nurse to administer the drug. She was observed acting strangely on the nights of the deaths, and high concentrations of Lidocaine were found in the patients' syringes. Moreover, syringes containing the drug and Lidocaine vials were discovered in the defendant's home.

Pretrial investigation revealed that 26 other patients had died at the defendant's first hospital while under the nurse's care. All had the same symptoms. The defendant, who waived her right to trial by jury, was found guilty of the 12 counts of murder. The nurse appealed the judgment of death.

The California Supreme Court upheld the convictions. The expert testimony about the levels of Lidocaine in the patients' tissue, coupled with the nurse's testimony concerning the symptoms prior to the deaths, confirmed that the patients died from overdoses given to them by the defendant. Testimony showed that the defendant was the only nurse on duty the night each patient was poisoned, and only the defendant had the opportunity to administer the fatal doses.

Nurse Sentenced for Diabolical Acts

From 1993 to 1995, Majors worked as a licensed practical nurse (LPN) in the intensive care unit (ICU) of a county hospital. He might have been a competent nurse, but he had one problem: An incredibly high number of elderly patients died under his watch. By 1995, after rumors started to circulate that he was euthanizing patients, the hospital suspended him, and the state board of nursing suspended his license.

In 1994, 100 of the 351 people admitted to the hospital's four-bed ICU died. A large percentage of those who died were elderly. In comparison, during the previous 4 years, an average of only 27 patients per year passed away, out of an average of 354 admitted to the ICU each year.

An analysis was conducted that showed Majors was present for more deaths than any other nurse, almost twice as many as the nearest contender. The hospital's president and chief executive officer, Ling, suspended Majors from work. Later, Ling asked the police to investigate. Majors was subsequently prosecuted.

Majors was sentenced to spend the rest of his life in prison for murdering six elderly patients, a crime the judge referred to as a paragon of evil at its most wicked. Majors had been entrusted with these people's care. In response, he committed diabolical acts that extinguished the frail lives of six people.[29]

Fatal Injection of Pavulon

In a case involving the defendant–registered nurse Angelo on the cardiac/intensive care unit at a Long Island hospital, the defendant was found guilty of second-degree murder for injecting two patients with the drug Pavulon. He was found guilty of the lesser charges of manslaughter and criminally negligent homicide in the deaths of two other patients. Angelo committed the murders in a bizarre scheme to revive the patients and be thought of as a hero.[30]

REMOVAL OF LIFE SUPPORT

Although there might be a duty to provide life-sustaining equipment in the immediate aftermath of cardiopulmonary arrest, there is no duty to continue its use when it has become futile and ineffective to do so in the opinion of qualified medical personnel. Two physicians in *Barber v. Superior Court*[31] were charged with the crimes of murder and conspiracy to commit murder. The charges were based on their acceding to requests of the patient's family to discontinue life-support equipment and intravenous tubes. The patient suffered a cardiopulmonary arrest in the recovery room after surgery. A team of physicians and nurses revived the patient and placed him on life-support equipment. The patient suffered severe brain damage, which placed him in a comatose and vegetative state from which, according to tests and examinations by other specialists, he was unlikely to recover. On the written request of the family, the patient was taken off life-support equipment. The family, his wife and eight children, made the decision together after consultation with the physicians. Evidence had been presented that the patient, before his incapacitation, had expressed to his wife that he would not want to be kept alive by a machine. There was no evidence indicating that the family was motivated in their decision by anything other than love and concern for the dignity of their loved one. The patient continued to breathe on his own. Showing no signs of improvement, the physicians again discussed the patient's poor prognosis with the family. The intravenous lines were removed, and the patient died sometime thereafter.

A complaint then was filed against the two physicians. The magistrate who heard the evidence determined that the physicians did not kill the deceased because their conduct was not the proximate cause of the patient's death. On motion of the prosecution, the superior court determined as a matter of law that the evidence required the magistrate to hold the physicians to answer and ordered the complaint reinstated. The court of appeals held that the physicians' omission to continue treatment, although intentional and with knowledge that the patient would die, was not an unlawful failure to perform a legal duty. The evidence amply supported the magistrate's decision. The court of appeals determined that the superior court erred in determining that the evidence required the magistrate to hold the physicians to answer.

PETTY THEFT

Health care organizations must be alert to the potential ongoing threat of theft by unscrupulous employees, physicians, patients, visitors, and trespassers. The theft of patient or resident valuables, supplies, and equipment is substantial and costs health care organizations millions of dollars each year.

The evidence presented in *People v. Lancaster*[32] was found to have provided a probable cause foundation for information charging felony theft of nursing home residents' money by the office manager. Evidence showed that on repeated occasions the residents' income checks were cashed or cash was otherwise received on behalf of residents; that the defendant, by virtue of her office, had sole responsibility for maintaining the residents' ledger accounts; and that cash receipts frequently were never posted to the residents' accounts.

In another case, there was sufficient evidence in *Miller v. Dunn*[33] to hold that a nurse assistant had misappropriated $15,000 from an 83-year-old nursing home resident. The record indicated that the funds were taken during those times the resident made visits to the hospital for respiratory problems. The patient had been diagnosed with dementia, and the resident's confusion was increasing. The nursing assistant actively procured the check in question filling in the date, amount, and her name as payee.

CRIMINAL HISTORY AND FALSE STATEMENTS

The record indicated that the physician in *Hoxie v. Ohio State Med. Bd.* had made false statements concerning his criminal history when he stated in a deposition that he had never been arrested. There was sufficient evidence presented to support permanent revocation of his license to practice medicine. Certified records held by the state of California indicated that the physician had been arrested or detained by the Los Angeles Police Department multiple times in 1970s and 1980s for possessing marijuana and PCP, for driving under the influence of alcohol and/or drugs and for driving under a suspended license. Although the physician asserted that documentation of his criminal past had been fabricated by police and was not credible, law enforcement investigation reports were generally admissible. The physician himself added to the reliability of the records by verifying all significant identifying information contained within the documents and records.[34]

Notes

1. 871 F.2d 105 (9th Cir. 1989).
2. 366 F.2d 167 (6th Cir. 1966).
3. 265 U.S. 182, 188 (1924).
4. 385 F.3d 1013 (C.A. 6, Ky. 2004).
5. 824 F.2d 780 (9th Cir. 1987).
6. 513 So. 2d 493 (La. Ct. App. 1987).
7. Id. at 495.
8. 322 S.E.2d 696 (N.C. Ct. App. 1985).
9. No. 02-6183 (C.A. 10, Okla. 2004).
10. Richard J. Gelles, Murray A. Strauss, & Suzabbe K. Steinmetz, Behind Closed Doors: Violence in the American Family (1981). Anchor Books, NY, New York.
11. 557 F. Supp. 289 (D. Colo. 1983).
12. Id. at 293.
13. 42 C.F.R. § 483.13 (1989).
14. Nurse's Aide Jailed for Punching Patient, *THE BALTIMORE SUN*, June 29, 1990, §D, at 2.
15. 486 So. 2d 101 (La. 1986).
16. Id. at 101, 104.
17. 493 N.W.2d 884 (Iowa Ct. App. 1992).
18. Id. at 887–888.
19. 551 A.2d 354 (Pa. Commw. Ct. 1988).
20. Id. at 355.
21. Id. at 357.
22. 501 N.Y.S.2d 997 (N.Y. Sup. Ct. 1986).
23. Id. at 1001.
24. Id.
25. 556 A.2d 1 (Pa. Commw. Ct. 1989).
26. 655 S.W.2d 522 (Mo. 1983).
27. Id.
28. 834 P.2d 1171 (Cal. 1992).
28. Majors v. Engelbrecht, 149 F.3d 709 (1998).
30. Collwell, The Verdict of Angelo, 50(103) NEWSDAY 1989, at 3.
31. 195 Cal. Rptr. 484 (Cal. Ct. App. 1983).
32. 683 P.2d 1202 (Colo. 1984)
33. 184 S.W.3d 122 (Mo. App. 2006).
34. No. 05AP-681 (Ohio App. 2006).

5

Contracts

One of the many areas of law that affects health care providers is contracts. The intention here is to give the reader an introduction to contracts, focusing on providing a general understanding of their concepts, elements, and importance as they pertain to health care organizations and professionals.

PURPOSE OF A CONTRACT

A *contract* is a special kind of agreement, either written or oral, that involves legally binding obligations between two or more parties. A contract serves to provide one or more of the parties with a legal remedy if another of the parties does not perform his or her obligations pursuant to the terms of the contract. The major purpose of a contract is to specify, limit, and define the agreements that are legally enforceable. A contract forces the participants to be specific in their understandings and expectations of each other. Contracts, particularly those in writing, serve to minimize misunderstandings and offer a means for the parties of a contract to resolve any disputes that might arise.

TYPES OF CONTRACTS

The following is a general description of the various types of contracts and a brief definition of each. Health care professionals should be knowledgeable of each as they are commonly used in the health care setting.

Express Contract

An *express contract* is one in which the parties have an oral or written agreement.

Both *written* and *oral* contracts are generally recognized and are equally legal and binding. A written contract is always desirable over a verbal contract.

Implied Contract

An *implied contract* is one that is inferred by law. It is based on the conduct of the parties, such as a handshake or similar conduct. Much of the litigation concerning excesses of corporate authority involves questions of whether a corporation has the implied authority—incidental to its express authority—to perform a questioned act. For example, even though its certificate of incorporation did not authorize such an act specifically, a hospital was permitted to construct a medical office building on land that had been donated for maintaining and carrying on a general hospital. The court, in recognizing a trend to encourage charitable hospitals to provide private offices for rental to staff members, held that such an act was within the implied powers of the hospital and that such offices aid in the work of a general hospital even though it went beyond the hospital corporation's express powers.[1]

Voidable Contract

A *voidable contract* is one in which one party, but not the other, has the right to escape from its legal obligations under the contract. It is considered to be a voidable contract at the option of that party. For example, a minor, not having the capacity to enter into a contract, can void the contract. However, the competent party to the contract may not void the contract.

ELEMENTS OF A CONTRACT

The law will enforce contracts only when they are executed between persons who are competent; that is, those with the legal and mental capacity to contract. Certain classes of persons, such as minors, the insane, and prisoners, traditionally have been considered to be unable to understand the consequences of their actions and have been deemed incompetent, or lacking in legal capacity, to make a binding contract. Whether contracts are executed in writing or agreed to orally, they must contain the following elements to be enforceable.

Offer/Communication

An *offer* is a promise by one party to do (or not to do) something if the other party agrees to do (or not do) something. Preliminary negotiations are not offers. An offer *must be communicated* to the other party so that it can be accepted or rejected.

Consideration

Consideration requires that each party to a contract give up something of value in exchange for something of value. No side can have a free way out or the ability to obtain something of value without providing something in exchange. Only when legal consideration has been given will a court treat the agreement as a contract. The adequacy or inadequacy of consideration, or the price paid, will not normally affect the formation of a contract.

Acceptance

Upon proper acceptance of an offer, a contract is formed. A valid acceptance requires the following:

- *Meeting of the minds*: Acceptance requires a meeting of the minds (mutual assent); in other words, the parties must understand and agree on the terms of the contract. This means that each side must be clear as to the details, rights, and obligations of the contract.
- *Definite and complete*: Acceptance requires mutual assent to be found between the parties. The terms must be so complete that both parties understand and agree to what has been proposed.
- *Duration*: Generally, the offeror (the one who makes the offer) may revoke an offer at any time prior to a valid acceptance. When the offeror does revoke the proposal, the revocation is not effective until the offeree (the person to whom the offer is made) receives it. When the offeree has

accepted the offer, any attempt to revoke the agreement is too late and is invalid.

- *Complete and conforming*: The acceptance must be a mirror image of the offer. In other words, the acceptance must comply with all the terms of the offer and not change or add any terms.

BREACH OF CONTRACT

A *breach of contract* occurs when there is a violation of one or more of the terms of the contract. The basic elements that a plaintiff must establish to be successful in a breach of contract lawsuit include the following: (1) a valid contract was executed; (2) the plaintiff performed as specified in the contract; (3) the defendant failed to perform as specified in the contract; and (4) the plaintiff suffered an economic loss as a result of the defendant's breach of contract.

Breach of Contract—Blood Transfusion

Harvey was diagnosed with blockage in his carotid artery. Dr. Strictland recommended surgery. In anticipation of surgery, Harvey signed written consent forms indicating that he refused to have blood or blood products given to him and that he fully understood the attendant risks. The day before his surgery, Harvey signed another consent form indicating that he did not give permission to use blood.

Surgery was performed. Harvey developed a blood clot and had a stroke while in the recovery room. Because Harvey was unconscious, hospital personnel located his mother in the waiting room and obtained her permission to perform a CT scan and an arteriogram. A second surgery was performed, and more blood clots were removed along the side of the carotid artery. Harvey was then moved to the intensive care unit (ICU). After an ICU nurse discovered Harvey was having difficulty breathing, the on-call emergency room physician intubated him. The next day, Harvey began bleeding from the surgical site at his neck. He had lost approximately 30% of his blood volume. When his hemoglobin level reached 8, Dr. Strictland recommended a blood transfusion. After first denying the transfusion because of Harvey's religious beliefs, Harvey's mother consented to the blood transfusion.

Harvey sued. Harvey relied upon the documents he signed expressing his desire not to be administered blood. It was for the jury to determine whether an express contract was created. The trial court's directed verdict for the surgeon was reversed on appeal, and the matter was remanded for a new trial.[2]

CORPORATE CONTRACTS

The ability of a corporation to enter into a contract is limited by its powers as contained in or inferred from its articles of incorporation (sometimes called a charter) or conferred upon it by general corporation law. Whenever a contract of any consequence is made with a corporation, appropriate corporate approval and authorization must be obtained. In the event that a contract is entered into with a corporation without the appropriate authority, the contract nevertheless can be ratified and made binding on the corporation by subsequent conduct or statements made on its behalf by its representatives.

When the chief executive officer (CEO) of an organization exceeds the limits of his or her authority, the question of whether the organization will be responsible for the CEO's acts might arise. If the actions of the governing body give rise to a third party's reasonable belief that the CEO acts with the authority of the organization, and such belief causes the third party to enter into an agreement with the CEO, expecting that the organization will be obligated under the contract, then the organization generally is responsible under the concept of apparent authority (the appearance of being the agent of another [employer or principal] with the power to act for the principal). However, if a third party deals with the CEO in the absence of indications of the CEO's authority created by the governing body and thereby unreasonably assumes that the CEO possesses the authority to bind the organization to a contract, then such third party deals with the CEO in an individual capacity and not as an agent of the organization. There are times when the CEO clearly can exceed the limitations of his or her authority, but the governing body subsequently can approve such actions through ratification by accepting any resulting responsibility as though it had been authorized previously.

If, for example, the governing body has imposed a limitation on equipment purchases that could be made without specific prior approval of the governing body, the price of the equipment would determine whether the governing body was bound under the contract. If the equipment was $26,000 and the limitation on purchases without specific governing body approval was $25,000, then the CEO would have no authority to bind the organization for the purchase of the equipment. The CEO generally would be liable to the supplier of the equipment.

PARTNERSHIPS

A *partnership* comprises two or more persons who agree to carry on a business for profit and to share profits and losses in some proportions. A partnership, unlike a corporation, can be created by the parties' actions without a written or oral agreement.

AGENTS

An *agent* is one who has the power to contract for and bind another person, who is known as the principal. Corporations can act only through agents (e.g., their officers).

Apparent Agent or Ostensible Agent

An *apparent or ostensible agent* is one who a third person believes is acting on behalf of the principal. If a hospital undertakes to provide physician services to a community, and the community reasonably believes that the physician is employed by the hospital to deliver services, then the hospital would generally be liable for the physician's negligent acts. For example, in *Jennison v. Providence St. Vincent Med. Ctr.*,[3] Jennison, having severe abdominal pain, was taken to the hospital emergency department. Unsure of the cause of Jennison's medical problems, Cook, Jennison's assigned physician, recommended surgery. Prior to surgery Cook asked Nunez, a member of an independent anesthesiology group at the hospital, to place a central venous catheter in Jennison.

An X-ray had been taken to confirm the correct placement of the central line. The X-ray showed that the tip of the central line had gone into the pericardial sac of Jennison's heart. A procedure had not been established to timely notify the treating physicians that the central line had been dangerously misplaced.

Upon the eventual discovery that the central line had been misplaced, it was pulled back to its proper position. Unfortunately fluids had already infused through the central line and into the space between Jennison's heart and pericardial sac. The pressure of the fluid against her heart kept it from filling adequately. Jennison's blood pressure dropped, and she went into cardiac arrest. The doctors attempted to remove the excess fluid. During the procedure, Jennison suffered a second cardiac arrest. The doctors were again able to resuscitate her. However, due to the lack of oxygen to her brain, Jennison suffered a severe brain injury.

The jury returned a verdict in favor of the plaintiffs, finding the hospital 100% negligent, and the hospital appealed.

The Court of Appeals of Oregon affirmed the findings of the trial court. The hospital presented itself as providing radiology services to the public. The public, looking to the hospital to provide such care, is unaware of and unconcerned with the technical complexities and nuances surrounding the contractual and employment arrangements between the hospital and the various medical personnel operating therein. Public policy dictates that the public has every right to assume and expect that the hospital is the medical provider it purports to be.

INDEPENDENT CONTRACTOR

An *independent contractor* is an individual who agrees to undertake work without being under the direct control or direction of another. Independent contractors are personally responsible for their own negligent acts. Whether a physician is an employee or an independent contractor is of primary importance in determining liability for damages. Generally, a health care organization is not liable for injuries resulting from negligent acts or omissions of independent physicians. There is no liability on the theory of respondeat superior, whereby a physician is an independent contractor as long as the physician is not an employee of the organization, is not compensated by the organization, maintains a private practice, and is chosen directly by his or her patients. The mere existence of an independent contractual relationship, however, is not sufficient to remove an organization from liability for the acts of certain of its professional personnel for which the independent contractor status is not readily known to the injured party.

Hospital Liable for Physician's Negligence

A hospital can be liable for a physician's negligence, even if the physician is under contract to provide services to the hospital. The appellate division of the New York State Supreme Court in *Mduba v. Benedictine Hospital*[4] held that the hospital was liable for the emergency department physician's negligence whether the physician was an independent contractor or, even if under contract, the physician was considered to be an independent contractor. The court held that the patient had no way of knowing of the existence of a contract and relied on the relationship between the hospital and the physician in seeking treatment in the emergency department.

LEGALITY OF OBJECT

To be a valid contract, the purpose or object of the contract must not be against state or federal policy and must not violate any statute, rule, or regulation. If the subject or purpose of the contract becomes illegal by some statute, rule, or regulation before actual formation of the contract, the parties no longer can form the contract.

CONDITIONS

A *condition* precedent is an act or event that must happen or be performed by one party before the other party has any responsibility to perform under the contract. An *express condition* is formally written into the contract in specific terms. An *implied condition* is one in which, although the parties might not have specifically mentioned the condition, it can reasonably be assumed that the parties intended the condition to be enforced.

PERFORMANCE

Performance is the act of doing what is required by a contract. Each party to a contract is bound to perform the promises according to the stipulated terms of a contract. The effect of successful performance by each party to a contract is to discharge the parties bound to the contract from any future contractual liability.

NONPERFORMANCE DEFENSES

Under some circumstances the law gives a person a right not to perform under a contract. Defenses permitting nonperformance of a contract include fraud, mistakes, duress, illegal contract, impossibility, and statute of limitations.

Fraud

A victim of fraud will not have to perform under a contract. Fraud occurs when one party intentionally misrepresents a material fact or term of the contract and intends that the other party rely on that misrepresentation. The second party must rely on the misrepresentation and suffer some damage before it will be excused from performing.

Mistake of Fact

Mistakes often occur in contracts. However, a party will be allowed to claim mistake as a defense in only certain instances. There are two types of mistakes: mistake of fact and mistake of law. A *mistake of fact* is an incorrect belief regarding a fact. Both parties must have made the mistake. If only one is in error (and it is not known to the other), mistake of fact is not a defense. *Mistake of law*, on the other hand, is an incorrect judgment of the legal consequences of known facts. If the parties to a suit make a mistake as to the law involved, they usually must accept their plight without any remedy.

Duress

Duress is the use of unlawful threats or pressure to force an individual to act against his or her will. An act performed under duress is not legally binding.

Illegal Contract

An *illegal contract* is a contract whose formation, object, or performance is against the law or contrary to public policy that no court would uphold or enforce. No individual can recover damages when a contract is formed for illegal purposes.

Impossibility

Contracts can become impossible to perform because (1) certain facts might have existed at the time the contract was executed or (2) they might have arisen subsequent to the formation of the contract. Contracts that are impossible to perform do not have to be carried out by the parties to a contract.

Statute of Limitations

A party who does not, within a period of time known as the statute of limitations, take action to enforce contract rights by suing for damages caused by a breach of the contract or taking other action can be barred from doing so.

REMEDIES

What can a party do when another has breached the contract and refuses to or cannot perform? The general rule is that legal redress will attempt to make the injured party whole again.

Specified Performance

When an aggrieved party has subsequently complied with his or her obligations pursuant to the agreed-upon terms of a contract, that party might seek specific performance as a remedy rather than monetary remuneration. The most satisfactory remedy available to an injured party might be to require specific performance by the other party to the contract.

Monetary Damages

Money damages, sometimes called compensatory damages, are awarded in an attempt to restore to the aggrieved party the money that it would have had if the other party had not breached the contract. This can include the cost of making a substitute contract with another party and the expense of delays caused by the breach.

General and Consequential Damages

General damages are those that can be expected to arise from a breach of a contract. They are foreseeable and common in the circumstances. *Consequential damages* are those that occur because of some unexpected, unusual, or strange development involved in the particular contract in dispute. The distinction between the two types is one of foreseeability. If it is found that the party who breached the contract could have foreseen the damages that followed, that person could be liable for consequential as well as general damages.

Duty to Mitigate Damages

When someone has breached a contract, the other party cannot stand idly by and let damages build indefinitely. Every injured party has a duty to mitigate (lessen) damages caused by the breach of another person or entity. Failure to do so will prevent the aggrieved party's full recovery of damages that could have been mitigated.

EMPLOYMENT CONTRACTS

An *employment contract* is an agreement between an employee and employer that specifies the terms of employment. The conditions of employment including wages, hours, and type of work are generally described in an employment contract. Depending on the level of employment and the responsibility of the new employee, the conditions of employment should include the terms of employment; the duties and responsibilities of the employee; compensation; confidentiality requirements (e.g., trade secrets and proprietary information); a noncompete clause; and provisions for termination of the agreement (e.g., an inability to perform one's duties and responsibilities).

A contract can be express or implied. Most employees work under employment contracts. For example, if an employee signs a document promising to abide by company policy and procedures, it likely constitutes an employment contract. Certain categories of employees (e.g., radiologists) often have the ability to negotiate their employment contracts. An employer's right to terminate an employee can be limited by express agreement with the employee or through a collective bargaining agreement to which the employee is a beneficiary.

The rights of employees have been expanding through judicial decisions in the different states. Court decisions have been based on verbal promises, historical practices of the employer, and documents such as employee handbooks and administrative policy and procedure manuals that describe employee rights.

Breaches of Contract: Repayment of Tuition Required

The registered nurse in *Sweetwater Hosp. Ass'n v. Carpenter*[5] was found to have breached her contract with the hospital under which the hospital agreed to pay for her schooling as a nurse anesthetist in exchange for her agreeing to work for the hospital for five years following completion of her studies. The nurse agreed that if she failed to work at the hospital following completion of her studies, she would be responsible for cash advances by the hospital plus interest. Upon completion of her studies, the nurse sought employment elsewhere because it appeared to her that there were no nurse anesthetist positions available at the hospital.

The contract provided that one of the considerations for the loan was that the defendant agree to become or remain an employee of the hospital. The contract did not state in what capacity the defendant would become or remain an employee. There was nothing in the language of the contract stating that the hospital had an obligation to offer the defendant a nurse anesthetist position.

In this case, there was no proof by the defendant that the hospital breached the contract. The defendant breached her own contract by taking a job elsewhere without specifically getting proof that she was not going to be offered a job by the hospital. The defendant did not present herself for employment at the hospital after graduation. She accepted a position elsewhere. Because she did not become employed at the hospital, she was not entitled to rely upon the forgiveness provisions contained in the contract. She was, therefore, obligated to repay the hospital.

No Express Agreement: Right to Terminate

No express agreement was found to exist in *O'Connor v. Eastman Kodak Co.*,[6] in which the court held that an employer had a right to terminate an employee at will at any time and for any reason or no reason. The plaintiff did not rely on any specific representation made to him during the course of his employment interviews nor did he rely on any documentation in the employee handbook, which would have limited the defendant's common-law right to discharge at will. The employee had relied on a popular perception of Kodak as a "womb-to-tomb" employer.

Restrictive Covenant Enforceable

The plaintiff–hospital, in *Sarah Bush Lincoln Health Ctr. v. Perket*,[7] sued its former director of physical medicine and rehabilitation to enforce a restrictive covenant in the employment contract precluding the director from accepting similar employment in the same county within one year of termination of employment. The parties to the complaint entered into a contract whereby the defendant was employed as the plaintiff's director of physical medicine. The contract provided that during the director's employment and for a period of one year thereafter, the director would not, directly or indirectly, invest in, own, manage, operate, control, be employed by, participate in, or be connected in any manner with the ownership, management, operation, or control of any person, firm, or corporation engaged in competition with the hospital in providing health services or facilities within Coles County, including the provision of services in a private office, without prior written consent of the hospital. Following the termination, the defendant engaged in the business of providing physical medicine and rehabilitation services in Coles County. The plaintiff argued that unless the defendant was enjoined, the hospital would suffer irreparable injury. The circuit court granted the hospital's motion for preliminary injunction. On appeal, the Illinois Appellate Court held that the grant of the preliminary injunction was proper and that the defendant was engaging in the business of providing physical medicine and rehabilitation services in Coles County. By hiring the defendant, the hospital was thereby bringing him in contact with a clientele that the hospital had established over a period of years. The hospital was naturally interested in protecting its clients from being taken over by the defendant as a result of these contacts.

Restrictive Covenant Not Enforceable

Not every restrictive covenant is enforceable; for example, a restrictive covenant in an employment contract between a hospital and neurosurgeon was found to be geographically too restrictive whereby the neurosurgeon was not to practice within a 30-mile radius of the hospital. This restriction was determined to be excessive. Such a restriction was considered to be detrimental to public interest in that the restricted area was plagued with a shortage of neurosurgeons.[8]

The reader should understand that employment contracts that contain a restrictive covenant between a physician and a hospital, although not favored, are not per se unreasonable and unenforceable. The trial court must determine whether the restrictive covenant protects the legitimate interests of the employer, imposes no undue hardship on the employee, and is not adverse to the public interest.[9]

Handbook Considered a Contract

For an employee handbook to constitute a contract, thereby giving enforceable rights to the employee, the following elements must be present:

1. A policy statement that clearly sets forth a promise that the employee can construe to be an offer.
2. The policy statement must be distributed to the employee, making him or her aware of the offer.
3. After learning about the offer and policy statement, the employee must "begin" or "continue" to work.

In *Watson v. Idaho Falls Consolidated Hospitals, Inc.*[10] a nurse's aide was awarded $20,000 for damages when the hospital, as employer, violated the provisions of its employee handbook in the manner in which it terminated her employment. Although the nurse's aide had no formal written contract, the employee handbook and the hospital policies and procedures manual constituted a contract in view of evidence to the effect that these documents had been intended to be enforced and complied with by both employees and management. Employees read and relied on the handbook as creating terms of an employment contract. They were required to sign for the handbook to establish receipt of a revised handbook that explained hospital policy, discipline, counseling, and termination. A policy-and-procedure manual placed on each floor of the hospital also outlined termination procedures.

Handbook Not a Contract Due to Disclaimer

The employee handbook in *Churchill v. Waters*[11] was not considered to be a contract because of a disclaimer in the handbook. A nurse brought a civil rights action against the hospital and hospital officials after her discharge. The federal district court held for the defendants, finding that the hospital employee handbook did not give the nurse a protected property interest in continued employment: "Absent proof that the handbook contained clear promises which indicated the intent to bind the parties, no contract was created."[12] The "handbook contained a disclaimer" expressly disavowing any attempt to be bound by it and stated that its contents were not to be considered conditions of employment. The handbook was presented as a matter of information only, and the language contained therein was not intended to constitute a contract between McDonough District Hospital and the employee. Although an employee handbook can delineate specific disciplinary procedures, that fact does not in and of itself constitute an enforceable contract.[13]

Termination of Contract Due to Insubordination

The physician in *Trieger v. Montefiore Med. Ctr.*[14] circulated a memorandum to department chairs at the hospital strongly criticizing management and urging his cochairs "to set things right and reclaim their prerogatives and responsibilities." The appellate court found that the trial court correctly determined that the memorandum was insubordinate and that it gave just cause for termination of the physician's employment contract. In addition, the physician's age discrimination claim was dismissed for lack of evidence sufficient to raise an issue of fact as to whether the hospital's reason for the doctor's dismissal, circulation of the insubordinate memorandum, was a pretext for discrimination. The doctor was terminated immediately after circulating the insubordinate memorandum, and there was no other evidence in the record to support the claim that the hospital's actions were pretextual.

MEDICAL STAFF BYLAWS: CONTRACT

Medical staff bylaws can be considered a contract. The plaintiff, Dr. Bass, in *Bass v. Ambrosius*,[15] alleged that the hospital's termination of his staff privileges violated its own bylaws. The hospital contended that its bylaws did not constitute a contract between itself and Bass, and, therefore, any violation of those bylaws would not support a breach-of-contract claim. The general rule that hospital bylaws can constitute a contract between the hospital and its staff is consistent with Wisconsin law that an employee handbook written and disseminated by the employer, and whose terms the employee has accepted, constitutes a contract between the employer and the employee. For example, in *Ferraro v. Koelsch*,[16] an employee handbook was management's statement of what the company offered its employees and what it expected from its employees in return. It thus contained the essential elements of a binding contract: the promise of employment on stated terms and conditions by the employer and the promise by the employee to continue employment under those conditions. The court noted that a promise for a promise, or the exchange of promises, constitutes consideration to support any contract of this bilateral nature.

The bylaws at issue in *Bass v. Ambrosius*, required by Wis. Admin. Code § HSS 124.12(5) and approved by the hospital's board of directors, have the same contractual elements as did the handbook in Ferraro. First, the bylaws state that they provide the rules that govern the physicians and dentists practicing at the hospital. Second, members of the hospital's medical–dental staff must continuously meet the qualifications, standards, and requirements set forth in the bylaws. Third, an appointment to the medical–dental staff confers only those privileges provided by the letter of appointment and the bylaws. Fourth, all applicants for appointment to the medical–dental staff must submit a signed application acknowledging the requirement to familiarize themselves with the bylaws. Each applicant for appointment to the medical–dental staff must submit a signed application attesting that he or she has read and agreed to accept and abide by the provisions and directives in the bylaws. Thus, Bass's application to the medical–dental staff acknowledged by his signature that he would conduct his professional activities according to the bylaws and rules and regulations of both the hospital and the medical–dental staff of the hospital. In a separate letter, part of the application process, Bass agreed to conduct his activities according to the bylaws of the hospital, as well as the bylaws and rules and regulations of the hospital's medical–dental staff. For its part, the hospital promised that the medical–dental staff would be guided and governed by rules and regulations consistent with the bylaws, and it promised that any adverse action against a member of the medical–dental staff would comply with various procedural safeguards. The bylaws constituted a contract between Bass and the hospital. Accordingly, Bass was entitled to an order holding that the hospital had to comply with its bylaws before it could terminate his staff privileges.

EXCLUSIVE CONTRACTS

An organization often enters into an exclusive contract with physicians or medical groups for the purpose of providing a specific service to the organization. Exclusive contracts generally occur within the organization's ancillary service departments (e.g., radiology, anesthesiology, and pathology). Physicians who seek to practice at organizations in these ancillary areas but who are not part of the exclusive group have attempted to invoke the federal antitrust laws to challenge these exclusive contracts. These challenges generally have been unsuccessful.

In *Jefferson Parish Hospital v. Hyde*,[17] the defendant hospital had a contract with a firm of anesthesiologists that required all anesthesia services for the hospital's patients be performed by that firm. Because of this contract, the plaintiff–anesthesiologist's application for admission to the hospital's medical staff was denied. Dr. Hyde commenced an action in the federal district court, claiming the exclusive contract violated Section 1 of the Sherman Antitrust Act. The district court rejected the plaintiff's complaint, but the US Court of Appeals for the Fifth Circuit reversed, finding the contract illegal per se. The Supreme Court reversed the Fifth Circuit, holding that the exclusive contract in question does not violate Section 1 of the Sherman Antitrust Act. The Supreme Court's holding was based on the fact that the defendant hospital did not possess "market power," and therefore patients were free to enter a competing hospital and to use another anesthesiologist instead of the firm. Thus, the court concluded that the evidence was insufficient to provide a basis for finding that the contract, as it actually operates in the market, had unreasonably restrained competition.

CONTRACTS AND NONCOMPETITIVE CLAUSES

The respondent–hospital in *Washington County Memorial Hospital v. Sidebottom*[18] employed the appellant–nurse practitioner from October 1993 through April 1998. Prior to beginning her employment, the nurse entered into an employment agreement with the hospital. The agreement included a noncompetition clause providing in part that the nurse, during the term of the agreement and for a period of 1 year after the termination of her employment, would not within a 50-mile radius directly or indirectly engage in the practice of nursing without the express direction or consent of the hospital. In February 1994, the nurse requested the hospital's permission to work for the Washington County Health Department doing prenatal nursing care. Because the hospital was not then doing prenatal care, the hospital gave her permission to accept that employment but reserved the ability to withdraw the permission if the services the nurse was providing later came to be provided by the hospital. In January 1996, the nurse and the hospital entered into a second employment agreement that continued the parties' employment relationship through January 9, 1998. This agreement included a noncompetition clause identical to the 1993 employment agreement. It also provided for automatic renewal for an additional 2 years unless either party gave written termination notice no less than 90 days prior to the expiration of the agreement.

On March 11, 1998, the nurse gave the hospital written notice of her resignation effective April 15. On April 16, the nurse began working as a nurse practitioner with Dr. Mullen at his office. The office was located within 50 miles of the hospital.

The Circuit Court, on October 16, prohibited the nurse from practicing nursing within a 50-mile radius of the hospital for a period of 1 year from April 15.

The noncompetition clause in the nurse's employment agreement was found to be clear and unambiguous. The nurse obtained legal advice before signing her original employment agreement and before resigning. The hospital notified the nurse before her last day that the noncompetition clause would be enforced. On appeal, the judgment of the circuit court was affirmed.

TRANSFER AGREEMENTS

Health care organizations should have a written transfer agreement in effect with other organizations to help ensure the smooth transfer of patients from one facility to another when the attending physician determines such appropriate. A *transfer agreement* is a written document that sets forth the terms and conditions under which a patient can be transferred to a facility that more appropriately provides the kind of care required by the patient. It also establishes procedures to admit patients of one facility to another when their condition warrants a transfer.

Transfer agreements should be written in compliance with and reflect the provisions of the many federal and state laws, regulations, and standards affecting health care organizations. The parties to a transfer agreement should be particularly aware of applicable federal and state regulations.

Agreements that will aid in bringing about the maximum use of the services of each organization and in ensuring the best possible care for patients should be established. The basic elements of a transfer agreement include: *identification of each party to the agreement*, including the name and location of each organization to the agreement; *purpose of the agreement; policies and procedures* for transfer of patients (Language in this section of the agreement should make it clear that the patient's physician makes the determination as to the patient's need for the facilities and services of the receiving organization. The receiving organization should agree that, subject to its admission requirements and availability of space, it will admit the patient from the transferring organization as promptly as possible.); *organizational responsibilities* for arranging and making the transfer (Generally, the transferring organization is responsible for making transfer arrangements. The agreement should specify who will bear the costs involved in the transfer.); *exchange of information* (The agreement must provide a mechanism for the interchange of medical and other information relevant to the patient.); *retention of autonomy* (The agreement should make clear that each organization retains its autonomy and that the governing bodies of each facility will continue to exercise exclusive legal responsibility and control over the management, assets, and affairs of the respective facilities. It also should be stipulated that neither organization assumes any liability by virtue of the agreement for any debts or obligations of a financial or legal nature incurred by the other.); *procedure for settling disputes* (The agreement should include a method of settling disputes that might arise over some aspect of the patient transfer relationship.); *procedure for modification or termination of the agreement* (The agreement should provide that it can be modified or amended by mutual consent of the parties. It also should provide for termination by either organization on notice within a specified time period.); *sharing of services* (Depending on the situation, cooperative use of facilities and services on an outpatient basis [e.g., laboratory and X-ray testing] can be an important element of the relationship between organizations. The method of payment for services rendered should be carefully described in the agreement.); *publicity* (The agreement should provide that neither organization will use the name of the other in any promotional or advertising material without prior approval of the other.); and *exclusive versus nonexclusive agreement* (It is advisable for organizations—when and where possible—to have transfer agreements with more than one organization. The agreement can include language to the effect that either party has the right to enter into transfer agreements with other organizations.).

INSURANCE CONTRACT

Insurance is a form of risk management used primarily to hedge against the risk of potential loss. In an *insurance contract*, the insurer has an obligation to indemnify the insured for losses caused by specified events. In return, the insured must pay a fixed premium during the policy period. As noted, the interpretation of an insurance contract can give rise to a legal action when the insurer refuses to indemnify the insured.

Notes

1. Hungerford Hosp. v. Mulvey, 225 A.2d 495 (Conn. 1966).
2. Harvey v. Strickland, 350 S.C. 303, 566 S.E.2d 529 (2002).
3. 25 P.3d 358 (2001).
4. 384 N.Y.S.2d 527 (N.Y. App. Div. 1976).
5. 2005 WL 249695 (Tenn. App. Ct. 2005).
6. 492 N.Y.S.2d 9 (N.Y. 1985).
7. 605 N.E.2d 613 (Ill. App. Ct. 1992).
8. Community Hosp. Group, Inc. v. More, No. A-75 September Term 2003 (N.J. 2005).
9. Pierson v. Medical Health Ctrs., 869 A.2d 901 (N.J. 2005).
10. 720 P.2d 632 (Idaho 1986).
11. 731 F. Supp. 311 (D. Ill. 1990).
12. Id. at 321–322.
13. Chesnick v. Saint Mary of Nazareth Hosp., 570 N.E.2d 545 (Ill. App. Ct. 1991).
14. 789 N.Y.S.2d 42 (N.Y. App. Div. 2005).
15. 520 N.W.2d 625 (Wis. App. 1994).
16. 368 N.W.2d 666, 668, 674 (1985).
17. 466 U.S. 2 (1984).
18. 7 S.W.3d 542 (Mo. App. 1999).

6

Civil Procedure and Trial Practice

This chapter in particular is valuable to readers in understanding the law and its application in the courtroom. Although many of the procedures leading up to and followed during a trial are discussed in this chapter, civil procedure and trial practice are governed by each state's statutory requirements. Cases on a federal level are governed by federal statutory requirements.

PLEADINGS

The pleadings of a case are the written statements of fact and law filed with a court by the parties to a lawsuit. Pleadings generally include such papers as a complaint, demurrer, answer, and bill of particulars.

A *complaint* is the first pleading filed by a plaintiff that initiates a lawsuit. It sets forth the relevant allegations of fact that give rise to one or more legal causes of action along with the damages requested. A *demurrer* is a pleading filed by a defendant challenging the legal sufficiency of a complaint. An *answer* to a complaint is a pleading that admits or denies the specific allegations set forth in a complaint and constitutes a general appearance by a defendant. A *bill of particulars* is a request for a written itemization of the claims, which a defendant can demand from the plaintiff to determine what the details of a claim are.

A defendant can also file a *cross-complaint* and bring other parties into a lawsuit by the process. If only questions of law are at issue, the judge will decide the case based on the pleadings alone. If questions of fact are involved, a trial is conducted to determine those facts.

Summons and Complaint

The parties to a controversy are the plaintiff and the defendant. The *plaintiff* is the person who initiates an action by filing a complaint; the *defendant* is the person against whom a lawsuit is brought. Many cases have multiple plaintiffs and defendants.

The first pleading filed with the court in a negligence action is the complaint. The *complaint* identifies the parties to a suit, states a cause of action, and includes a demand for damages. It is filed by the plaintiff and is the first statement of a case by the plaintiff against the defendant. In some jurisdictions, a complaint must accompany a summons (an announcement to the defendant that a case has been commenced). The essential elements contained in a complaint are: (1) a short statement of the grounds on which the court's jurisdiction depends (the court's authority to hear the case); (2) a statement of the claim demonstrating that the pleader is entitled to relief; and (3) a demand for judgment for the relief to which the plaintiff deems him- or herself entitled. All these elements apply to any counterclaim, cross claim, or third-party claim.

The complaint can be served on the defendant either with the summons or within a prescribed time after the summons has been served. Specific formalities must be observed in the service of a summons so that appropriate jurisdiction over a defendant is obtained. Such formalities dictate the manner in which a summons is to be delivered, the time period within which service must be effected, and the geographic limitations within which service must be made.

Improper service of a summons occurred on March 14, 1989, when the sheriff attempted to serve the writ on the defendant by leaving a copy with the receptionist at the hospital where he had worked. The defendant had terminated his relationship with the hospital on February 22, 1988. The plaintiff's attempted service of the writ of summons was defective because the defendant was not affiliated with the hospital at which service was attempted. A copy of the complaint was left with a nurse on the intensive care unit of the hospital where the defendant was then a patient. The intensive care unit of a hospital, however, cannot be deemed the defendant–patient's place of residence, nor can it be said that the defendant–patient resides there.[1]

Demurrer

Upon receiving the plaintiff's complaint, the defendant can file preliminary objections prior to answering the complaint. A *demurrer*, for example, can be filed by one of the parties to a lawsuit claiming that the evidence presented by the other party is insufficient to sustain an issue or case.

Answer

After service of a complaint, a response is required from the defendant in a document called the answer. In the answer, the defendant responds to each of the allegations contained in the complaint by stating his or her defenses and by admitting to or denying each of the plaintiff's allegations. If the defendant fails to answer the complaint within the prescribed time, the plaintiff can seek judgment by default against the defendant. However, in certain instances, a default judgment will be vacated if the defendant can demonstrate an acceptable excuse for failing to answer.

Personal appearance of the defendant to respond to a complaint is not necessary. To prevent default, the defendant's attorney responds to the complaint with an answer. The defense attorney attempts to show through evidence that the defendant is not responsible for the negligent act claimed by the plaintiff to have occurred. The answer generally consists of a denial of the charges made and specifies a defense or argument justifying the position taken. The defense can show that the claim is unfounded because: (1) the period within which a suit must be instituted has run out; (2) there is contributory negligence on the part of the plaintiff; (3) any obligation has been paid; (4) a general release was presented to the defendant; or (5) the contract was illegal and therefore canceled by mutual agreement. The original answer to the complaint is filed with the court having jurisdiction over the case, and a copy of the answer is provided to the plaintiff's attorney.

Counterclaim

In some cases, the defendant can file a counterclaim. For example, the plaintiff might have sued an organization for personal injuries and property damage caused by the negligent operation of an organization's ambulance. The organization might file a counterclaim on grounds that its driver was careful and that it was the plaintiff who was negligent and is liable to the organization for damage to the ambulance.

Bill of Particulars

The defense attorney can request a bill of particulars, seeking more specific and detailed information than is provided in the complaint. If a counterclaim has been filed, the plaintiff's attorney can request a bill of particulars from the defense attorney. More specifically, a bill of particulars for a malpractice suit might request, for example, from the plaintiff's attorney: (1) the date and time of day when the alleged malpractice occurred; (2) if the claim involves misdiagnosis or failure to diagnose correctly, failure to perform a test or diagnostic procedure, failure to medicate, treat, or operate, or a contraindicated test given or a contraindicated test or surgical procedure performed; (3) administration of a medicine or treatment or performance of a test or surgical procedure in a manner contrary to accepted standards of medical practice; (4) where the alleged malpractice occurred; (5) the commissions and/or omissions constituting the malpractice that is alleged to have occurred; (6) how the alleged malpractice occurred; (7) a listing of injuries claimed to have been caused by the defendant's alleged malpractice; (8) a listing of any witnesses to the alleged malpractice; (9) the length of time the plaintiff was confined to bed; and (10) the weekly earnings of the plaintiff.

DISCOVERY AND EXAMINATION BEFORE TRIAL

Discovery is the process of investigating the facts of a case before trial. The objectives of discovery are to: (1) obtain evidence that might not be obtainable at the time of trial; (2) isolate and narrow the issues for trial; (3) gather knowledge of the existence of additional evidence that might be admissible at trial; and (4) obtain leads to enable the discovering party to gather further evidence.

Discovery can be obtained on any matter that is not privileged and that is relevant to the subject matter involved in the pending action. The parties to a lawsuit have the right to discovery and to examine witnesses before trial. *Examination before trial* (EBT) is one of several discovery techniques used to enable the parties of a lawsuit to learn more regarding the nature and substance of each other's case. An EBT consists of oral testimony under oath and includes cross-examination. A deposition, taken at an EBT, is the testimony of a witness that has been recorded in a written format. Testimony given at a deposition becomes part of the permanent record of the case. Each question and answer is transcribed by a court stenographer and can be used at the subsequent trial. Truthfulness and consistency are important because answers from an EBT that differ from those given at trial will be used to attack the credibility of the witness.

ATTORNEY–CLIENT PRIVILEGE

Confidential communications made by a client and an attorney to one another are protected by attorney–client privilege. There are three elements required to successfully assert attorney–client privilege:

1. Both parties must agree that the attorney–client relationship does or will exist.

2. The client must seek advice from that attorney in his or her capacity as a legal advisor.
3. Communication between the attorney and client must be identified to be confidential.

INCIDENT AND INVESTIGATIVE REPORTS

Hospital incident and investigation reports are generally not protected from discovery. The burden rests upon the hospital to demonstrate that incident and investigation reports are protected from discovery under attorney–client privilege and work–product doctrine. *Attorney–client privilege* is intended to ensure that a client remains free from apprehension that consultations with a legal advisor will be disclosed. Such privilege further encourages a client to talk freely with his or her attorney so that he or she can receive quality advice. Likewise, with regard to the work–product doctrine, not even the most liberal of discovery theories can justify unwarranted inquiries into the files and the mental impressions of an attorney. Courts are required to protect the integrity and fairness of the fact-finding process by requiring full disclosure of all relevant facts connected with the impending litigation while, at the same time, promoting full and frank consultation between a client and a legal advisor by removing the fear of compelled disclosure of information.

If in connection with an accident or an event, a business entity, in the ordinary course of business, conducts an investigation for its own purposes, the resulting investigative report is producible in civil pretrial discovery. The distinction between whether a defendant's in-house report was prepared in the ordinary course of business or was work product in anticipation of litigation is an important one. The fact that a defendant anticipates the contingency of litigation resulting from an accident or event does not automatically qualify an in-house report as work product. *A document that is not privileged does not become privileged by the mere act of sending it to an attorney.*

PREPARATION OF WITNESSES

The manner in which a witness handles questioning at a deposition or trial is often as important as the facts of the case. Each witness should be well prepared before testifying. Preparation should include a review of all pertinent records. Helpful guidelines for witnesses undergoing examination in a trial or a court hearing include the following:

- Review the records (e.g., medical records and other business records) from which you might be questioned.
- Do not be antagonistic in answering the questions. The jury might already be somewhat sympathetic toward a particular party to the lawsuit; antagonism might only serve to reinforce such an impression.
- Be organized in your thinking and recollection of the facts regarding the incident.
- Answer only the questions asked.
- Explain your testimony in simple, succinct terminology.
- Do not overdramatize the facts you are relating.
- Do not allow yourself to become overpowered by the cross-examiner.
- Be polite, sincere, and courteous at all times.
- Dress appropriately and be neatly groomed.
- Pay close attention to any objections your attorney might have as to the line of questioning being conducted by the opposing counsel.
- Be sure to have reviewed any oral deposition in which you might have participated during an EBT.
- Be straightforward with the examiner. Any answers designed to cover up or cloud an issue or fact will, if discovered, serve only to discredit any previous testimony that you might have given.

- Do not show any visible signs of displeasure regarding any testimony with which you are in disagreement.
- Be sure to have questions that you did not hear repeated and questions that you did not understand rephrased.
- If you are not sure of an answer, indicate that you are not sure or that you just do not know the answer.

MOTIONS

The procedural steps that occur before trial are specifically classified as pretrial proceedings. After the pleadings have been completed, many states permit either party to move for a *judgment on the pleadings*. When this motion is made, the court will examine the entire case and decide whether to enter judgment according to the merits of the case as indicated in the pleadings. In some states, the moving party is permitted to introduce sworn statements showing that a claim or defense is false or a sham. This procedure cannot be used when there is substantial dispute concerning the facts presented by the affidavits.

PRETRIAL CONFERENCE

In many states, a pretrial conference will be ordered at the judge's initiative or on the request of one of the parties to the lawsuit. The *pretrial conference* is an informal discussion during which the judge and the attorneys eliminate matters not in dispute, agree on the issues, and settle procedural matters relating to the trial. Although it is not the purpose of the pretrial conference to compel the parties to settle the case, it often happens that cases are settled at this point.

MOTION TO DISMISS

A defendant can make a motion to dismiss a case, alleging that the plaintiff's complaint, even if believed, does not set forth a claim or cause of action recognized by law. A motion to dismiss can be made before, during, or after a trial. Motions made before a trial can be made on the basis that the court lacks jurisdiction, that the case is barred by the statute of limitations, that another case is pending involving the same issues, and other similar matters. A motion during trial can be made after the plaintiff has presented his or her case on the grounds that the court has heard the plaintiff's case and the defendant is entitled to a favorable judgment as a matter of law. In the case of a motion made by the defendant at the close of the plaintiff's case, the defendant normally will claim that the plaintiff has failed to present a *prima facie case* (i.e., that the plaintiff has failed to establish the minimum elements necessary to justify a verdict even if no contrary evidence is presented by the defendant). After a trial has been completed, either party can move for a directed verdict on the grounds that he or she is entitled to such verdict as a matter of law.

SUMMARY JUDGMENT

Either party to a suit might believe that there are no triable issues of fact and only issues of law to be decided. In such event, either party can make a motion for summary judgment. This motion asks the court to rule that there are no facts in dispute and that the rights of the parties can be determined as a matter of law, on the basis of submitted documents, without the need for a trial. Although the courts are reluctant to look favorably on motions for summary judgment, they will grant them if the circumstances of a particular case warrant it.

The plaintiff in *Thomas v. New York University Med. Ctr.*,[2] while under general anesthesia, slid off the operating table during a surgical procedure. The plaintiff's head was pulled out of a head-stabilizing device, causing his head to be lacerated by one of the pins. The plaintiff suffered trauma to his neck and required mechanical assistance to breathe for 6 days following the accident. The Supreme Court, Appellate Division, on motion by the plaintiff, determined that summary judgment on the issue of liability was warranted. It could easily be reasoned that anesthetized patients do not fall from operating tables in the absence of negligence. The defendants, who were in joint and exclusive control of plaintiff, failed to explain their conduct in the operating room, and their failure to do so mandated summary judgment.

NOTICE OF TRIAL

The examination before trial can reveal sufficient facts that would discourage the plaintiff from continuing the case, or it might encourage one or both parties to settle out of court. When a decision to go forward is reached, the case is placed on the court calendar. Postponement of the trial can be secured with the consent of both parties and the consent of the court. A case may not be postponed indefinitely without being dismissed by the court. If one party is ready to proceed and another party seeks a postponement, a valid excuse must be shown. Should a defendant fail to appear at trial, the judge can pass judgment against the defendant by default. A case also can be dismissed if the plaintiff fails to appear at trial.

MEMORANDUM OF LAW

A memorandum of law (or trial brief) presents to the court the nature of the case, cites case decisions to substantiate arguments, and aids the court regarding points of law. Trial briefs are prepared by both the plaintiff's and the defendant's attorneys. A trial brief is not required, but it is a recommended strategy. It provides the court with a basic understanding of the position of the party submitting the brief before the commencement of the trial. It also focuses the court's attention on specific legal points that might influence the court in ruling on objections and on the admissibility of evidence in the course of the trial.

THE COURT

A case is heard in the court that has jurisdiction over the subject of controversy. The judge decides questions of law and is responsible for ensuring that a trial is conducted properly in an impartial atmosphere that is fair to both parties of a lawsuit. The judge informs the jury of what the defendant's conduct should have been, thereby making a determination of the existence of a legal duty.

The judge decides whether evidence is admissible, charges the jury (defines the jurors' responsibility in relation to existing law), and may take a case away from the jury (by directed verdict or making a judgment notwithstanding the verdict) when he or she believes that there are no issues for the jury to consider or that the jury has erred in its decision. This right of the judge with respect to the role of the jury narrows the jury's responsibility with regard to the facts of the case. The judge maintains order throughout the trial, determines issues of procedure, and is generally responsible for the conduct of the trial.

THE JURY

The right to a trial by jury is a constitutional right, but an individual may waive the right to a jury trial. If this right is waived, the judge acts as judge and jury, becoming the trier of facts and deciding issues of law.

Members of the jury are selected from a jury list. They are summoned to court by a paper known as the summons. Impartiality is a prerequisite of all jurors. The number of jurors who sit at trial is 12 in common law. If there are fewer than 12, the number must be established by statute.

Counsel for both parties of a lawsuit question each prospective jury member for impartiality, bias, and prejudicial thinking. This process is referred to as the *voir dire*, the examination of jurors. When members of the jury are selected, they are sworn in to try the case.

The jury makes a determination of the facts that occurred, evaluating whether the plaintiff's damages were caused by the defendant's negligence and whether the defendant exercised due care. The jury makes a determination of the particular standard of conduct required in all cases in which the judgment of reasonable people might differ. The jury must pay close attention to the evidence presented by both sides to a suit to render a fair and impartial verdict. Jurors who fall asleep during the trial can be replaced with an alternate juror, as was the case in *Richbow v. District of Columbia*.[3]

The jury also determines the extent of damages, if any, and the degree to which the plaintiff's conduct might have contributed to his or her injury, thereby mitigating the responsibility of the defendant (contributory negligence).

A Jury Decision

A New York City jury awarded $26 million to a boy injured during surgery. What was it that so disturbed the jury that caused it to grant such a huge award? According to an article written by an alternate juror, who invited the jurors to his home three weeks after the trial:

> The defense lawyers were on their feet objecting they didn't want the jury to see Stephen. But that just raised a question for us: If his injuries were as slight as the defense had been insisting, why the resistance? The judge agreed that it was proper for Stephen to appear at his own trial, and the rear doors to the courtroom were opened.
>
> Most of the jurors had begun to cry. But we were also angry. The defense lawyers it seemed, had been trying to put one over on us, claiming that Stephen was a normal teenage boy with a few minor handicaps.
>
> For seven weeks, the jury had sat in that courtroom listening to the defense lawyers belittle Stephen's problems. We saw the doctors refuse to acknowledge Stephen's handicaps or to accept responsibility for them. To the jury at least, it seemed that the doctors had made mistakes, refused to admit them, and then tried to cover them up.[4]

SUBPOENAS

A *subpoena* is a legal order requiring the appearance of a person and/or the presentation of documents to a court or administrative body. Attorneys, judges, and certain law enforcement and administrative officials, depending on the jurisdiction, may issue subpoenas. Subpoenas generally include: a reference number; names of plaintiff and defendant; date, time, and place to appear; name, address, and telephone number of opposing attorney; and documents requested if a subpoena is for records.

Some jurisdictions require the service of a subpoena at a specified time in advance of the requested appearance (e.g., 24 hours). In other jurisdictions, no such time limitation exists. A court clerk, sheriff, attorney, process server, or other person as provided by state statute can serve a subpoena.

A *subpoena ad testificandum* orders the appearance of a person at a trial or other investigative proceeding to give testimony. Witnesses have a duty to appear and can suffer a penalty for contempt of court should they fail to appear. They may not deny knowledge of a subpoena if they simply refused to accept it. The court can issue a bench warrant, ordering the appearance of a witness in court, if a witness fails to answer a subpoena. Failure to appear may be excused if extenuating circumstances exist.

A subpoena for records, known as a *subpoena duces tecum*, is a written command to bring records, documents, or other evidence described in the subpoena to a trial or other investigative proceeding. The subpoena is served on one who is able to produce such records. Disobedience in answering a subpoena duces tecum is considered to be contempt of court and carries a penalty of a fine or imprisonment.

BURDEN OF PROOF

The *burden of proof in a criminal case* requires that the evidence presented against the defendant must be beyond a reasonable doubt. Note the terminology: reasonable doubt—not all doubt. The burden of proof in a criminal case lies with the prosecution. In a civil suit, the evidence presented need only tip the scales of justice.

The *burden of proof in a civil case* is the obligation of the plaintiff to persuade the jury regarding the truth of his or her case. A preponderance of the credible evidence must be presented for a plaintiff to recover damages. Credible evidence is evidence that, in the light of reason and common sense, is worthy of belief. A preponderance of credible evidence requires that the prevailing side of the case carries more weight than the evidence on the opposing side.

In a negligence case the burden of proof requires that the plaintiff's attorney show that the defendant violated a legal duty by not following an acceptable standard of care and that the plaintiff suffered injury because of the defendant's breach. If the evidence presented does not support the allegations made, the case is dismissed. Where a plaintiff, who has the burden of proof, fails to sustain such burden, the case can be dismissed despite the failure of the defendant to present any evidence to the contrary on his or her behalf. The burden of proof in some states shifts from the plaintiff to the defendant when it is obvious that the injury would not have occurred unless there was negligence.

STATUTORY VIOLATION

Violation of a statute can constitute direct evidence of negligence, or it simply can voice a duty that is owed to a particular class of persons who are protected by the statute or regulation. For example, assume a regulation specifies a nurse–patient ratio of no less than one registered nurse for two patients on intensive care units. This regulation is an expression of the duty imposed on the facility to provide adequate nursing care to patients. Patients are, therefore, a class of persons identified within the regulation who are to have the benefits of the protection to be gained by having a predetermined minimum standard nurse–patient ratio.

POLICY AND PROCEDURE VIOLATIONS

Policies and procedures of a health care organization are established for day-to-day operations. If a violation of a facility's policy and procedures causes injury to one whom the policy or procedure is designed to protect, such violation can give rise to evidence for negligent conduct.

RES IPSA LOQUITUR

Res ipsa loquitur ("the thing speaks for itself" or "circumstances speak for themselves") is the legal doctrine that shifts the burden of proof from the plaintiff to the defendant. It is an evidentiary device that allows the plaintiff to make a case legally adequate to go to the jury on the basis of well-defined circumstantial evidence even though direct evidence is lacking. This does not mean that the plaintiff has proven fully the defendant's negligence. It merely shifts the burden of going forward to the defendant who must argue to dismiss the circumstantial evidence presented as "speaking for itself."

An inference of negligence is permitted from the mere occurrence of an injury when the defendant owed a duty and possessed the sole power of preventing the injury by exercise of reasonable care. For example, the presence of severe burns on a patient's body after being bathed by an employee raises the question of negligence without the need for expert testimony. Negligence is considered so obvious that expert testimony is not necessary. It lies within a layperson's realm of knowledge that people generally do not suffer burns from a bath. That alone is sufficient to require a defendant to come forward with a rebuttal. The three elements necessary to shift the burden of proof from the plaintiff to the defendant under the doctrine of res ipsa loquitur are as follows: (1) The event would not normally have occurred in the absence of negligence; (2) the defendant must have had exclusive control over the instrumentality that caused the injury; and (3) the plaintiff must not have contributed to the injury.

For example, the oxygen mask discussed in *Gold v. Ishak*[5] caught fire during surgery. In performing surgery, the physician used an electrocautery unit provided by the hospital. At some point during surgery the oxygen mask caught on fire and the patient was injured. A claim of negligent treatment was presented to a medical review panel, which concluded that the medical providers had complied with the requisite standard of care. The plaintiff then filed a complaint against the medical providers for medical malpractice. The trial court refused to apply the doctrine of res ipsa loquitur.

On appeal, the trial court was found to have erred by refusing to apply the doctrine of res ipsa loquitur. The evidence presented at trial, as described here, clearly shows that the elements necessary for the inference of res ipsa loquitur had been established.

1. The injuring instrumentality was under the management or exclusive control of the medical providers.
2. A fire under these circumstances is such that in the ordinary course of things would not have occurred if the medical providers had used proper care in relation to the electrocautery unit and oxygen mask.
3. Expert testimony is not required because a fire occurring during surgery where an instrument that emits a spark is used near a source of oxygen is not beyond the realm of the layperson to understand. It is easily understandable to the common person that careless use of the two could cause a fire and result in bodily injury.

OPENING STATEMENTS

During the opening statement, the plaintiff's attorney attempts to prove the wrongdoing of the defendant by presenting credible evidence favorable to his or her client. The opening statement by the plaintiff's attorney provides in summary: (1) the facts of the case; (2) what the attorney intends to prove by means of a summary of the evidence to be presented; and (3) a description of the damages to his or her client. Opening statements are prepared so that each jury member can sympathize with the plaintiff, relate to the injustice, and then see it happening to themselves. The opening statement must be concise and to the point.

The defense attorney makes his or her opening statement indicating the position of the defendant and the points of the plaintiff's case he or she intends to refute. The defense attorney explains the facts as they apply to the case for the defendant.

EXAMINATION OF WITNESSES

After conclusion of the opening statements, the judge calls for the plaintiff's witnesses. An officer of the court administers an oath to each witness, and direct examination begins. The attorney obtains information from each witness in the form of questions. On cross-examination by the defense, an attempt is made to challenge or discredit the plaintiff's witness. Redirect examination by the plaintiff's attorney can follow the cross-examination, if so desired. The plaintiff's attorney may at this time wish to have his or her witness review an important point that the jury might have forgotten during cross-examination. The plaintiff's attorney may ask the same witness more questions in an effort to overcome the effect of the cross-examination. Recross-examination can take place, if necessary, for the defense of the defendant.

A sampling of preliminary questions that a physician might expect to be asked can take the following form:

- Please state your name, residence, and any prior residences.
- Where did you attend medical school?
- Are you licensed in this state?
- Where did you serve your internship?
- Where did you serve your residency?
- Is your practice general or special?
- Are you board certified in one or more specialties?
- How does a physician obtain board certification?
- Are you presently practicing medicine?
- How long have you been in practice?
- During your _______ years of practice, have you had occasion to treat a good number of personal injury cases?
- On or about _______ did you have occasion to see the patient on a professional basis?
- Where? Describe the patient's condition at the time.
- What, if anything, did you do on that occasion?
- Have you been the attending physician since that date?
- Describe the nature of the examination that you made on the patient and any others from time to time since then.
- Did you see the patient daily, several times a day at first?
- Did you continue to see the patient? How often?
- Of what, generally, did your treatment consist?
- From your examination and treatment of the patient, did you determine what injuries were sustained?
- As a result of your examination, did you find it necessary to seek consultation from another physician or specialist?
- Did there come a time when you found it necessary to transfer the patient to another health care facility?

The credibility of a witness can be impeached if prior statements are inconsistent with later statements or if there is bias in favor of a party or prejudice against a party to a lawsuit. Either attorney to a lawsuit can ask the judge for permission to recall a witness.

After all the witnesses of the plaintiff have testified, the defense can call its witnesses, and the process of direct, cross, redirect, and recross-examination is repeated until the defense rests.

EVIDENCE

Evidence consists of the facts proved or disproved during a lawsuit. The law of evidence is a body of rules under which facts are proved. The rules of evidence govern the admission of items of proof in a lawsuit. A fact can be proven by either circumstantial or direct evidence. Evidence must be competent, relevant, and material to be admitted at trial.

Direct Evidence

Direct evidence is proof offered through direct testimony. It is the jury's function to receive testimony presented by witnesses and to draw conclusions in the determination of the facts of a case.

Demonstrative Evidence

Demonstrative evidence is proof furnished by things themselves. It is considered to be the most trustworthy and preferred type of evidence. It consists of tangible objects to which testimony refers (e.g., medical supplies, instruments, equipment) that can be requested by a jury. Demonstrative evidence is admissible in court if it is relevant, has probative value, and serves the interest of justice. It is not admissible if it will prejudice, mislead, confuse, offend, inflame, or arouse the sympathy or passion of the jury. Other forms of demonstrative evidence include photographs, motion pictures, X-ray films, drawings, human bodies as exhibits, pathology slides, fetal monitoring strips, safety committee minutes, infection committee reports, medical staff bylaws, rules and regulations, nursing policy and procedure manuals, census data, and staffing patterns. The plaintiff's attorney uses all pertinent evidence to reconstruct chronologically the care and treatment rendered.

When presenting photographs as a form of evidence, the photographer or a reliable witness who is familiar with the object photographed must testify that the picture is an accurate representation and a fair likeness of the object portrayed. The photograph must not exaggerate a client's physical condition. Such exaggeration could unfairly prejudice a jury. Photographs can be valuable legal evidence when they illustrate graphically the nature and extent of a medical injury. Motion pictures also are valuable evidence. The same principles that apply to photographs apply to motion pictures. Motion pictures must be accurately portrayed. The cutting and/or splicing of videos are suspect and might have no probative value. Videotape is admissible in court, assuming the matter being taped, the time of the taping, and the manner in which such taping took place can be authenticated.

Imaging films are considered to be pictures of the interior of the object portrayed and are admissible under the same requirements as photographs and motion pictures. Competent evidence must be offered to show that the films are those of the patient, the object, or body part under consideration; that the films were made in a recognized manner, taken by a competent technician; and that they were interpreted by a competent physician trained to read the films. The value of films is that they illustrate fractures, foreign objects, and so forth.

Where an issue as to personal injuries is involved, an injured person may be permitted to exhibit to the jury the wound or injury, or the member or portion of his body upon which such wound or injury was inflicted, and if relevant, the exhibition is allowable in the discretion of the court where there is no reason to expect that the sympathy of the jury will be excited. The human body is considered to be the best evidence as to the nature and extent of the alleged injury/ injuries. If there is no controversy about either the nature or the extent of an injury, presenting such evidence could be considered prejudicial, and an objection can be made as to its presentation to a jury.

Demonstrations are permitted in some instances to illustrate the extent of injuries. The resident in *Hendricks v. Sanford*[6] developed serious bed sores on her back. The defendant objected to the offer of the plaintiff to display her back to the jury. The court found that the plaintiff's injuries, which had healed, were completely relevant as evidence. Even though the injuries had healed and a skin graft had been performed, a declivity of about three and a half inches in diameter and about the depth of a shallow ashtray was still discernible on the plaintiff's back.

Documentary Evidence

Documentary evidence is written information that is capable of making a truthful statement (e.g., drug manufacturer inserts, autopsy reports, birth certificates, and medical records). Documentary evidence must satisfy the jury as to authenticity. Proof of authenticity is not necessary if the opposing party accepts its genuineness. In some instances (e.g., wills), witnesses are necessary. In the case of documentation, the original of a document must be produced unless it can be demonstrated that the original has been lost or destroyed, in which case a properly authenticated copy may be substituted.

A sampling of preliminary questions that a witness might be asked on entering a medical record into evidence includes the following:

- Please state your name.
- Where are you employed?
- What is your position?
- What is your official title?

- Did you receive a subpoena for certain records?
- Did you bring those records with you?
- Can you identify these records?
- Did you retrieve the records yourself?
- Are these the complete records?
- Are these the original records or copies of the originals?
- How were these records prepared?
- Are these records maintained under your care, custody, and control?
- Were these records made in the regular course of business?
- Was the record made at the time the act, condition, or event occurred or transpired?
- Is this record regularly kept or maintained?

A manufacturer's drug insert or manual describing the proper use of medical equipment is generally admissible in court as evidence. In *Mueller v. Mueller*,[7] a physician was sued by a patient who charged that she had suffered a deterioration of bone structure and ultimately a collapsed hip as a result of the administration of cortisone over an extended period of time. The jury decided that the physician's prolonged use of cortisone was negligent, and the physician appealed. The appeals court held that the manufacturer's recommendations are not only admissible but also essential in determining a physician's possible lack of proper care.

Judicial Notice Rule

The *judicial notice* rule prescribes that well-known facts (e.g., that fractures need prompt attention and that two X-rays of the same patient might show different results) need not be proven, but, rather, they are recognized by the court as fact. If a fact can be disputed, the rule does not apply.

The use of X-rays as a diagnostic aid in cases of fracture can be considered a matter of common knowledge to which a court, in the absence of expert testimony, can take judicial notice. Should a patient have a serious fall and a fracture is indicated, under the foregoing rule, it is a matter of common knowledge that the ordinary physician in good standing, in the exercise of ordinary care and diligence, would have ordered X-rays.

Hearsay Evidence

Hearsay evidence is based on what another has said or done and is not the result of the personal knowledge of the witness. Hearsay consists of written and oral statements. When a witness testifies to the utterance of a statement made outside court and the statement is offered in court for the truth of the facts that are contained in the statement, this is hearsay and therefore objectionable.

If a statement is offered not as proof of the facts asserted in the statement but rather only to show that the statement was made, the statement can come into evidence. For example, if it is relevant that a conversation took place, the testimony relating to the conversation may be entered as evidence. The purpose of that testimony would be to establish that a conversation took place and not to prove what was said during the course of the conversation. If testimony is based on personal knowledge, it would be admissible as evidence.

Because of the ability to challenge hearsay evidence successfully, which rests on the credibility of the witness as well as on the competency and veracity of other persons not before the court, it is admitted as evidence in a trial under very strict rules.

There are many exceptions to the hearsay rule that allow testimony that ordinarily would not be admitted. Included in the list of exceptions are admissions made by one of the parties to the action, threats made by a victim, dying declarations, statements to refresh a witness's recollection if he or she is unable to remember the facts known earlier, business records, medical records, and other official records (e.g., certified copies of birth and death records). If hearsay evidence is admitted without objection, its probative value is for the jury to determine.

Medical Books as Hearsay Evidence

Medical books are considered hearsay because the authors are not generally available for cross-examination. Although medical books are not admissible as evidence, a physician may testify as to how he or she formed an opinion and what part textbooks played in forming that opinion. During cross-examination, medical experts may be asked to comment on statements from medical books that contradict their testimony.

Expert Testimony

It is the jury's function to receive testimony presented by witnesses and draw conclusions in the determination of facts. The law recognizes that a jury is composed of ordinary men and women and that some fact-finding will involve subjects beyond their knowledge. When a jury cannot otherwise obtain sufficient facts from which to draw conclusions, an expert witness who has special knowledge, skill, experience, or training can be called on to submit an opinion. The expert witness assists the jury when the issues to be resolved in the case are outside the experience of the average juror.

Laypeople are quite able to render opinions about a great variety of general subjects, but for technical questions the opinion of an expert is necessary. At the time of testifying, each expert's training, experience, and special qualifications will be explained to the jury. The experts will be asked to give an opinion concerning hypothetical questions based on the facts of the case. Should the testimony of two experts conflict, the jury will determine which expert opinion to accept. Expert witnesses can be used to assist a plaintiff in proving the wrongful act of a defendant or to assist a defendant in refuting such evidence. In addition, expert testimony may be used to show the extent of the plaintiff's damages or to show the lack of such damages. To qualify as an expert witness in a specified area, that person must have the appropriate training, experience, and qualifications necessary to explain and/or answer questions based on the facts of a particular case.

Not all negligence cases require testimony from an expert witness. Citing *Donovan v. State*, "If a doctor operates on the wrong limb or amputates the wrong limb, a plaintiff would not have to introduce expert testimony to establish that the doctor was negligent. On the other hand, highly technical questions of diagnoses and causation which lie beyond the understanding of a layperson require introduction of expert testimony."[8]

Admissibility

Expert testimony concerning what a reasonable patient wanted to know and what doctors think patients wanted know was found to be admissible in an informed consent case. Thus, where the patient sued the physician for medical malpractice, alleging information he had given her over the telephone, relating to her report of abdominal pain and nausea several months after stomach surgery, did not allow her to make an intelligent decision to seek emergency room treatment. Expert testimony by doctors who had extensive experience interacting with patients was found to be relevant concerning the amount and kinds of information that patients generally want in late night phone calls, and was relevant to establish whether the physician had given the patient as much information as a reasonable patient would want to know.[9]

DEFENSES AGAINST PLAINTIFF'S ALLEGATIONS

When a plaintiff's case has been established, the defendant may put forward a defense against the claim for damages. The defendant's case is presented to discredit the plaintiff's cause of action and prevent recovery of

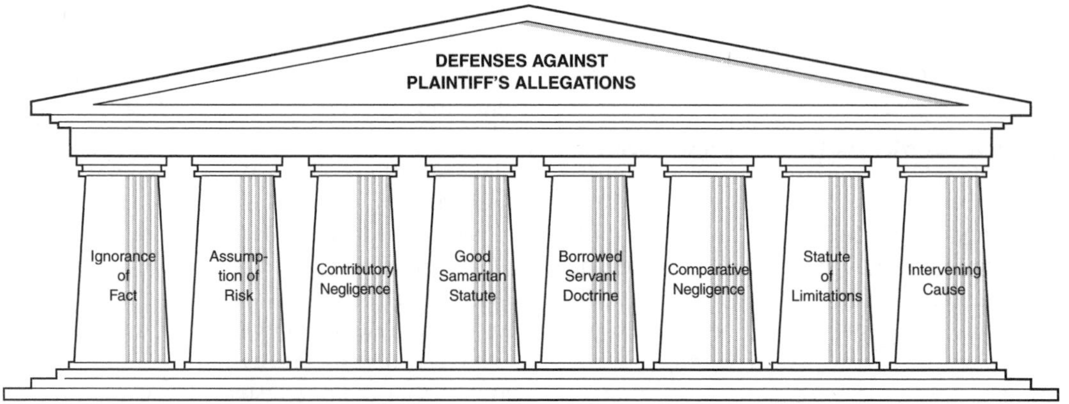

Figure 6-1 Pillars: Defenses Against Recovery

damages. This section covers the defenses available to defendants in a negligence suit. These are principles of law that can relieve a defendant from liability.

Ignorance of Fact and Unintentional Wrongs

Ignorance of the law is not a defense; otherwise an individual would be rewarded by pleading ignorance. Arguing that a negligent act is unintentional is no defense. If such a defense were acceptable, all defendants would use it.

Assumption of a Risk

Assumption of a risk is knowing that a danger exists and voluntarily accepting the risk by exposing oneself to it, aware that harm might occur. Assumption of a risk can be implicitly assumed, as in alcohol consumption, or expressly assumed, as in relation to warnings found on cigarette packaging.

This defense provides that the plaintiff expressly has given consent in advance, relieving the defendant of an obligation of conduct toward the plaintiff and taking the chances of injury from a known risk arising from the defendant's conduct. For example, one who agrees to care for a patient with a communicable disease and then contracts the disease would not be entitled to recover from the patient for damages suffered. In taking the job, the individual agreed to assume the risk of infection, thereby releasing the patient from all legal obligations.

The following two requirements must be established for a defendant to be successful in an assumption of a risk defense:

1. The plaintiff must know and understand the risk that is being incurred.
2. The choice to incur the risk must be free and voluntary.

The patient in *Faile v. Bycura*[10] was awarded $75,000 in damages on her allegations that a podiatrist used inappropriate techniques during an unsuccessful attempt to treat her heel spurs. On appeal, it was held that the trial court erred in striking the podiatrist's defense of assumption of a risk. Evidence established that the patient signed consent forms that indicated the risks of treatment as well as alternative treatment modalities.

Contributory Negligence

Contributory negligence occurs when a person does not exercise reasonable care for his or her own safety. As a general proposition, if a person has knowledge of a dangerous situation and disregards the danger, then that person is contributorily negligent. Actual knowledge of the danger of injury is not necessary for a person to be contributorily negligent. It is sufficient if a reasonable person should have been aware of the possibility of the danger.

In some jurisdictions, contributory negligence, no matter how slight, is sufficient to defeat a plaintiff's claim. Generally, the defense of contributory negligence has been recognized in a medical malpractice action when the patient has: (1) failed to follow a medical instruction, (2) refused or neglected prescribed treatment, or (3) intentionally given erroneous, incomplete, or misleading information that is the basis for medical care or treatment of the patient.

The elements necessary to establish contributory negligence are: (1) the plaintiff's conduct fell below the required standard of personal care, and (2) there is a causal connection between the plaintiff's careless conduct and the plaintiff's injury. Thus, the defendant contends that some, if not all, liability is attributable to the plaintiff's own actions.

The rationale for contributory negligence is based on the principle that all persons must be both careful and responsible for their acts. A plaintiff is required to conform to the broad standard of conduct of the reasonable person. The plaintiff's negligence will be determined and governed by the same tests and rules as the negligence of the defendant. A person incurs the risk of injury if he or she knew of a danger, understood the risk involved, and voluntarily exposed him- or herself to such danger.

Good Samaritan Statutes

Various states have enacted Good Samaritan laws, which relieve physicians, nurses, dentists, and other health care professionals, and, in some instances, laypersons, from liability in certain emergency situations. Good Samaritan legislation encourages health care professionals to render assistance at the scene of emergencies. The language that grants immunity also supports the conclusion that the physician, nurse, or layperson who is covered by the act will be protected from liability for ordinary negligence in rendering assistance in an emergency.

Under most statutes, immunity is granted only during an emergency or when rendering emergency care. The concept of emergency usually refers to a combination of unforeseen circumstances that require spontaneous action to avoid impending danger. Some states have sought to be more precise regarding what constitutes an emergency or accident. According to the Alaska statute 09.65.090(a), the emergency circumstances must suggest that the giving of aid is the only alternative to death or serious bodily injury.

Apparently, this provision was inserted to emphasize that the actions of a Good Samaritan must be voluntary. To be legally immune under the Good Samaritan laws, a physician or nurse must render help voluntarily and without expectation of later pay.

Statute Applicable: Due Care Rendered

The daughter of a deceased patient in *Dunlap v. Young*[11] had brought a wrongful death action against Emergency Medical Services (EMS) personnel for the death of her mother. The critically ill patient died after receiving care for respiratory distress in the ambulance while en route to the hospital. Under the Good Samaritan statute, an Illinois court found that EMS personnel were not negligent in their treatment of the decedent. They had acted promptly to get the patient to the hospital. Although EMS personnel had failed to intubate the patient, she had been provided with oxygen and assisted respiration.

Statute Not Applicable: Preexisting Duty to Care

The plaintiff, Kearney, suffered a life-threatening injury and was taken by ambulance to the emergency department of Kodiak Island Hospital (KIH), where he was examined by the on-call emergency department physician, a family practitioner. It was determined that a surgical consultation was necessary, and Dr. Deal, a surgeon with staff privileges at the hospital, was called. After ordering certain tests, Deal was of the opinion that Kearney could not survive a transfer to Anchorage. Deal then performed emergency surgery that lasted over 9 hours, ending the following morning.

The plaintiff was eventually transferred to Anchorage. His condition worsened, and he suffered loss of circulation and tissue death in both legs. The plaintiff alleged that KIH was negligent in failing to properly evacuate him to Anchorage. Kearney reached a settlement totaling $510,000. He also brought an action against Deal for negligent acts. Deal moved for summary judgment claiming to be immune from suit under the Good Samaritan statute.

The trial court denied Deal's motion for summary judgment, ruling that the Good Samaritan statute was not applicable to Deal because he was acting under a preexisting duty to render emergency care to Kearney. Deal petitioned for review, and his petition was granted.

The superior court held that the immunity provided by the Good Samaritan statute is unavailable to physicians with a preexisting duty to respond to emergency situations. The court concluded that Deal was under a preexisting duty in the instant case by virtue of his contract with KIH, the duty being part of the consideration that Deal gave to KIH in exchange for staff privileges at the hospital. The court further found that the Good Samaritan statute did not apply to Deal in any event because the actions allegedly constituting malpractice occurred during the follow-up care and treatment given Kearney after surgery. By then, the court reasoned, Deal had become Kearney's treating physician and was no longer responding to an emergency situation. Deal appealed to the Alaska Supreme Court.

The Alaska Supreme Court held that the Good Samaritan statute does not extend immunity to physicians who have preexisting duty to render emergency care.

The legislature clearly intended this provision to encourage health care providers, including medical professionals, to administer emergency medical care, whether in a hospital or not, to persons who are not their patients, by immunizing them from civil liability. The clear inference of this recommendation is that the statute would not cover those with a preexisting duty to care.[12]

Borrowed Servant Doctrine

The *borrowed servant doctrine* is a special application of the doctrine of respondeat superior and applies when an employer lends an employee to another for a particular employment. Although an employee remains the servant of the employer, under the borrowed servant doctrine, the employer is not liable for injury negligently caused by the servant while in the special service of another. For example, in certain situations, a nurse employed by a hospital can be considered the employee of the physician. In these situations, the physician is the special or temporary employer and is liable for the negligence of the nurse. To determine whether a physician is liable for the negligence of a nurse, it must be established that the physician had the right to control and direct the nurse at the time of the negligent act. If the physician is found to be in exclusive control, and if the nurse is deemed to be the physician's temporary special employee, the hospital is not generally liable for the nurse's negligent acts.

Captain of the Ship Doctrine

In the context of the operating room, the application of the borrowed servant doctrine generally is referred to as the captain of the ship doctrine. Historically, under this doctrine, the surgeon was viewed as being the one in command in the operating room. Today's courts, however, recognize that surgeons do not always have the right to control all persons within the operating room. An assignment of liability based on the theory of who had actual control over the patient more realistically reflects the actual relationship that exists in a modern operating room. For example, summary dismissal in *Thomas v. Raleigh*[13] was properly ordered for those portions of a patient's medical malpractice action that sought to hold a surgeon vicariously liable for throat injuries suffered by his patient because of the negligent manner in which an endotracheal tube was inserted during the administration of anesthesia. The patient's allegations that the surgeon exercised control over the administration of anesthesia were rebutted by evidence to the contrary. Liability of the surgeon could not be premised on the captain of the ship doctrine because that doctrine would not be recognized in West Virginia, where the surgery took place.

Comparative Negligence

A defense of *comparative negligence* provides that the degree of negligence or carelessness of each party to a lawsuit must be established by the finder of fact and that each party then is responsible for his or her proportional share of any damages awarded. For example, when a plaintiff suffers injuries of $10,000 from an accident, and when the plaintiff is found 20% negligent and the defendant 80% negligent, the defendant would be required to pay $8000 to the plaintiff. Thus, with comparative negligence, the plaintiff can collect for 80% of the injuries, whereas an application of contributory negligence would deprive the plaintiff of any monetary judgment. This doctrine relieves the plaintiff from the hardship of losing an entire claim when a defendant has been successful in establishing that the plaintiff contributed to his or her own injuries. A defense that provides that the plaintiff will forfeit an entire claim if he or she has been contributorily negligent is considered to be too harsh a result in jurisdictions that recognize comparative negligence.

Statute of Limitations

The *statute of limitations* refers to legislatively imposed time constraints that restrict the period of time after the occurrence of an injury during which a legal action must be commenced. Should a cause of action be initiated later than the period of time prescribed, the case cannot proceed. Many technical rules are associated with statutes of limitations. Statutes in each state specify that malpractice suits and other personal injury suits must be brought within fixed periods of time. An injured person who is a minor or is otherwise under a legal disability may, in many states, extend the period within which an action for injury may be filed. Computation of the period when the statute begins to run in a particular state may be based on any of the following factors:

- the date that the physician terminated treatment
- the time of the wrongful act
- the time when the patient should have reasonably discovered the injury
- the date that the injury was discovered
- the date when the contract between the patient and the physician ended

The running of the statute will not begin if fraud (the deliberate concealment from a patient of facts that might present a cause of action for damages) is involved. The cause of action begins at the time fraud is discovered.

The statute of limitations does not generally begin to run in those cases where a patient is unaware that an act of malpractice has occurred. Such is the case when foreign objects are left in a patient during surgery. A New Hampshire patient in *Shillady v. Elliot Community Hospital*[14] sued the hospital for negligence in treatment that was administered 31 years earlier. A needle had been left in the patient's spine after a spinal tap in 1940. In 1970, an X-ray showed the needle. The patient had suffered severe pain immediately after the spinal tap, which had decreased over the intervening years to about three "spells" a year. The court held that the 6-year statute of limitations does not begin "until the patient learns or in the exercise of reasonable care and diligence should have learned of its presence."[15] Therefore, the defendant's motion to dismiss the case on the grounds that the statute of limitations had run out was not granted.

Intervening Cause

Intervening cause arises when the act of a third party, independent of the defendant's original negligent conduct, is the proximate cause of an injury. If the negligent act of a third party is extraordinary under the circumstances and unforeseeable as a normal and probable consequence of the defendant's negligence, then the third party's negligence supersedes that of the defendant and relieves the defendant of liability.

In *Cohran v. Harper*,[16] a patient sued a physician, charging him with malpractice for an alleged staphylococcus infection that she received from a hypodermic needle used by the physician's nurse. The grounds of negligence included an allegation that the physician failed to properly sterilize the hypodermic needle that was used to administer penicillin. Evidence showed that a prepackaged sterilized needle and syringe were used. There was inadequate proof that the physician or his nurse negligently contaminated the needle and syringe. The court found that even if there was evidence that the needle was contaminated and that the patient's ailment was caused thereby, there was no evidence that either the physician, his nurse, or anyone in his office knew, or by the exercise of ordinary care could have discovered, that the prepackaged needle and syringe were so contaminated. The defense of *intervening cause* would have been an adequate defense against recovery of damages if it had been established that the needle was contaminated when packaged by the manufacturer.

SOVEREIGN IMMUNITY

Sovereign immunity refers to the common-law doctrine by which federal and state governments historically have been immune from liability for harm suffered from the tortious conduct of employees. For the most part, both federal and state governments have abolished sovereign immunity.

Action was brought on behalf of a minor in *Steele v. United States*,[17] who received treatment at a US Army hospital and suffered injury because of the optometrist's failure to refer the child to an ophthalmologist for examination. The US district court held that it was probable that an ophthalmologist would have diagnosed the child's problem and prevented the loss of his right eye. Recovery was permitted against the United States under the FTCA.

CLOSING STATEMENTS

After completion of the plaintiff's case and the defendant's defense, the judge calls for closing statements. The defense proceeds first, followed by the plaintiff. *Closing statements* provide attorneys with an opportunity to summarize for the jury and the court what they have proven. They may point out faults in their opponent's case and emphasize points they want the jury to remember.

If there appears to be only a question of law at the end of a case, a motion can be made for a directed verdict. The court will grant the motion if there is no question of fact to be decided by the jury. A directed verdict also may, for example, be made on the grounds that the plaintiff has failed to present sufficient facts to prove his or her case or that the evidence fails to establish a legal basis for a verdict in the plaintiff's favor.

JUDGE'S CHARGE TO JURY

After the attorneys' summations, the court charges the jury before the jurors recess to deliberate. Because the jury determines issues of fact, it is necessary for the court to instruct the jury with regard to applicable law. This is done by means of a charge. The charge defines the responsibility of the jury, describes the applicable law, and advises the jury of the alternatives available to it. As an example, statements from the trial judge's oral charge to the jurors in *Estes Health Care Centers v. Bannerman*,[18] in which a nursing facility resident died after transfer to a hospital after suffering burns in a bath, included:

> The complaint alleges the defendant Jackson Hospital undertook to provide hospital and nursing care to the deceased, and that the defendant negligently failed to provide proper hospital and nursing care to the plaintiff's intestate.
>
> The defendants in response to these allegations . . . have each separately entered pleas of the general issue or general denial. Under the law, a plea of the general issue has the effect of placing the burden of proof on the plaintiffs to reasonably satisfy you from the evidence, the truth of those things claimed by them in the bill of the complaint. The defendants carry no burden of proof.
>
> As to the defendant Jackson Hospital, the duty arises in that in rendering services to a patient, a hospital must use that degree of care, skill, and diligence used by hospitals generally in the community under similar circumstances.
>
> Negligence is not actionable unless the negligence is the proximate cause of the injury. The law defines proximate cause as that cause which is the natural and probable sequence of events and without the intervention of any new or independent cause, produces the injury, and without which such injury would not have occurred. For an act to constitute actionable negligence, there must not only be some causal connection between the negligent act complained of and the injury suffered, but connection must be by natural and unbroken sequence, without intervening sufficient causes, so that but for the negligence of the defendant, the injury would not have occurred.
>
> If one is guilty of negligence which concurs or combines with the negligence of another, and the two combine to produce injury, each negligent person is liable for the resulting injury. And the negligence of each will be deemed the proximate cause of the injury. Concurrent causes may be defined as two or more causes which run together and act contemporaneously to produce a given result or to inflict an injury. This does not mean that the causes of the acts producing the injury must necessarily occur simultaneously, but they must be active simultaneously to efficiently and proximately produce a result.
>
> In an action against two or more defendants for injury allegedly caused by combined or concurring negligence of the defendants, it is not necessary to show negligence of all the defendants in order for recovery to be had against one or more to be negligent. If you are reasonably satisfied from the evidence in this case that all the defendants are negligent and that their negligence concurred and combined to proximately cause the injury complained by the plaintiffs, then each defendant is liable to the plaintiffs.[19]

When a charge given by the court is not clear enough on a particular point, it is the obligation of the attorneys for both sides to request clarification of the charge. When the jury retires to deliberate, the members are reminded not to discuss the case except among themselves.

JURY DELIBERATION AND DETERMINATION

After the judge's charge, the jury retires to the jury room to deliberate and determine the defendant's liability. The jury members return to the courtroom upon reaching a verdict, and their determinations are presented to the court.

If a verdict is against the weight of the evidence, a judge may dismiss the case, order a new trial, or set his or her own verdict. At the time judgment is rendered, the losing party has an opportunity to motion for a new trial.

AWARDING DAMAGES

Monetary damages generally are awarded to individuals in cases of personal injury and wrongful death. Damages generally are fixed by the jury and are nominal, compensatory, hedonic, or punitive.

- *Nominal damages* are awarded as a mere token in recognition that wrong has been committed when the actual amount of compensation is insignificant.
- *Compensatory damages* are estimated reparation in money for detriment or injury sustained (including loss of earnings, medical costs, and loss of financial support).
- *Hedonic damages* are those damages awarded to compensate an individual for the loss of enjoyment of life. Such damages are awarded because of the failure of compensatory damages to compensate an individual adequately for the pain and suffering that he or she has endured as a result of a negligent wrong.
- *Punitive damages* are additional money awards authorized when an injury is caused by gross carelessness or disregard for the safety of others.

Plaintiff's Schedule of Damages

Plaintiffs seek recovery for a great variety of damages. The following are typical: personal injuries; permanent physical disabilities; permanent mental disabilities; past and future physical and mental pain and suffering sustained and to be sustained; loss of enjoyment of life; loss of consortium where a spouse is injured in an accident; loss of child's services where a minor child is injured in the accident; medical and other health expenses reasonably paid or incurred or reasonably certain to be incurred in the future; past and future loss of earnings sustained and to be sustained; and permanent diminution in the plaintiff's earning capacity. The following cases illustrate the types of damages sought by plaintiffs.

Damages/Future Pain and Suffering

In *Luecke v. Bitterman*,[20] an award of $490,000 for future pain and suffering was found reasonable with respect to a 20-year-old patient who, as a result of a physician's negligent application of liquid nitrogen to remove a wart, suffered a 12- by 4-inch third-degree burn. The burn resulted in a scar on the right buttock extending to the back of the thigh. The plaintiff suffered excruciating pain and posttraumatic stress disorder.

Punitive Damages/Mighty Engine of Deterrence

Punitive damages are awarded over and above that which is intended to compensate the plaintiff for economic losses resulting from the injury. Punitive damages cover such items as physical disability, mental anguish, loss of a spouse's services, physical suffering, injury to one's reputation, and loss of companionship. Punitive damages were referred to as that mighty engine of deterrence in *Johnson v. Terry*.[21]

The court in *Henry v. Deen*[22] held that allegations of gross and wanton negligence incidental to wrongful death in the plaintiff's complaint gave sufficient notice of a claim against the treating physician and physician's assistant for punitive damages. The original complaint, which alleged that the treating physician, the physician's assistant, and the consulting physician agreed to create and did create false and misleading entries in the patient's medical record, was sufficient to allege a civil conspiracy. The decision of the lower court was reversed, and the case was remanded for further proceedings.

In *Estes Health Care Centers v. Bannerman*, discussed earlier, the court stated:

> While human life is incapable of translation into a compensatory measurement, the amount of an award of punitive damages may be measured by the gravity of the wrong done, the punishment called for by the act of the wrongdoer, and the need to deter similar wrongs in order to preserve human life.[23]

In *Payton Health Care Facilities, Inc. v. Estate of Campbell*,[24] a punitive damage award in the amount of $1.7 million for the wrongful death of a patient from infected decubitus ulcers was found to be justified. The treating physician had agreed to a settlement prior to trial in the amount of $50,000. The deceased, a stroke victim, had been admitted to the Lakeland Health Care Center for nursing and medical care. While at the center, the patient developed several severe skin ulcers that eventually necessitated hospitalization in Lakeland General Hospital. The patient's condition deteriorated to such a state that further treatment was inadequate to prolong his life. Expert testimony had been presented that indicated that the standard of care received by the patient while at the nursing facility was an outrageous deviation from acceptable standards of care. There was sufficient evidence of the willful and wanton disregard for rights of others to permit an award of punitive damages against the companies who owned and managed the nursing facility. The cause of death was determined to be bacteremia with sepsis, because of extensive infected necrotic decubitus ulcers, that the patient developed at the nursing facility.

Punitive Damages for Failure to Diagnose Inappropriate

Punitive damages in *Brooking v. Polito*[25] were determined to be inappropriate in an action alleging failure to timely diagnose pancreatic cancer. It was undisputed that the defendants performed various tests on the decedent, which included blood tests, CAT scans, an MRI, and ultrasound. The tests had been analyzed, and the patient was treated accordingly.

Damages for Surviving Spouse and Children

Damages may be awarded given evidence of a patient's pain and the mental anguish of the surviving husband and children. In *Jefferson Hospital Association v. Garrett*,[26] damages in the amount of $180,000 were found not to be excessive given evidence of the patient's pain and the mental suffering of the surviving spouse and children.

Damages for Emotional Distress

The court of appeals in *Haught v. Maceluch*[27] held that under Texas law the mother was entitled to recover for her emotional distress, even though she was not conscious at the time her child was born. The mother had brought a medical malpractice action, alleging that the physician was negligent in the delivery of her child, causing her daughter to suffer permanent brain injury. The district court entered judgment of $1,160,000 for the child's medical expenses and $175,000 for her lost future earnings. The court deleted a jury award of $118,000 for the mother's mental suffering over her daughter's impaired condition. On appeal, the court of appeals permitted recovery, under Texas law, for mental suffering. The mother was conscious for more than 11 hours of labor and was aware of the physician's negligent acts, his absence in a near-emergency situation, and the overadministration of the labor-inducing drug Pitocin.

Damages Not Excessive

In determining excessiveness, the courts often consider the severity of the injury, whether the injury is manifested by objective physical evidence or whether it is revealed only by the subjective testimony, whether the injury is permanent, whether the plaintiff can continue with his or her employment, and the size of out-of-pocket expenses.[28]

The plaintiff in *Burge v. Parke*[29] suffered a laceration of his right foot on April 2 and was taken to St. Margaret's Hospital. A physician in the emergency department cleaned and stitched the laceration and released the patient with instructions to keep the foot elevated. Even though reports prepared by the fire medic who arrived on the scene of the accident and by ambulance personnel indicated the chief complaint as being a fracture of the foot, no X-rays were ordered in the emergency department. The admitting clerk had typed a statement on the admission form indicating possible fracture of the right foot. However, a handwritten note stated the chief complaint as being a laceration of the right foot. The patient returned to the hospital later in the day with his mother, complaining of pain in the right foot. His mother asked if X-rays had been taken. The physician said that it was not necessary. The wound was redressed, and the patient was sent home again with instructions to keep the foot elevated. The pain continued to worsen, and the patient was taken to see another physician on April 5. X-rays were ordered, and an orthopedic surgeon called for a consultation diagnosed three fractures and compartment syndrome, a swelling of tissue in the muscle compartments. The swelling increased pressure on the blood vessels, thus decreasing circulation, which tends to cause muscles to die.

Approximately one half pint of clotted blood was removed from the wound. By April 11, the big toe had to be surgically removed. It was alleged that the emergency department physician failed to obtain a full medical history, to order the necessary X-rays, and to diagnose and treat the fractures of the foot. As a result, the patient ultimately suffered loss of his big toe. The Macon County Circuit Court awarded damages totaling $450,000 for loss of a big toe, and the physician appealed. The Alabama Supreme Court found the damages not to have been excessive.

A medical malpractice action was brought against the employer of a physician, alleging that the physician's failure to properly treat an abscess some three weeks after an infant received a live polio vaccine resulted in suppression of the infant's immune system and the infant's contraction of paralytic polio. The jury in the circuit court returned a $16 million verdict in favor of the plaintiffs, and the defendant appealed. The case was transferred from the court of appeals to the state supreme court.[30]

The Missouri Supreme Court held that there was no basis for a new trial on the grounds of excessiveness of the $16 million verdict. There is no formula for determining the excessiveness of a verdict. Each case must be decided on its own facts to determine what is fair and reasonable. A jury is in the best position to make such a determination. The trial judge could have set aside the verdict if a determination was made that passion and prejudice brought about an excessive verdict. The size of the verdict alone does not establish passion and prejudice. The appellant failed to establish that the verdict was: (1) glaringly unwarranted and (2) based on prejudice and passion. Compensation of a plaintiff is based on such factors as the age of the patient, the nature and extent of injury, diminished earnings capacity, economic condition, and awards in comparable cases. A jury is entitled to consider such intangibles that do not lend themselves to precise calculation, such as past and future pain, suffering, effect on lifestyle, embarrassment, humiliation, and economic loss.

Damages Excessive

A jury verdict totaling $12,393,130 was considered an excessive award in *Merrill v. Albany Medical Center*,[31] in which damages were sought with respect to the severe brain damage sustained by a 22-month-old infant as the result of oxygen deprivation. This occurred when the infant went into cardiac arrest during surgery for removal of a suspected malignant tumor from her right lung. Reduction of the amount to $6,143,130 was considered to be appropriate.

Damages Capped

The trial court in *Judd v. Drezga*[32] was found to have properly limited a brain-damaged infant's recovery of quality-of-life damages to $250,000. The Idaho cap on damages was designed to reduce health care costs, increase the availability of medical malpractice insurance, and secure the continued availability of health care resources—all legitimate legislative goals given the clear social and economic evil of rising health care costs and a shortage of qualified health care professionals. In attempting to meet its goals, the legislature had not unreasonably or arbitrarily limited recovery. Rather, it had chosen to place a limit on the recovery of noneconomic quality-of-life damages—one area where legislation had been shown to actually and substantially further these goals. Applying each individual test, the open courts, uniform operation of laws, and due-process provisions of the constitution were not offended by the damage cap. Additionally, neither the right to a jury trial nor the constitutional guarantee of separation of powers were offended by the cap.

Joint and Several Liability

The doctrine of joint and several liability permits the plaintiff to bring suit against all persons who share responsibility for his or her injury. The doctrine allows the plaintiff to recover monetary damages from any one of or all the defendants. Any one defendant, even though partially responsible for the plaintiff's injury, can be required to pay the full judgment awarded by the jury. Awards tend to fall in greater amounts on defendants with the better insurance. This is the deep-pockets concept: Whoever has the most pays the greater percentage of the award.

APPEALS

An appellate court reviews a case on the basis of the trial record as well as written briefs and, if requested, concise oral arguments by the attorneys. A brief summarizes the facts of a case, testimony of the witnesses, laws affecting the case, and arguments of counsel. The party making the appeal is the appellant. The party answering the appeal is the appellee. After hearing oral arguments, the court takes the case under advisement until such time as the judges consider it and agree on a decision. An opinion then is prepared explaining the reasons for a decision.

Grounds for appeal can result from one or more of the following: the verdict was excessive or inadequate in the lower court; evidence was rejected that should have been accepted; inadmissible evidence was permitted; testimony that should have been admissible was excluded; the verdict was contrary to the weight of the evidence; the court improperly charged the jury; the jury was confused by jury instructions; and/or the jury verdict is the result of bias, prejudice, and/or passion.

Notice of appeal must be filed with the trial court, the appellate court, and the adverse party. The party wishing to prevent execution of an adverse judgment until such time as the case has been heard and decided by an appellate court also should file a stay of execution.

The appellate court may modify, affirm, or reverse the judgment or reorder a new trial on an appeal. The majority ruling of the judges in the appellate court is binding on the parties of a lawsuit. If the appellate court's decision is not unanimous, the minority may render a dissenting opinion. Further appeal may be made, as set by statute, to the highest court of appeals. If an appeal involves a constitutional question, it eventually might be appealed to the US Supreme Court.

When the highest appellate court in a state decides a case, a final judgment results, and the matter is ended. The instances when one may appeal the ruling of a state court to the US Supreme Court are rare. A federal question must be involved, and even then the Supreme Court must decide whether it will hear the case. A federal question is one involving the US Constitution or a statute enacted by Congress, so it is unlikely that a negligence case arising in a state court would be reviewed and decided by the Supreme Court.

EXECUTION OF JUDGMENTS

When the amount of damages has been established and all the appeals have been heard, the defendant must comply with the judgment. If he or she fails to do so, a court order can be executed requiring the sheriff or other judicial officer to sell as much of the defendant's property as necessary, within statutory limitations, to satisfy the plaintiff's judgment.

Notes

1. Collins v. Park, 621 A.2d 996 (Pa. Super. Ct. 1993).
2. 725 N.Y.S.2d 35 (2001).
3. 600 A.2d 1063 (D.C. 1991).
4. STEVE COHEN, Malpractice, NEW YORKER MAGAZINE, Oct. 1, 1990, at 43, 47.
5. 720 N.E.2d 1175 (Ind. App. 1999).
6. 337 P.2d 974 (Or. 1959).
7. 221 N.W.2d 39 (S.D. 1974).
8. 445 N.W.2d 763 (Iowa 1989).
9. Marsingill v. O'Malley, 128 P.3d 151 (Alas. 2006).
10. 346 S.E.2d 528 (S.C. 1986).
11. 187 SW.3d 828 (2006).
12. Deal v. Kearney, 851 P.2d 1353 (Alaska 1993).
13. 358 S.E.2d 222 (W. Va. 1987).
14. 320 A.2d 637 (N.H. 1974).
15. Id.
16. 154 S.E.2d 461 (Ga. Ct. App. 1967).
17. 463 F. Supp. 321 (D. Alaska 1978).
18. 411 So. 2d 109 (Ala. 1982).
19. 657 N.Y.S.2d 419 (N.Y. App. Div. 1997).
20. 658 N.Y.S.2d 34 (N.Y. App. Div. 1997).
21. No. 537-907 (Wis. Cir. Ct. Mar. 18, 1983).
22. 310 S.E.2d 326 (N.C. 1984).
23. 411 So. 2d 109, 113 (Ala. 1982).
24. 497 So. 2d 1233 (Fla. Dist. Ct. App. 1986).
25. 16 A.D.3d 898, 791 N.Y.S.2d 686 (N.Y. App. Div. 2005).
26. 804 S.W.2d 711 (Ark. 1991).
27. 681 F.2d 291 (5th Cir. 1982).
28. Tesauro v. Perrige, 650 A.2d 1079 (Pa. Super. 1994).
29. 510 So. 2d 538 (Ala. 1987).
30. Callahan v. Cardinal Glennon Hosp., 863 S.W.2d 852 (Mo. 1993).
31. 512 N.Y.S.2d 519 (N.Y. App. Div. 1987).
32. 103 P.3d 135, 2004 UT 91 (Utah 2004).

7

CORPORATE STRUCTURE AND LIABILITY

This chapter introduces the health care professional to the responsibilities, as well as legal risks, of health care organizations and their governing bodies. Health care organizations are incorporated under state law as freestanding for-profit or not-for-profit corporations. Each corporation has a governing body (e.g., board of directors) that has ultimate responsibility for the operation of the organization. The existence of this authority creates certain duties and liabilities for governing boards and their individual members. The governing body is legally responsible for establishing and implementing policies regarding the management and operation of the organization. Responsibility for the day-to-day operations of an organization is generally accomplished by appointing a chief executive officer.

Not-for-profit health care organizations are usually exempt from federal taxation under Section 501(c)(3) of the Internal Revenue Code of 1986, as amended. Such federal exemption usually entitles the organization to an automatic exemption from state taxes as well. Such tax exemption not only relieves the organization from the payment of income taxes and sales taxes but also permits the organization to receive contributions from donors, who then may obtain charitable deductions on their personal income tax returns.

Although health care organizations can operate as sole proprietorships or partnerships, most function as corporations. Thus, an important source of law applicable to governing boards and to the duties and responsibilities of their members is found in state incorporation laws. These duties include holding meetings, establishing policies, being financially scrupulous, providing adequate insurance, and paying taxes, as might be required.

AUTHORITY OF HEALTH CARE CORPORATIONS

Health care corporations—governmental, charitable, or proprietary—have certain powers expressly or implicitly granted to them by state statutes. Generally, the authority of a corporation is expressed in the law under which the corporation is chartered and in the corporation's articles of incorporation. The existence of this authority creates certain duties and liabilities for governing bodies and their individual members. Members of the governing body of an organization have both express and implied corporate authority.

Express Corporate Authority

Express corporate authority is the power specifically delegated by statute. A health care corporation derives its authority to act from the laws of the state in which it is incorporated. The articles of incorporation set forth the purpose(s) of the corporation's existence and the powers the corporation is authorized to exercise to carry out its purposes.

Implied Corporate Authority

Implied corporate authority is the right to perform any and all acts necessary to exercise a corporation's expressly conferred authority and to accomplish the purpose(s) for which it was created. Generally, implied corporate authority arises from situations in which such authority is required or suggested as a result of a need for corporate powers not specifically granted in the articles of incorporation. A governing body, at its own discretion, can enact new bylaws, rules, and regulations; purchase or mortgage property; borrow money; purchase equipment; select employees; adopt corporate resolutions that delineate decision-making responsibilities; and so forth. These powers can be enumerated in the articles of incorporation and, in such cases, would be categorized as express rather than implied corporate authority.

Duty to Appoint Competent Physicians

Hospitals have an implied duty to patients to select competent physicians who, although they are independent practitioners, would be providing in-hospital care to their patients. Hospitals are in the best position to protect their patients and consequently have an independent duty to select competent independent physicians seeking staff privileges.

The surgeon in *Purcell & Tucson General Hospital v. Zimbelman*[1] performed inappropriate surgery because of his misdiagnosis of the patient's ailment. Prior malpractice suits against the surgeon revealed that the hospital had reason to know or should have known that the surgeon apparently lacked the skill to treat the patient's condition. The court held that the hospital had a clear duty to select competent physicians; to regulate the privileges granted to staff physicians; to ensure that privileges are conferred only for those procedures for which the physician is trained and qualified; and to restrict, suspend, or require supervision when a physician has demonstrated an inability to perform certain procedures. The hospital assumed the duty of supervising the competence of its physicians. The department of surgery was acting for and on behalf of the hospital in fulfilling this duty. If the department is negligent in not taking action against the surgeon or recommending to the governing body that action be taken, the hospital would be negligent. The court noted that it is reasonable to conclude that if the hospital had taken some action against the surgeon, the patient would not have been injured.

Ultra Vires Acts

A governing body can be held liable for acting beyond its scope of authority, which is either expressed (e.g., in its articles of incorporation) or implied in law. Acts of this nature are referred to as *ultra vires acts*. The governing body acts in and on behalf of the corporation. If any action is in violation of a statute or regulation, it is illegal. An example of an illegal act would be the "known" employment of an unlicensed person in a position that by law requires a license. The state, through its attorney general, has the power to prevent the performance of an ultra vires act by injunction.

Governing bodies should have their corporate charters reviewed periodically by legal counsel to ensure that their express powers are consistent with the organization's mission, operations, and development plans.

CORPORATE ORGANIZATION AND COMMITTEE STRUCTURE

Ultimate responsibility for the functioning of a health care corporation rests with the governing body. Ideally, the governing body generally includes representation from both the community and the organization's medical staff. The business of the governing body is generally conducted through a variety of committees. Some of those committees are described here.

Executive Committee

The executive committee is a working group of the governing body that has delegated authority to act on behalf of the full board when it is not in session. The committee must act within the scope and authority assigned by the governing body. The duties and responsibilities of the committee should be delineated in the corporate bylaws. The functions of the executive committee generally include acting as a liaison between management and the full board, reviewing and making recommendations on management proposals, and performing special assignments as may be delegated by the full board from time to time. Business transacted and actions taken by the executive committee should be reported at regular sessions of the governing body and ratified. The executive committee generally has all the powers of the governing body, except such powers as the governing body may be prohibited from delegating in accordance with applicable laws.

Bylaws Committee

The bylaws committee reviews and recommends bylaw changes to the governing body. Bylaws generally are amended or rescinded by a majority vote of the governing body.

Finance Committee

The finance committee is responsible for overseeing the financial affairs of the organization and making recommendations to the governing body. This committee is responsible for directing and reviewing the preparation of financial statements, operating budgets, major capital requests, and so on. The governing body must approve actions of the finance committee.

Nominating Committee

The nominating committee is generally responsible for developing and recommending to the governing body criteria for governing body membership. The requirements for membership on a governing body generally include a willingness to devote the time and energy necessary to fulfill the commitment as a board member; residence in the community or an identifiable association with the community served; demonstration of a knowledge of local health care issues; possession of the traits of good moral character and maturity; and professional, as well as appropriate, life experiences necessary to make managerial decisions in the health care setting.

Planning Committee

The planning committee is responsible for recommending to the governing body the use and development of organizational resources as they relate to the mission and vision of the organization. Specifically, the planning committee oversees: the development of short-term and long-range goals; acquisition of major equipment; addition of new services based on identified community need; program development; and the preparation of progress reports to the full board.

Patient Care Committee

The patient care committee reviews the quality of patient care rendered in the organization and makes recommendations for the improvement of such care. The committee is generally responsible for developing a process to identify patient and family needs and expectations and to establish a process to continuously improve customer relations.

Audit and Regulatory Compliance Committee

The audit and regulatory compliance committee is responsible for the assessment of various functions and control systems of the organization and for providing management with analysis and recommendations regarding activities reviewed. Health care organizations must be vigilant in conducting their financial affairs. An effective audit committee can be helpful in uncovering and thwarting poor or inept financial decision making. The committee should include members from the governing body and internal auditing staff. Responsibilities of the committee include: developing corporate auditing policies and procedures; recommending independent auditors to the governing body; reviewing the credentials of the independent auditors and facilitating change in auditors as might be deemed appropriate; reviewing with independent auditors the proposed scope and general extent of their auditing duties and responsibilities; reviewing the scope and results of the annual audit with the independent auditors and the organization's management staff; setting, overseeing, reviewing, and acting on the recommendations of the internal audit staff; reviewing the internal accounting practices of the corporation, including policies and procedures; reviewing and evaluating financial statements (e.g., income statements, balance sheets, cash flow reports, investment accounts); promoting the prevention, detection, deterrence, and reporting of fraud; reviewing the means for safeguarding assets, and, as appropriate, the existence of such assets; ensuring that financial reporting functions are in keeping with generally accepted accounting principles; and reviewing the reliability and integrity of financial and operating information.

SARBANES-OXLEY ACT

The Sarbanes-Oxley Act of 2002, commonly called SOX or SARBOX, was enacted as a response to the misconduct committed by executives in companies such as Enron, World Com, and Tyco, resulting in investor losses exceeding half a trillion dollars. To protect investors in public companies and improve the accuracy and reliability of corporate disclosures, SOX requires top executives of public corporations to vouch for the financial reports of their companies. The act encourages self-regulation and the need to promote due diligence; select a leader with morals and core values; examine incentives; constantly monitor the organization's culture; build a strong, knowledgeable governing body; continuously search for conflicts of interest in the organization; focus attention on processes and controls that support accurate financial reporting through documented policies and procedures; and establish strong standards of conduct and a code of ethics that encourages employees to report unethical or fraudulent behavior without fear of retribution.

The act covers issues such as establishing a public company accounting oversight board, auditor independence, corporate responsibility, and enhanced financial disclosure.

Major provisions of SOX include: certification of financial reports by CEOs and CFOs; ban on personal loans to any executive officer and director; accelerated reporting of trades by insiders; prohibition on insider trades during pension fund blackout periods; public reporting of CEO and CFO compensation and profits; inside audit board independence; criminal and civil penalties for securities violations; obligation to have an internal audit function, which will need to be certified by external auditors; significantly longer jail sentences and larger fines for corporate executives who knowingly misstate financial statements; and codes of ethics and standards of conduct for executive officers and board members.

Although not-for-profit organizations are not legally required to adopt SOX, the accountability and financial reporting requirements are being adopted by many hospitals.

DOCTRINE OF *RESPONDEAT SUPERIOR*

Respondeat superior (let the master respond) is a legal doctrine holding employers liable, in certain cases, for the wrongful acts of their agents (employees). This doctrine has also been referred to as vicarious liability, whereby an employer is answerable for the torts committed by employees. In the health care setting, an organization, for example, is liable for the negligent acts of its employees, even though there has been no wrongful conduct on the part of the organization. For liability to be imputed to the employer:

1. A master–servant relationship must exist between the employer and the employee; and
2. The wrongful act of the employee must have occurred within the scope of his or her employment.

The question of liability frequently rests on whether persons treating a patient are independent agents (responsible for their own acts) or employees of the organization. The answer to this depends on whether the organization can exercise control over the particular act that was the proximate cause of the injury. The basic rationale for imposing liability on an employer developed because of the employer's right to control the physical acts of its employees. It is not necessary that the employer actually exercise control, only that it possesses the right, power, or authority to do so.

When filing a lawsuit, the plaintiff's attorney generally names both the employer and employee. This occurs because the employer is generally in a better financial condition to cover the judgment. The employer is not without remedy if liability has been imposed against the organization due to an employee's negligent act. The employer can seek indemnification from the employee.

Independent Contractor

An *independent contractor* relationship is established when the principal has no right of control over the manner in which the agent's work is to be performed. The independent contractor therefore is responsible for his or her own negligent acts. However, some cases indicate that an organization can be held liable for an independent contractor's negligence. For example, in *Mehlman v. Powell*,[2] the court held that a hospital can be found vicariously liable for the negligence of an emergency department physician who was not a hospital employee but who worked in the emergency department in the capacity of an independent contractor. The court reasoned that the hospital maintained control over billing procedures, maintained an emergency department in the main hospital, and represented to the patient that the members of the emergency department staff were its employees, which might have caused the patient to rely on the skill and competence of the staff.

Corporate Officer/Director

An officer or a director of a corporation is not personally liable for the torts of corporate employees. To incur liability, the officer or the director ordinarily must be shown to have in some way authorized, directed, or participated in a tortious act. The administrator of the estate of the deceased in *Hunt v. Rabon*[3] brought a malpractice action against hospital trustees and others for the wrongful death of the decedent during an operation at the hospital. A contractor had incorrectly crossed the oxygen and nitrous oxide lines of a newly installed medical gas system leading to the operating room. The trustees filed a pleading claiming that the facts of the case were not sufficient for an action against them individually as trustees. The South Carolina Supreme Court held that the allegations presented were insufficient to hold the trustees liable for the wrongs alleged.

CORPORATE NEGLIGENCE

A corporation is treated no differently from an individual. If a corporation has a duty and fails in the exercise of that duty, it has the same liability to the injured party as an individual would have.

Corporate negligence occurs when a health care corporation fails to perform those duties it owes directly to a patient or to anyone else to whom a duty might extend. If such a duty is breached and a patient is injured as a result of that breach, the organization can be held culpable under the theory of corporate negligence.

Darling—A Benchmark Case

The benchmark case in the health care field, which has had a major impact on the liability of health care organizations, was decided in 1965 in *Darling v. Charleston Community Memorial Hospital*.[4] The court enunciated a corporate negligence doctrine under which hospitals have a duty to provide an adequately trained medical and nursing staff. A hospital is responsible, in conjunction with its medical staff, for establishing policies and procedures for monitoring the quality of medicine practiced within the hospital.

The Darling case involved an 18-year-old college football player who was preparing for a career as a teacher and coach. The patient, a defensive halfback for his college football team, was injured during a play. He was rushed to the emergency department of a small, accredited community hospital where the only physician on emergency duty that day was Dr. Alexander, a general practitioner. Alexander had not treated a major leg fracture in 3 years.

The physician examined the patient and ordered an X-ray that revealed that the tibia and the fibula of the right leg had been fractured. The physician reduced the fracture and applied a plaster cast from a point three or four inches below the groin to the toes. Shortly after the cast had been applied, the patient began to complain continually of pain. The physician split the cast and continued to visit the patient frequently while the patient remained in the hospital. The emergency department physician did not call in any specialist for consultation.

After 2 weeks, the student was transferred to a larger hospital and placed under the care of an orthopedic surgeon. The specialist found a considerable amount of dead tissue in the fractured leg. During a period of 2 months, the specialist removed increasing amounts of tissue in a futile attempt to save the leg until it became necessary to amputate the leg eight inches below the knee. The student's father did not agree to a settlement and filed suit against the emergency department physician and the hospital. Although the physician later settled out of court for $40,000, the case continued against the hospital.

The documentary evidence relied on to establish the standard of care included the rules and regulations of the Illinois Department of Public Health under the Hospital Licensing Act; the standards for hospital accreditation, today known as The Joint Commission; and the bylaws, rules, and regulations of Charleston Hospital. These documents were admitted into evidence without objection. No specific evidence was offered that the hospital failed to conform to the usual and customary practices of hospitals in the community.

The trial court instructed the jury to consider those documents, along with all other evidence, in determining the hospital's liability. Under the circumstances in which the case reached the Illinois Supreme Court, it was held that the verdict against the hospital should be sustained if the evidence supported the verdict on any one or more of the 20 allegations of negligence. Allegations asserted that the hospital was negligent in its failure to: (1) provide a sufficient number of trained nurses for bedside care—in this case, nurses who were capable of recognizing the progressive gangrenous condition of the plaintiff's right leg and (2) failure of its nurses to bring the patient's condition to the attention of the administration and staff so that adequate consultation could be secured.

Although these generalities provided the jury with no practical guidance for determining what constitutes reasonable care, they were considered to be relevant to aid the jury in deciding what was feasible and what the hospital knew or should have known concerning its responsibilities for patient care.

Evidence relating to the hospital's failure to review Alexander's work, to require consultation or examination by specialists, and to require proper nursing care was found to be sufficient to support a verdict for the patient. Judgment was eventually returned against the hospital in the amount of $100,000. The Illinois Supreme Court held that the hospital could not limit its liability as a charitable corporation to the amount of its liability insurance.

> [T]he doctrine of charitable immunity can no longer stand . . . a doctrine which limits the liability of charitable corporations to the amount of liability insurance that they see fit to carry permits them to determine whether or not they will be liable for their torts and the amount of that liability, if any.[5]

In effect, the hospital was liable as a corporate entity for the negligent acts of its employees and physicians. Among other things, the Darling case indicates the importance of instituting effective credentialing and continuing medical evaluation and review programs for all members of a professional staff.

JOINT LIABILITY

Joint liability is based on the concept that all joint or concurrent tort-feasors are actually independently at fault for their own wrongful acts. Both a hospital and its physicians can be held jointly liable for damages suffered by patients. In *Gonzales v. Nork & Mercy Hospital*,[6] the hospital was found negligent for failing to protect the patient, a 27-year-old man, from acts of malpractice by an independent, privately retained physician. The patient had been injured in an automobile accident and was operated on by Dr. Nork, an orthopedic surgeon. The plaintiff's life expectancy was reduced as a result of an unsuccessful and allegedly unnecessary laminectomy. It was found that the hospital knew or should have known of the surgeon's incompetence because the surgeon previously had performed many operations either unnecessarily or negligently. In such cases the defendant produced false and inadequate findings as well as false-positive myelograms. He deceived his patients with this information and caused them to undergo surgery. Evidence was presented showing that the surgeon had performed more than three dozen similar operations unnecessarily or in a negligent manner. Even if the hospital was not aware of the surgeon's acts of negligence, an effective monitoring system should have been in place for monitoring his abilities. Consequently, the surgeon and hospital were jointly liable for damages suffered.

DUTIES OF HEALTH CARE CORPORATIONS

Governing body members are considered by law to have the highest measure of accountability. They have a fiduciary duty that requires acting primarily for the benefit of the corporation. The general duties of a governing body are both implied and express. The duty to supervise and manage is applicable to the trustees just as it is to the managers of any other business corporation. In both instances, there is a duty to act as a reasonably prudent person would act under similar circumstances.

Appoint a CEO

The governing body is responsible for appointing a CEO to act as an agent in the management of the organization. The individual selected as CEO must possess the competence and the character necessary to maintain satisfactory standards of patient care within the organization. The responsibilities and authority of the CEO should be expressed in an appropriate job description, as well as in any formal agreement or contract that the organization has with the CEO. Some state health codes describe the responsibilities of administrators in broad terms. They generally provide that the CEO/administrator shall be responsible for the overall management of the organization; enforcement of any applicable federal, state, and local regulations, as well as the organization's bylaws, policies, and procedures; appointment of, with the approval of the governing body, a qualified medical director; liaison between the governing body and staff (including both employed and appointed members of the professional staff); and appointment of an administrative person to act during the CEO's absence from the organization.

Comply with Laws and Regulations

The governing body in general and its agents (assigned representatives) in particular are responsible for compliance with federal, state, and local laws regarding the operation of the organization. Depending on the scope of the wrong committed and the intent of the governing body, failure to comply could subject board members and/or their agents to civil liability and, in some instances, to criminal prosecution.

Failure to comply with applicable statutory regulations can be costly. This was the case in *People v. Casa Blanca Convalescent Homes*,[7] in which there was evidence of numerous and prolonged deficiencies in resident care. The nursing home's practice of providing insufficient personnel constituted not only illegal practice but also unfair business practice. The trial court was found to have properly assessed a fine of $2,500 for each of 67 violations, totaling $167,500, where the evidence showed that the operator of the nursing home had the financial ability to pay that amount.

The Joint Commission Standards

The governing body, if accredited by The Joint Commission, is responsible for compliance with applicable standards promulgated by The Joint Commission. Noncompliance could cause an organization to lose accreditation, which in turn would provide grounds for third-party reimbursement agencies (e.g., Medicare) to refuse payment for treatment rendered to patients.

Provide Timely Treatment

Health care organizations can be held liable for delays in treatment that result in injuries to their patients. For example, the patient in *Heddinger v. Ashford Memorial Community Hospital*[8] filed a malpractice action against a hospital and its insurer, alleging that a delay in treating her left hand resulted in the loss of her little finger. Medical testimony presented at trial indicated that if proper and timely treatment had been rendered, the finger would have been saved. The US District Court entered judgment on a jury verdict for the plaintiff in the amount of $175,000. The hospital appealed, and the US Court of Appeals held that even if the physicians who attended the patient were not employees of the hospital but were independent contractors, the risk of negligent treatment was clearly foreseeable by the hospital.

Avoid Self-Dealing and Conflicts of Interest

Governing body members must refrain from self-dealing and avoid conflict of interest situations. Each board member should submit in writing all outstanding voting shares (where applicable) or any relationships or transactions in which the director might or could have a conflict of interest. Membership on the governing body or its committees should not be used for private gain. Board members are expected to disclose potential conflict of interest situations and withdraw from the boardroom at the time of voting on such issues. Board members who suspect a conflict of interest situation have a right and a duty to raise pertinent questions regarding any potential conflict. Conflict of interest is presumed to exist when a board member or a firm with which he or she is associated can benefit or lose from the passage of a proposed action.

Provide Adequate Staff

Staffing shortages for both hospitals and nursing homes continue to plague the health care industry. Because the quality of care provided by nursing homes is the subject of much scrutiny, American families face difficult decisions about whether to move a loved one into such a setting.

Under federal law, nursing facilities must have sufficient nursing staff to provide nursing and related services adequate to attain and maintain the highest practicable physical, mental, and psychosocial well-being of each resident, as determined by resident assessments and individual plans of care. As nursing facilities are increasingly filled with older, disabled residents with ever-increasing complex care needs, the demands for highly educated and trained nursing personnel continue to grow.

> Many medical and regulatory investigators who work in nursing homes every day characterize the number of wrongful deaths in terms such as "massive" and "pervasive," based on their daily experience. Most of the deaths can be traced to an inadequate number of nurses and aides to provide life-sustaining care. The US Department of Health and Human Services reported to Congress in 2002 that 9 out of 10 nursing homes have staffing levels too low to provide adequate care.[9]

Deficient Nursing Care

The nursing facility in *Our Lady of the Woods v. Commonwealth of Kentucky Health Facilities*[10] was closed because of deficiencies found during an inspection of the facility, the most serious of which was the lack of continuous nursing care on all shifts. The court held that evidence that the nursing facility lacked continuous services required by regulation was sufficient to sustain an order to close the facility. The appellants in this case had been notified of the deficiencies and were ordered to correct them. Many witnesses testified concerning the deficiencies, and even the administrator admitted to the most serious violation—lack of continuous nursing services.

Timely Response to Patient Calls

Health care organizations must provide for adequate staffing. The Court of Appeal in *Leavitt v. St. Tammany Parish Hospital*[11] held that the hospital owed a duty to respond promptly to patient calls for help. The hospital breached its duty by having less-than-adequate staff on hand and by failing to at least verbally answer an assistance light to inquire what the patient needed.

Postoperative Care

The patient in *Czubinsky v. Doctors Hospital*,[12] recovering from anesthesia, went into cardiac arrest and sustained permanent damages. The court of appeals held that the injuries sustained by the patient were the direct result of the hospital's failure to properly monitor and render aid when needed in the immediate postoperative period. The registered nurse assigned to the patient had a duty to remain with her until the patient was transferred to the recovery room. The nurse's absence was the proximate cause of the patient's injuries. Failure of the hospital to provide adequate staff to assist the patient in the immediate postoperative period was an act in dereliction of duty—a failure that resulted in readily foreseeable permanent damages.

Deficient Care Given

In *Montgomery Health Care Facility v. Ballard*,[13] three nurses testified that the nursing facility was understaffed. One nurse testified that she asked her supervisor for more help but did not get it. The estate of a nursing home resident, who had expired as the result of multiple infected bedsores, brought a malpractice action against the nursing home. First American Health Care, Inc., is the parent corporation of the Montgomery Health Care Facility. The trial court entered a judgment on a jury verdict against the home, and an appeal was taken. The Alabama Supreme Court held that reports compiled by the Alabama Department of Public Health concerning deficiencies found in the nursing home were admissible as evidence. Evidence showed that the care given to the deceased was deficient in the same ways as noted in the survey and complaint reports, which indicated that deficiencies in the home included:

> [I]nadequate documentation of treatment given for decubitus ulcers; 23 patients found with decubitus ulcers, 10 of whom developed those ulcers in the facility; dressings on the sores were not changed as ordered; nursing progress notes did not describe patients' ongoing conditions, particularly with respect to descriptions of decubitus ulcers; ineffective policies and procedures with respect to sterile dressing supplies; lack of nursing assessments; incomplete patient care plans; inadequate documentation of doctor's visits, orders or progress notes; A.M. care not consistently documented; inadequate documentation of turning of patients; incomplete "activities of daily living" sheets; "range of motion" exercises not documented; patients found wet and soiled with dried fecal matter; lack of bowel and bladder retaining programs; incomplete documentation of ordered force fluids. . . .[14]

From a corporate standpoint, the parent corporation of the nursing facility could be held liable for the nursing facility's negligence, where the parent company controlled or retained the right to control the day-to-day operations of the home. The defendants argued that the punitive damage award of $2 million against the home was greater than what was necessary to meet society's goal of punishing them. The Alabama Supreme Court, however, found the award not to be excessive. "The trial court also found that because of the large number of nursing home residents vulnerable to the type of neglect found in Mrs. Stovall's case, the verdict would further the goal of discouraging others from similar conduct in the future."[15]

Provide Adequate Facilities and Equipment

Health care organizations are under a duty to exercise reasonable care to furnish adequate equipment, appliances, and supplies for use in the diagnosis or treatment of patients. Equipment furnished by an organization should be fit for the purposes and uses intended. Within its duty to provide adequate facilities and equipment, the governing body must exercise reasonable care and skill in supervising and managing facility property. This obligation includes protecting property from destruction and loss.

Health care organizations must be designed, constructed, equipped, and maintained to provide a safe, healthy, functional, sanitary, and comfortable environment for patients, employees, and the public. Buildings and equipment should be maintained and operated to prevent fire and other hazards to personal safety. Patient rooms should be designed and equipped for adequate nursing care, comfort, and privacy. Mechanical, electric, and patient care equipment should be maintained in a safe operating condition.

Driftwood Convalescent Hospital, operated by Western Medical Enterprises, Inc., in *Beach v. Western Medical Enterprises, Inc.*,[16] was fined $2,500 in civil penalties because of nonfunctioning hallway lights and the facility's failure to provide the required type and amount of decubitus preventive equipment necessary for resident care as required by the California

Health and Safety Code. The regulations required that equipment necessary for care to patients, as ordered or indicated, be provided.

Provide Adequate Insurance

The duty of the governing body is to purchase insurance against different risks. Organizations face as much risk of losing their tangible and intangible assets through judgments for negligence as they do through fires or other disasters. When this is true, the duty to insure against the risks of fire is as great as the duty to insure against the risks of negligent conduct.

Be Financially Scrupulous

Health care organizations searching for alternate sources of income must do so scrupulously and not find themselves in what could be construed as questionable corporate activities. Such was the case in *Smith v. van Gorkum*[17] where the board of directors authorized the sale of its company through a cash-out merger for a tendered price per share nearly 50% over the market price. Although that might sound like a good deal, the governing body did not make any inquiry to determine whether it was the best deal available. In fact, it made no decision during a hastily arranged, brief meeting in which it relied solely on the CEO's report regarding the desirability of the move. The Delaware Supreme Court held that the board's decision to approve a proposed cash-out merger was not a product of informed business judgment and that it acted in a grossly negligent manner in approving amendments to the merger proposal.

Require Competitive Bidding

Many states have developed regulations requiring competitive bidding for work or services commissioned by public organizations. The fundamental purpose of this requirement is to eliminate or at least reduce the possibility that such abuses as fraud, favoritism, improvidence, or extravagance will intrude into an organization's business practices. Contracts made in violation of a statute are considered to be illegal and could result in personal liability for board members, especially if the members become aware of a fraudulent activity and allow it to continue.

Provide a Safe Environment

Health care corporations are liable for injuries to both patients and employees rising from environmental hazards. For example, the license of a nursing facility operator was revoked in *Erie Care Center, Inc. v. Ackerman*[18] on findings of uncleanliness, disrepair, inadequate record keeping, and nursing shortages. The court held that although violation of a single public health regulation might have been insufficient in and of itself to justify revocation of the nursing home's operating license, multiple violations, taken together, established the facility's practice and justified revocation.

Fire Hazards

Hospitals have a duty to protect patients from fire hazards. As was the case, for example, in *Stacy v. Truman Medical Center*,[19] where the patients' families brought wrongful death actions against the medical center and one of its nurses. The wrongful death actions resulted from a fire in the decedents' room at the medical center. On the day of the fire, Ms. Stacy visited her brother, Stephen Stacy. When she arrived, Stephen, who suffered from head injuries and was not supposed to walk around, was sitting in a chair smoking a cigarette with the permission of one of the nurses. No one told Ms. Stacy not to allow her brother to smoke. Stacy also lit a cigarette and because she did not see an ashtray in the room, she used a juice cup and a plastic soup tray for her ashes. At approximately 5:00 p.m., a nurse came in and restrained Stephen in his chair with ties to prevent him from sliding out of the chair. Before Stacy left, she lit a cigarette, held it to Stephen's mouth, and extinguished it in the soup tray.

Shortly after 5:00 p.m., a fire started in a wastebasket in the room. There was no smoke detector in the room. Another patient, Wheeler, was in the bed next to the windows. When Ms. Schreiner, the nurse in charge, discovered the fire, she did not think Wheeler was in immediate danger. She unsuccessfully tried to untie Stephen from his restraints. Then she attempted to put out the fire by smothering it with a sheet. When her attempts to extinguish the fire failed, she ran to the door of the room and yelled for help, which alerted Nurses Cominos and Rodriguez. After calling for help, Ms. Schreiner resumed her attempts to smother the flames with bed linens. Subsequently, she and others grabbed Stephen by the legs and pulled him and his chair toward the hallway. In the process, Stephen's restraints burned through, and he slid from the chair to the floor. Schreiner and her assistants pulled him the remaining few feet out of the room and into the hallway. Schreiner tried to get back into the room but was prevented by the intense smoke, flames, and heat.

After initially entering the room, both Rodriguez and Cominos returned to the nurse's station to sound alarms and to call security; neither attempted to remove Wheeler from the room. Both ran directly past a fire extinguisher, but neither grabbed it before returning to the room. After Stephen was removed from the room, Cominos entered the room with a fire extinguisher and tried to rescue Wheeler. Because of the intense smoke and heat, however, she was unable to reach Wheeler. Wheeler died in the room from smoke inhalation. Stephen survived for several weeks and then died as a result of complications from infections secondary to burns.

The medical center's policy in case of fire provided for the removal of patients from the room and out of immediate danger first. In its fire-training programs, the medical center used the acronym of "RACE" to supply a chronology of steps to take in case of a fire.

R—Rescue or remove the patient first.
A—An alarm should be sounded second.
C—Contain the fire third.
E—Extinguish the fire last.

The medical center's written smoking policy at the time of the fire stated: "No smoking shall be permitted in the Truman Medical Center Health Care Facility except in those areas specifically designated and posted as smoking areas." The smoking policy further stated: "In the event violations of this policy are observed, the person violating the policy must be requested to discontinue such violation." Nurse Cominos admitted that she was a supervisor and that she violated this portion of the smoking policy on the date of the fire by observing smoking and the use of a juice cup for an ashtray.

The Missouri Supreme Court held that a causal connection between the medical center's negligence and the patients' deaths was sufficiently established. The *medical center owed a duty* of reasonable care to all of its patients. There was evidence that the fire started in the trash can from discarded smoking materials.

Duty to Prevent Falls

Falls are frequent occurrences in health care settings. They can occur anywhere from the time of arrival to the time of departure. Falls can be reduced by maintaining a safe environment and providing ongoing staff and patient education.

Duty to Safeguard Patient Valuables

A health care facility can be held liable for the negligent handling of a patient's valuables. Patients should be encouraged to have a trusted individual take their personal belongings and valuables home when such is feasible.

CEO/ADMINISTRATOR

The CEO is responsible for the supervision of the administrative staff and managers who assist in the daily operations of the organization. The CEO derives authority from the owner or governing body. CEOs, as is the case with governing body members, can be personally liable for their own acts of negligence that injure others.

MEDICAL STAFF

The governing body is responsible for ensuring that medical staff bylaws, rules, and regulations include: application requirements for clinical privileges and admission to the medical staff; a process for granting emergency staff privileges; requirements for medical staff consultations; a peer-review process; a process for auditing medical records; a process for addressing disruptive physicians and substance abuse; and a process for instituting corrective action (disciplinary actions can take the form of a letter of reprimand, suspension, or termination of privileges).

CORPORATE REORGANIZATION

Traditionally, hospitals have functioned as independent, freestanding corporate entities or as units or divisions of multihospital systems. Until recently, a freestanding hospital functioned as a single corporate entity with most programs and activities carried out within such entity to meet increasing competition.

Dependence on government funding and related programs (e.g., Medicare, Medicaid, and Blue Cross) and the continuous shrinkage occurring in such revenues have forced hospitals to seek alternative sources of revenue. Greater competition from nonhospital sources also has contributed to this need to seek alternative revenue sources. It has become apparent that traditional corporate structures might no longer be appropriate to accommodate both normal hospital activities and those additional activities undertaken to provide alternative sources of revenue.

The typical hospital is incorporated under state law as a freestanding for-profit or not-for-profit corporation. The corporation has a governing body. Such governing body has an overall responsibility for the operation and management of the hospital with a necessary delegation of appropriate responsibility to administrative employees and the medical staff.

Not-for-profit hospitals are usually exempt from federal taxation under Section 501(c)(3) of the US Internal Revenue Code of 1986 as amended. Such federal exemption usually entitles the organization to an automatic exemption from state taxes as well. Such tax exemption not only relieves the hospital from the payment of income taxes, sales taxes, and the like, but also permits the hospital to receive contributions from donors who then can obtain charitable deductions on their personal tax returns.

Given the need to obtain income and to meet competition, hospitals often consider establishing business enterprises. They also might consider other nonbusiness operations, such as the establishment of additional nonexempt undertakings (e.g., hospices and long-term care facilities). Because hospitals have resources including the physical plant, administrative talent, and technical expertise in areas that are potentially profitable, the first option usually considered is direct participation by the hospital in health-related business enterprises. There are, however, regulatory and legal pressures that present substantial impediments, including: risk of loss of tax-exempt status if a substantial portion of the corporation's activities are related to nonexempt activities and costs not associated with patient care must be deducted from costs submitted to third-party payers for reimbursement. The "carving out" of these costs can be detrimental to the hospital unless alternative revenues are found.

Certificate of Need

Generally, hospitals may not add additional programs or services nor may they expend monies for the acquisition of capital in excess of specified threshold limits without first obtaining approval from appropriate state regulatory agencies. The process by which this approval is granted generally is referred to as the certificate of need (CON) process.

The National Health Planning and Resources Development Act of 1974, Public Law No. 93-641, sought to encourage state review of all plans calling for the construction, expansion, or renovation of health facilities or services by conditioning receipt of certain federal funds on the establishment of an approved state CON program. Most states responded to this law by instituting state CON programs that complied with federal standards. Although the federal law is now history, CON programs remain in effect in a dwindling number of states. Some states continue to maintain control over Medicaid expenditures for hospital and nursing home care by controlling the number of beds through the CON process. This process can be lengthy and expensive. Further, it might not always result in approval of the request to offer the new program or service or to make the capital expenditure.

Notes

1. 500 P.2d 335 (Ariz. Ct. App. 1972).
2. 46 U.S.I.W. 2227 (Md. 1977).
3. 272 S.E.2d 643 (S.C. 1980).
4. 211 N.E.2d 253 (Ill. 1965).
5. Id. at 260.
6. No. 228566 (Cal. Super. Ct. Sacramento Co. 1976).
7. 206 Cal. Rptr. 164 (Cal. Ct. App. 1984). 24. 734 F.2d 81 (1st Cir. 1984).
8. 734 F.2d 81 (1st Cir. 1984).
9. Nation's Nursing Homes Are Quietly Killing Thousands, Andrew Schneider and Phillip O'Connor, St. Louis Post-Dispatch, October 12, 2002,
10. 655 S.W.2d 14 (Ky. Ct. App. 1982).
11. 396 So.2d 406 (La. Ct. App. 1981).
12. 188 Cal. Rptr. 685 (Cal. Ct. App. 1983).
13. 565 So. 2d 221, 224 (Ala. 1990).
14. 28. Id. at 223–224.
15. Id. at 226.
16. 171 Cal. Rptr. 846 (Cal. Ct. App. 1981).
17. 488 A.2d 858 (Del. 1985).
18. 449 N.E.2d 486 (Ohio Ct. App. 1982).
19. 836 S.W.2d 911 (Mo. 1992).

8

MEDICAL STAFF

This chapter provides an overview of medical staff organization, the credentialing process, and a review of cases focused on the legal risks of physicians. The cases presented highlight those areas in which physicians tend to be most vulnerable to lawsuits.

MEDICAL STAFF ORGANIZATION

The medical staff is an integral part of a health care organization with defined responsibilities under its bylaws. The medical staff is formally organized with officers, committees, and bylaws. The responsibilities of a variety of medical staff committees are described here.

- *Executive committee*: The executive committee oversees the activities of the medical staff. It is responsible for recommending to the governing body such things as medical staff structure, a process for reviewing credentials and appointing members to the medical staff, a process for delineating clinical privileges, a process for peer review, a mechanism by which medical staff membership can be terminated, and a mechanism for fair hearing procedures. The executive committee reviews and acts on the reports of medical staff departmental chairpersons and designated medical staff committees. Actions requiring approval of the governing body are forwarded to the governing body for approval.
- *Bylaws committee*: The functioning of the medical staff is described in its bylaws, rules, and regulations, which must be reviewed and approved by the organization's governing body. Bylaws must be kept current, and the governing body must approve recommended changes. The bylaws describe the various membership categories of the medical staff (e.g., active, courtesy, consultative, and allied professional staff) as well as the process for obtaining privileges.

- *Blood and transfusion committee*: The blood and transfusion committee develops blood usage policies and procedures. It is responsible for monitoring transfusion services and reviewing indications for transfusions, blood ordering practices, each transfusion episode, and transfusion reactions.
- *Credentials committee*: The credentials committee oversees the application process for medical staff applicants, requests for clinical privileges, and reappointments to the medical staff. The committee makes its recommendations to the medical executive committee.
- *Infection control committee*: The infection control committee is generally responsible for the development of policies and procedures for investigating and preventing infections.
- *Medical records committee*: The medical records committee develops policies and procedures as they pertain to the management of medical records. The committee determines the format of complete medical records and reviews medical records for accuracy, completeness, legibility, and timely completion. The committee ensures that medical records reflect the condition and progress of the patient, including the results of all tests and therapy given, and makes recommendations for disciplinary action as necessary.
- *Pharmacy and therapeutics committee*: The pharmacy and therapeutics committee is generally charged with developing policies and procedures relating to the selection, procurement, distribution, handling, use, and safe administration of drugs, biologicals, and diagnostic testing material. The committee oversees the development and maintenance of a drug formulary. The committee oversees the tracking of medication errors and adverse drug reactions; the management, control, and effective and safe use of medications through monitoring and evaluation; the monitoring of problem-prone, high-risk, and high-volume medications utilizing parameters such as appropriateness, safety, effectiveness, medication errors, food–drug interactions, drug–drug interactions, drug–disease interactions, and adverse drug reactions.
- *Tissue committee*: The tissue committee reviews all surgical procedures. Surgical case reviews address the justification and indications for surgical procedures.
- *Utilization review committee*: The utilization review committee monitors and evaluates utilization issues such as medical necessity and appropriateness of admission and continued stay, as well as delay in the provision of diagnostic, therapeutic, and supportive services. The utilization review committee ensures that each patient is treated at an appropriate level of care. Objectives of the committee include timely transfer of patients requiring alternate levels of care; promotion of the efficient and effective use of the organization's resources; adherence to quality utilization standards of third-party payers; maintenance of high-quality, cost-effective care; and identification of opportunities for improvement.

Medical Director

The medical director serves as a liaison between the medical staff and the organization's governing body and management. The medical director should have clearly written agreements with the organization, including duties, responsibilities, and compensation arrangements. The responsibilities of a medical director include enforcing the bylaws of the governing body and medical staff and monitoring the quality of medical care in the organization.

MEDICAL STAFF PRIVILEGES

Medical staff privileges are restricted to those professionals who fulfill the requirements as described in an organization's medical staff bylaws. Although cognizant of the importance of medical staff membership, both the medical staff and the governing body must meet their obligation to maintain standards of good medical practice in dealing with matters of staff appointment, credentialing, and the disciplining of physicians for such things as disruptive behavior, incompetence, psychological problems, criminal actions, and substance abuse.

Appointment to the medical staff and medical staff privileges should be granted only after there has been a thorough investigation of the applicant. The delineation of clinical privileges should be discipline-specific and based on appropriate predetermined criteria (e.g., education, training, and experience) that adhere to national standards.

Credentialing and Privileging Process

The purpose of the appointment process is to evaluate the competency of the applicant to determine whether he or she is qualified for appointment to the medical staff. The following sections describe the appointment process.

- *Application*: The medical staff application should provide pertinent information regarding the applicant's medical school; internship; residency; privileges requested; availability to provide on-call emergency department coverage; other hospital staff appointments; previous disciplinary actions against the applicant; unexplained breaks in work history; and voluntary and/or involuntary limitations or relinquishment of staff privileges.
- *Medical staff bylaws*: Each member of the organization's medical staff should be required to sign a statement attesting to the fact that the medical staff bylaws have been read and that the physician agrees to abide by the bylaws and other policies and procedures that might be adopted from time to time.
- *Physical and mental status review*
- *Consent for release of information*
- *Certificate of insurance*: The applicant should provide evidence of professional liability insurance.
- *State licensure*: A physician's right to practice medicine is subject to the licensing laws contained in the statutes of the state in which the physician resides.
- *National Practitioner Data Bank*: The National Practitioner Data Bank (NPDB) was created by Congress as a national repository of information with the primary purpose of facilitating a comprehensive review of physicians' and other health care practitioners' professional credentials. The National Practitioner Data Bank must be queried as to information in its files that might pertain to medical staff applicants. Health care organizations must query the data bank every 2 years on the renewal of clinical privileges of health care practitioners.
- *References*: Both written and oral references should be obtained from previous organizations with which the applicant has been affiliated.
- *Applicant review process*: The applicant review process includes receipt and review of all documents prior to the interview; explanation of unaccounted-for breaks or gaps in education or employment; review of any disciplinary action or misconduct investigation that has been initiated or is pending against the applicant by any licensing body; review of the applicant's license to practice medicine in any state, looking for any denials, limitations, suspensions, or revocations; determining if the applicant ever withdrew an application or resigned from any medical staff to avoid disciplinary action; determining if the applicant has ever been named as a defendant in a criminal proceeding; determining if the applicant has back-up coverage for his or her practice; determining if the applicant has reviewed and is willing to abide by the medical staff bylaws, rules, and regulations, and, where applicable, departmental rules and

regulations; and determining if the applicant has any physical or mental impairments that could affect his or her ability to practice medicine.

- *Delineation of clinical privileges*: The delineation of clinical privileges is the process by which the medical staff determines precisely what procedures a physician is authorized to perform. This determination is based on predetermined criteria as to what credentials are necessary to competently perform the privileges requested.
- *Governing body responsibility*: The governing body has ultimate responsibility for granting medical staff privileges.
- *Appeal process*: An appeal process should be described in the medical staff bylaws to cover issues such as the denial of professional staff privileges, grievances, and disciplinary actions. The governing body should reserve the right to hear any appeals and be the final decision maker within the organization. A physician whose privileges are either suspended or terminated must exhaust all remedies provided in a hospital's bylaws, rules, and regulations before commencing a court action.
- *Reappointments*: The medical staff must provide an effective mechanism for monitoring and evaluating the quality of patient care and the clinical performance of physicians. For problematic physicians, consideration should be given to privileges with supervision, a reduction in privileges, suspension of privileges with purpose (e.g., suspension pending further training), or termination of privileges.

Screening for Competency

Failure to properly screen a medical staff applicant's credentials can lead to liability for injuries suffered by patients as a result of that omission. This was the case in *Johnson v. Misericordia Community Hospital*,[1] where the patient brought a malpractice action against the hospital and its liability insurer for alleged negligence in granting orthopedic privileges to a physician who performed an operation to remove a pin fragment from the patient's hip. The Wisconsin Court of Appeals found the hospital negligent for failing to scrutinize the physician's credentials before approving his application for orthopedic privileges. The hospital failed to adhere to procedures established under both its own bylaws and state statute. The measure of quality and the degree of quality control exercised in a hospital are the direct responsibilities of the medical staff. Hospital supervision of the manner of appointment of physicians to its staff is mandatory, not optional. On appeal by the hospital, the Wisconsin Supreme Court affirmed the appellate court's decision, finding that if the hospital had exercised ordinary care, it "would not" have appointed the physician to the medical staff.

PHYSICIAN SUPERVISION AND MONITORING

The medical staff is responsible to the governing body for the quality of care rendered by members of the medical staff. The landmark decision in this area occurred in *Darling v. Charleston Community Memorial Hospital*,[2] in which it was decided that the hospital's governing body has a duty to establish a mechanism for the medical staff to evaluate, counsel, and, when necessary, take action against an unreasonable risk of harm to a patient arising from the patient's treatment by a physician. Physician monitoring is best accomplished through a system of peer review. Most states provide statutory protection from liability for peer-review activities when they are conducted in a reasonable manner and without malice.

DISRUPTIVE PHYSICIANS

Disruptive physicians can have a negative impact on an organization's staff and ultimately affect the quality of patient care. Having the right policies in place as they relate to conflict resolution is a must for an effective working environment. Criteria other than academic credentials (e.g., a physician's ability to work with others) should be considered before granting medical staff privileges. That factor was considered by the court in *Ladenheim v. Union County Hospital District*,[3] which held that the physician's inability to work with other members of the staff was sufficient grounds to deny him staff privileges. The physician's record was replete with evidence of his inability to work effectively with other members of the hospital staff. As stated in *Huffaker v. Bailey*,[4] most courts have found that the ability to work smoothly with others is reasonably related to the objective of ensuring patient welfare. A staff member who, because of personality characteristics or other problems, is incapable of getting along with others could severely hinder the effective treatment of patients.

MISREPRESENTATION OF CREDENTIALS

There was reliable, probative, and substantial evidence in *Graor v. State Medical Board* to support the Ohio State Medical Board's decision to permanently revoke a physician's license for misrepresenting his credentials by claiming that he was board certified in internal medicine.[5]

LIMITATIONS ON REQUESTED PRIVILEGES

A physician–pediatrician obtained associate staff privileges at a hospital in 1997. She later applied for full privileges through the hospital's credentials committee. Concern was raised about her alleged difficulty with the intubation of children. As a result, action on the pediatrician's request for full privileges was deferred. In May of 1998, the credentials committee recommended full privileges with the exception of neonatal resuscitation. After several in-hospital appeals, the pediatrician filed a lawsuit. The court determined that there was substantial evidence to support the hospital's suspension of the pediatrician's resuscitation privileges.[6]

MISDIAGNOSING UNCONSCIOUS PATIENT

In *Ramberg v. Morgan*,[7] a police department physician, at the scene of an accident, examined an unconscious man who had been struck by an automobile. The physician concluded that the patient's insensibility was a result of alcohol intoxication, not the accident, and ordered the police to remove him to jail instead of the hospital. The patient subsequently died, and the autopsy revealed massive skull fractures. The court found that any physician should reasonably anticipate the presence of head injuries especially in those instances where a person is struck by a car. Although a physician does not ensure the correctness of the diagnosis or treatment, a patient is entitled to such thorough and careful examination as his or her condition and attending circumstances permit, with such diligence and methods of diagnosis as usually are approved and practiced by medical people of ordinary or average learning, judgment, and skill in the community or similar localities.

FAILURE TO RESPOND TO EMERGENCY CALL

Physicians on call in an emergency department are expected to respond to requests for emergency assistance when such is considered necessary. Failure to respond is grounds for negligence should a patient suffer injury as a result of a physician's failure to respond.

Issues of fact in *Dillon v. Silver*[8] precluded summary dismissal of an action charging that a woman's death from complications of an ectopic pregnancy occurred because of a gynecologist's refusal to treat her despite a request for aid by a hospital emergency department physician. Although the gynecologist contended that no physician–patient relationship had ever arisen, the hospital bylaws not only mandated that the physician accept all patients referred to him, but also stated that the emergency department physician had authority to decide which service physician should be called and required the on-call service physician to respond to such a call.

DELAY IN TREATMENT

A physician might be liable for failing to respond promptly if it can be established that such inaction caused a patient's injury. A patient afflicted with lung cancer was awarded damages in *Blackmon v. Langley* because of the failure of the examining physician to inform the patient in a timely manner that a chest X-ray showed a lesion in his lung.[9] The lesion eventually was diagnosed as cancerous. The physician contended that because the evidence showed the patient had less than a 50% chance of survival at the time of the alleged negligence, he could not be the proximate cause of injury. The Arkansas Supreme Court found that the jury was properly entitled to determine that the patient suffered and lost more than would have been the case had he been notified promptly of the lesion.

INADEQUATE HISTORY AND PHYSICAL EXAMINATION

The history and physical examination is the beginning point for preparing a patient's treatment plan. The often written note in a patient's medical record that, for example, references a patient's family history as "unremarkable" or "noncontributory" raises a red flag as to the thoroughness of the history and physical. Failure to obtain an adequate family history and perform an adequate physical examination violates a standard of care owed to the patient. This was the case in *Solomon v. Connecticut Medical Examining Board,*[10] where there was substantial evidence to support disciplinary action against a physician where the record indicated that the physician failed to: adequately document patient histories; perform adequate physical examinations; fully assess each patient's condition; or order appropriate laboratory tests or secure appropriate consultations.

The physician's practice of medicine was determined by the board to pose a threat to the health and safety of any person. The board concluded that there was a basis on which to subject the physician to disciplinary action.

FAILURE TO USE PATIENT DATA GATHERED

The medical record is a tool for communicating between disciplines. The attending physician is responsible for reviewing entries entered into the record and coordinating the patient's overall plan of care. The physician is responsible for pulling the threads and making sense out of all the data collected regarding the patient's ongoing care. Someone must take the lead, and that lead must come from the physician.

Critical information that is gathered often gets lost in the record. Providers are responsible for assuring that the information critical to a patient's care is readily available to all caregivers in the opening pages of the record and not buried in the bowels of the record. Provider mistakes often occur because of the unwieldy, unorganized, and voluminous amount of information gathered on the patient. Caregivers, however, who fail to use the information collected when assessing patient needs might find themselves in a lawsuit. Take, for example, the patient who advised her physician that she was allergic to latex and the hospital inserted a latex catheter into the patient. As a result, the patient developed interstitial cystitis (IC). Expert testimony was sufficient to establish to a reasonable degree of medical certainty that the catheter "caused" the patient's injury (chronic bladder disorder).[11]

Patients should be ever watchful and repeat information important to their care needs. Patients cannot assume that information given will be both heard and recorded in the medical record. Even if the information is given, heard, and recorded in the patient's medical record, there are no assurances that the information will be read by other caregivers and acted upon or used appropriately in his or her care.

CHOICE OF TREATMENT: DIFFERING OPINIONS

A physician will not be held liable for exercising his or her judgment in applying a course of treatment supported by a reputable and respected body of medical experts even if another body of expert medical opinion would favor a different course of treatment. The *two schools of thought doctrine* is only applicable in medical malpractice cases in which there is more than one method of accepted treatment for a patient's disease or injury. Under this doctrine, a physician will not be liable for medical malpractice if he or she follows a course of treatment supported by reputable, respected, and reasonable medical experts.

A physician's care and treatment does not constitute negligence simply because the outcome of a particular case is unsuccessful. A physician cannot be required to guarantee the results of his or her treatment. The mere fact that an adverse result might occur following treatment is not in and of itself evidence of professional negligence.

FAILURE TO ORDER DIAGNOSTIC TESTS

A plaintiff who claims that a physician failed to order proper diagnostic tests must show: (1) it is standard practice to use a certain diagnostic test under the circumstances of the case; (2) the physician failed to use the test and therefore failed to diagnose the patient's illness; and (3) the patient suffered injury.

Failure to order diagnostic tests resulted in the misdiagnosis of appendicitis in *Steeves v. United States*.[12] In this case, physicians failed to order the appropriate diagnostic tests for a child who was referred to a Navy hospital with a diagnosis of possible appendicitis. Judgment in this case was entered against the United States, on behalf of the US Navy, for medical expenses and for pain and suffering. The child had been referred to the hospital by an Air Force dispensary, where a lab test indicated a high white blood cell count. A consultation sheet had been given to the mother, indicating the possible diagnosis. The physician who examined the child at the Navy hospital performed no tests, failed to diagnose the patient's condition, and sent him home at 5:02 p.m., some 32 minutes after his arrival on July 21. The child was returned to the emergency department on July 22 at about 2:30 a.m. only to be sent home again by an intern who diagnosed the boy's condition as gastroenteritis. Once again, no diagnostic tests were ordered. The boy was returned to the Navy hospital on July 23, at which time diagnostic tests were performed. The patient was subsequently operated on and found to have a ruptured appendix. Holding the Navy hospital liable for the negligence of the physicians who acted as its agents, the court pointed out that a wrong diagnosis will not in and of itself support a verdict of liability in a lawsuit. However, a physician must use ordinary care in making a diagnosis. Only where a patient is examined adequately is there no liability for an erroneous diagnosis. In this instance, the physicians' failure to perform further laboratory tests the first two times the child was brought to the emergency department was found to be a breach of good medical practice.

FAILURE TO REVIEW LAB TESTS

A physician's failure to review test results on a timely basis can be the proximate cause of a patient's injuries. As in *Smith v. U.S. Department of Veterans Affairs*,[13] the plaintiff, Smith, was taken to the VA hospital, where Dr. Rizk was assigned as Smith's attending physician. Smith developed an acute problem with his respiration and level of consciousness. During his stay, Smith began to complain of pain in his shoulders and neck. A rheumatology consultation was requested. Various tests were ordered, including an erythrocyte sedimentation rate (ESR).

A medical student noted that Smith was having difficulty breathing and called for a pulmonary consultation. Smith began complaining that his neck and back hurt and that he had no feeling in his legs and feet. A medical student noted that the result of Smith's ESR was 110 (more than twice the normal rate for a man his age). His white blood count was 18.1, also well above the normal rate. A staff member noted on the medical record that Smith had been unable to move his extremities for about 5 days. A psychiatric resident noted that Smith had been incontinent for 3 days and had a fever of 101.1 degrees.

Smith was taken to University Hospital for magnetic resonance imaging of his neck. Imaging revealed a mass subsequently identified as a spinal epidural abscess. By the time it was excised, it had been pressing on his spinal cord too long for any spinal function to remain below vertebrae four and five.

Smith filed a lawsuit alleging that the physicians' failure to promptly review his test results was the proximate cause of his paralysis. The US District Court agreed.

An elevated ESR generally accounts for one of three problems: infection, cancer, or a connective tissue disorder. Most experts agreed that at the very least a repeat ESR should have been ordered. The VA's care of the plaintiff fell below the reasonable standard of care. The fact that the tests were ordered mandates the immediate review of the results. Although it cannot be known with certainty what would have occurred had the ESR been read and acted upon, it is certain that the plaintiff had a chance to fully recover from his infection.

Failure to review the results of the plaintiff's ESR constituted negligence that led to a failure to make an early diagnosis of the plaintiff's epidural abscess and was the proximate cause of the patient's eventual paralysis. Given that a high ESR can manifest in a very serious illness, it was foreseeable that ignoring a high ESR could lead to serious injury.

IMAGING STUDIES/RADIOLOGY

Malpractice lawsuits often involve allegations of misdiagnosis and can be the result of the failure to order appropriate imaging tests; misinterpretation of an imaging study; failure to consult with a radiologist; failure to review imaging studies; delay in relaying test results; and failure to relay imaging results. Although the following cases describe many of these issues, they are not exhaustive of the problems that can arise in imaging-related lawsuits.

Failure to Order Appropriate X-Rays

Failure to order a proper set of X-rays is as legally risky as the failure to order X-rays. In *Betenbaugh v. Princeton Hospital*,[14] the plaintiff had been taken to the hospital because she injured her lower back. One of the defendant–physicians directed that an X-ray be taken of her sacrum. No evidence of a fracture was found. When the patient's pain did not subside, the family physician was consulted. He found that the films taken at the hospital did not include the entire lower portion of the spine and sent her to a radiologist for further study. On the basis of additional X-rays, a diagnosis of a fracture was made, and the patient was advised to wear a lumbosacral support. Two months later, the fracture was healed. The radiologist who had taken X-ray films on the second occasion testified that it was customary to take both an anterior–posterior and a lateral view when making an X-ray examination of the sacrum. In his opinion, the failure at the hospital to include the lower area of the sacrum was a failure to meet the standard required. There was sufficient evidence to support findings that the physicians and the hospital were negligent by not having taken the appropriate X-rays and that such negligence was the proximate cause of the patient's additional pain and delay in recovery.

Imaging Misinterpretation Leads to Death

The deceased, Jane Fahr, in *Setterington v. Pontiac General Hospital*,[15] was concerned about a lump in her thigh. She had a CT scan taken at the hospital in August 1987. The radiologist, Dr. Mittner, did not mention that the lump could be cancerous. In reliance on the radiologist's report, Dr. Sanford, the plaintiff's treating physician, regarded the condition as a hematoma and believed that a biopsy was not warranted. In late January 1988, Fahr returned to the hospital for another CT scan because the lump seemed to be enlarging. The radiologist, Dr. Khalid, did not include the possibility of a malignant tumor in his report. As a result, Sanford continued to believe that Fahr had a hematoma. In early September 1988, Fahr returned to Sanford, who had another CT scan performed. Dr. Kayne, the radiologist, found an enlarged hematoma. In a follow-up discussion with Sanford, Kayne assured Sanford that the lump did not appear to be dangerous or invasive. As a result, Sanford concluded that Fahr had a hematoma with a leaking blood vessel. In October 1988, the tumor was biopsied and the cancer diagnosed. By December 1988, chest scans revealed metastasis. Fahr died on July 6, 1990, at the age of 32.

A malpractice action was filed against Sanford and the hospital, alleging that they failed to timely diagnose and treat Fahr.

The jury found that the radiologists were agents of the defendant hospital and they breached the standard of care. The breach was a proximate cause of Fahr's death. The jury returned a verdict for the plaintiff. The trial court denied the defendant's motion for a new trial.

The evidence as to the malpractice of Khalid and Kayne was supported by the jury's finding that they were professionally negligent. Kayne failed to diagnose the cancer in September 1988. With a proper diagnosis, there could have been a full month or more of treatment before metastasis was visible in December. As to Khalid, whose malpractice was 7 months earlier, the conclusion is even stronger.

Failure to Consult with a Radiologist

The internist in *Lanzet v. Greenberg*[16] failed to consult with the radiologist after his conclusion that the patient suffered from congestive heart failure. This factor most likely contributed to the death of the patient while on the operating table.

Failure to Read X-Rays

The patient in *Tams v. Lotz*[17] had to undergo a second surgical procedure to remove a laparotomy pad that had been left in the patient during a previous surgical procedure. The trial court was found to have properly directed a verdict with respect to the patient's assertion that the surgeon who performed the first operation failed to read a postoperative X-ray report, which allegedly would have put him on notice both that the pad was present and that there was a need for emergency surgery to remove the pad, therefore averting the need to remove a portion of the patient's intestine.

Delay in Reporting Critical Tests

A delay in reporting critical test results can result in a negligence suit, as is noted in the following case. The patient's[18] CT scan revealed an aneurysm of the thoracic aorta. The deceased patient underwent emergency surgery, and the surgeons found a ruptured aneurysm of the thoracic aorta. The hospital had the responsibility of seeing to it that the findings of the grossly abnormal chest X-rays were conveyed to the attending physician on an emergent basis. There was evidence that the hospital's failure to ensure that the X-ray reading was promptly relayed to the attending physician was a proximate cause of the patient's death.

Failure to Communicate X-Ray Results

The court of appeals in *Washington Healthcare Corp. v. Barrow*[19] held that evidence was sufficient to sustain a finding that the hospital was negligent in failing to provide a radiology report demonstrating pathology on patient Barrow's lung in a timely manner. An X-ray of the patient taken on April 4, 1982, disclosed a small nodular density in her right lung. Within a year, the cancerous nodule had grown to the size of a softball.

A medical student who worked for Dr. Oweiss, the defendant, testified that she received no such report while working for the physician, thus accounting for 19 days after the X-ray was taken. Dr. Odenwald, who dictated the patient's report on April 4, 1982, stated that X-ray reports usually are dictated, typed, and mailed the same day. The jury could have determined that if the report did not reach Oweiss by April 23, then it did not reach him by May 3. The patient's record eventually was found; however, it was not in the patient's regular folder. One could infer that the record therefore was negligently filed.

Questions also arise as to why Oweiss did nothing to follow up on the matter in ensuing months. Oweiss testified that he did receive the report by May 3, 1982, and that he informed Mrs. Barrow of its contents. Barrow stated that although her folder was on the physician's desk at the time of her visit, he did not relay to her any information regarding an abnormal X-ray. Oweiss, however, was severely impeached at trial, and the jury chose not to believe him. Considering the entire record, there was reasonable probability that WHC was negligent and that Oweiss had not received the report.

Failure to Timely Diagnose

A medical malpractice action against a hospital through its interventional radiologists and other medical employees failed to timely diagnose and treat the patient's internal bleeding, which is alleged to have occurred during the performance of an angioplasty that resulted in a hematoma around the patient's spinal cord causing paralysis and subsequent loss of use of his limbs. The trial court was found to have erred in directing a verdict against the plaintiff where excluded expert testimony was sufficient to establish evidence of a national standard of care and breach of that standard. The expert had 40 years of experience as a board certified general surgeon.[20]

John Ritter Case

More recently, in a well-publicized case, actor John Ritter was allegedly misdiagnosed in a California hospital as suffering from a heart attack. It was later determined that he had a tear in his aorta, which led to his death. The plaintiffs, having reached a $14 million settlement with the hospital, continued with a $67 million suit against defendant–physicians, a radiologist and a cardiologist who treated Ritter in the hospital's emergency department. The plaintiffs alleged that a radiologist did not warn Ritter 2 years earlier that he had an enlarged aorta and that there was inadequate follow-up on this finding. It was also alleged that on the night of his death, an X-ray test was ordered but somehow not performed. It was alleged by the plaintiffs' experts that the X-ray would have been helpful in diagnosing Ritter's condition and have led to the correct treatment. Defense attorneys argued that, even if the order was performed, it is unlikely that Ritter's condition would have been diagnosed by an X-ray and that a CT scan or MRI would have been more helpful. However, the defendants argued that time was critical and the decision was made to treat Ritter for a heart attack. Further, the defendants argued that even if the correct diagnosis had been made in the emergency department, it is unlikely that he would have survived. The trial took on the classic battle of the plaintiffs' versus the defendants' experts. In the end, the plaintiffs failed to prove their case. It was determined that if Ritter had followed up with his family physician at the request of the radiologist, following a complete body scan in 2001, he would have at least increased his chances to be alive today.

FAILURE TO OBTAIN SECOND OPINION

Dr. Goodwich, an obstetrician and gynecologist, in *Goodwich v. Sinai Hospital*,[21] had clinical practice patterns that were subject to question by his peers on a wide variety of medical matters. Dr. Goldstein (chairman of the department of obstetrics and gynecology) met with him on several occasions in 1988 regarding those concerns. It was suggested to Goodwich that he obtain second opinions from board-certified OB/GYNs. He orally agreed to do so. This agreement was presented to Goodwich in writing on two occasions in 1988. Goodwich failed to comply with the agreement, and Goldstein held a second meeting with him and his attorney in February 1990.

Due to continued noncompliance, the Medical Executive Committee (MEC) met and suspended Goodwich's privileges for 3 months. The suspension of Goodwich's privileges was reported to the Maryland State Board of Physicians and the National Practitioner Data Bank.

Goodwich appealed the MEC decision to two different physician panels and the hospital's governing board. Both physician panels and the governing board affirmed the MEC's decision to abridge Goodwich's privileges. Goodwich then sued the hospital. The court of special appeals held that the record was replete with documentation of questionable patient management and continual failure to comply with second-opinion agreements.

FAILURE TO REFER

A physician has a duty to refer his or her patient whom he or she knows or should know needs referral to a physician familiar with and clinically capable of treating the patient's ailments. To recover damages, the plaintiff must show that the physician deviated from the standard of care and that the failure to refer resulted in injury.

The California Court of Appeals found that expert testimony is not necessary where good medical practice would require a general physician to suggest a specialist's consultation.[22] The court ruled that because specialists were called in after the patient's condition grew worse, it is reasonable to assume that they could have been called in sooner. The jury was instructed by the court that a general practitioner has a duty to suggest calling in a specialist if a reasonably prudent general practitioner would do so under similar circumstances.

A physician is in a position of trust, and it is his or her duty to act in good faith. If a preferred treatment in a given situation is outside a physician's field of expertise, it is his or her duty to advise the patient.

In *Doan v. Griffith*,[23] an accident victim was admitted to the hospital with serious injuries, including multiple fractures of his facial bones. The patient contended that the physician was negligent in not advising him at the time of discharge that his facial bones needed to be realigned by a specialist before the bones became fused. As a result, his face became disfigured. Expert testimony demonstrated that the customary medical treatment for the patient's injuries would have been to realign his fractured bones surgically as soon as the swelling subsided and that such treatment would have restored the normal contour of his face. The appellate court held that the jury reasonably could have found that the physician failed to provide timely advice to the patient regarding his need for further medical treatment and that such failure was the proximate cause of the patient's condition.

PRACTICING OUTSIDE FIELD OF COMPETENCY

A physician must practice within his or her field of expertise or competence. The standard of care required in a malpractice case will be that of the specialty in which a physician is treating, whether or not he or she has been credentialed in that specialty.

In a California case, *Carrasco v. Bankoff*,[24] a small boy suffering third-degree burns over 18% of his body was admitted to a hospital. During his initial confinement, there was little done except to occasionally dress and redress the burned area. At the end of a 53-day confinement, the patient suffered hypergranulation of the burned area and muscular-skeletal dysfunction. The surgeon who treated him was not a board-certified plastic surgeon and apparently not properly trained in the management of burn cases. At trial, the patient's medical expert, a plastic surgeon who assumed responsibility for care after the first hospitalization, outlined the accepted medical practice in cases of this nature. The first surgeon acknowledged this accepted practice. The court held that there was substantial evidence to permit a finding of professional negligence because of the defendant surgeon's failure to perform to the accepted standard of care and that such failure resulted in the patient's injury.

TIMELY DIAGNOSIS

A physician can be liable for reducing a patient's chances for survival. The timely diagnosis of a patient's condition is as important as the need to accurately diagnose a patient's injury or disease. Failure to do so can constitute malpractice if a patient suffers injury as a result of such failure.

MISDIAGNOSIS

Misdiagnosis is the most frequently cited injury event in malpractice suits against physicians. Although diagnosis is a medical art and not an exact science, early detection can be critical to a patient's recovery. Misdiagnosis can involve the diagnosis and treatment of a disease different from that which the patient actually suffers or the diagnosis and treatment of a disease the patient does not have. Misdiagnosis in and of itself will not necessarily impose liability on a physician, unless deviation from the accepted standard of care and injury can be established.

FAILURE TO FORM A DIFFERENTIAL DIAGNOSIS

A case before the Mississippi Supreme Court, *Hill v. Stewart*,[25] involved a patient who became ill and was admitted to the hospital. The physician was advised of the patient's recent weight loss, frequent urination, thirst, loss of vision, nausea, and vomiting. Routine laboratory tests were ordered including a urinalysis but not a blood glucose test. On the following day, a consultant diagnosed the patient's condition as severe diabetic acidosis. Treatment was given, but the patient failed to respond to the therapy and died. The attending physician was sued for failing to test for diabetes and for failing to diagnose and treat the patient on the first day in the hospital. The attending physician said in court that he suspected diabetes and admitted that when diabetes is suspected, a urinalysis and a blood sugar test should be performed. An expert medical witness testified that failure to do so would be a departure from the skill and care required of a general practitioner. The expert also stated that the patient in this case probably would have had a good chance of survival if treated properly. The state supreme court determined that there was sufficient evidence presented to permit the case to go to the jury for decision.

When a physician concludes that a particular test is indicated, it should be performed and evaluated as soon as practicable. Delay might constitute negligence. The law imposes on a physician the same degree of responsibility in making a diagnosis as it does in prescribing and administering treatment.

FAILURE TO READ NURSING NOTES

A physician can breach his or her duty of care by failing to read nursing notes. In *Todd v. Sauls*,[26] Mr. Todd was admitted to Rapides General Hospital on October 3, 1988, and the next day, Dr. Sauls performed bypass surgery. Postoperatively, Todd sustained a heart attack. During the following days, Todd did not ambulate well and suffered a weight loss of 19.5 pounds.

On October 17, the medical record indicated that Todd's sternotomy wound and the midlower left leg incision were reddened, and his temperature was 99.6. Sauls did not commonly read the nurses' notes but instead preferred to rely on his own observations of the patient. In his October 18 notes, he indicated that there was no drainage. The nurses' notes, however, show that there was drainage at the chest tube site. Contrary to the medical records showing that Todd had a temperature of 101.2 degrees, Sauls noted that the patient was afebrile.

On October 19, Sauls noted that Todd's wounds were improving and he did not have a fever. Nurses' notes indicated redness at the surgical wounds and a temperature of 100 degrees. No white blood count had been ordered. Again on October 20, the nurses' notes indicated a wound redness and a temperature of 100.8 degrees. No wound culture had yet been ordered. Dr. Kamil, one of Todd's treating physicians, noted that Todd's nutritional status needed to be seriously confronted and suggested that Sauls consider supplemental feeding. Despite this, no follow-up to his recommendation appears, and the record is void of any action by Dr. Sauls to obtain a nutritional consult.

Todd was transferred to the intensive care unit on October 21 because he was gravely ill. The nurses' notes for the following day describe the chest tube site as draining foul-smelling bloody purulence. The patient's temperature was recorded to have reached 100.6 degrees. This is the first time that Sauls had the test tube site cultured. On October 23, the culture report from the laboratory indicated a staph infection, and Todd was started on antibiotics for treatment of the infection.

On October 25, at the request of family, Todd was transferred to St. Luke's Hospital. At St. Luke's, Dr. Leatherman, an internist and invasive cardiologist, treated Todd. Dr. Zeluff, an infectious disease specialist, examined Todd's surgical wounds and prescribed antibiotic treatment. Upon admission to St. Luke's, every one of Todd's surgical wounds was infected. Despite the care given at St. Luke's, Todd died on November 2, 1988. The family filed a malpractice suit against the surgeon. The district court entered judgment on a jury verdict for the defendant, and the plaintiff appealed claiming the surgeon breached his duty of care owed to the patient by failing to: (1) aggressively treat the surgical wound infections; (2) read the nurses' observations of infections; and (3) provide adequate nourishment, allowing the patient's body weight to rapidly waste away.

The Louisiana Court of Appeal held that Sauls committed medical malpractice when he breached the standard of care he owed to Todd. Sauls's testimony convinced the court that he failed to aggressively treat the surgical wound infections, that he chose not to take advantage of the nurses' observations of infection, and that he allowed Todd's body weight to waste away, knowing that extreme vigilance was required because of Todd's already severely impaired heart. Sauls's medical malpractice exacerbated an already critical condition and deprived Mr. Todd of a chance of survival.

MEDICATION ERRORS

As noted in the following cases, the negligent administration of medications is often due to errors, such as the wrong medication, the wrong patient, the wrong dosage, and the wrong route.

Wrong Dosage

Expert testimony in *Leal v. Simon*[27] a medical malpractice action, supported the jury's determination that the physician had been negligent when he reduced the dosage of a resident's psychotropic medication, Haldol. The resident, a 36-year-old individual who had been institutionalized his entire life, was a resident in an intermediate care facility. Expert medical testimony showed that the physician failed to familiarize himself with the resident's history, failed to secure the resident's complete medical records, and failed to wean the resident slowly off the medication.

Abuse in Prescribing Medications

The board of regents in *Moyo v. Ambach*[28] determined that a physician prescribed methaqualone with gross negligence to 20 patients. The board of regents found that the physician did not prescribe methaqualone in good faith or for sound medical reasons. His abuse in prescribing controlled substances constituted the fraudulent practice of medicine. Expert testimony established that it was common knowledge in the medical community that methaqualone was a widely abused and addictive drug. Methaqualone should not have been used for insomnia without first trying other means of treatment. On appeal, the court found that there was sufficient evidence to support the board's finding.

Medications Aggravate Preexisting Condition

Damages were awarded in *Argus v. Scheppegrell*[29] for the wrongful death of a teenage patient with a preexisting drug addiction. It was determined that the physician wrongfully supplied the patient with prescriptions for controlled substances in excessive amounts, with the result that the patient's preexisting drug addiction worsened, causing her death from a drug overdose. The Louisiana Court of Appeal held that the suffering of the patient caused by drug addiction and deterioration of her mental and physical condition warranted an award of \$175,000. Damages of \$120,000 were to be awarded for the wrongful death claims of the parents, who not only suffered during their daughter's drug addiction caused by the physician who wrongfully supplied the prescription, but also were forced to endure the torment of their daughter's slow death in the hospital.

FAILURE TO FOLLOW DIFFERENT COURSE OF TREATMENT

Failure of an attending physician to recognize recommendations by consulting physicians—who determine a different diagnosis and recommend a different course of treatment in a particular case—can result in liability for damages suffered by the patient. This was the case in *Martin v. East Jefferson General Hospital*[30] in which the attending physician continued to treat the patient for a viral infection despite three other physicians' diagnoses of lupus and their recommendations that the attending physician treat the patient for collagen vascular disease. The trial court found that lupus had been more probable than not the cause of the patient's death and that her chances of recovery had been destroyed by the physician's failure to rule out that diagnosis.

If a consulting physician has suggested a diagnosis with which the treating physician does not agree, it would be prudent to consider obtaining the opinion of a second consultant who could either confirm or disprove the first consultant's theory. Failure to diagnose and properly treat a suspected illness is an open door to liability.

FAILURE TO PROVIDE INFORMED CONSENT

The doctrine of informed consent is a theory of professional liability independent from malpractice. A physician's duty to disclose known dangers associated with a proposed course of treatment is imposed by law. The patient in *Leggett v. Kumar*[31] was awarded \$675,000 for pain and disfigurement resulting from a mastectomy procedure. The physician in this case failed to advise the patient of treatment alternatives. He also failed to perform the surgery properly.

It is the physician's role to provide the necessary medical facts and the patient's role to make the subjective decision concerning treatment based on his or her understanding of those facts. Before subjecting a patient to a course of treatment, the physician has a duty to disclose information that will enable the patient to evaluate options available and the risks attendant to a specific procedure. A failure to disclose known and existing risks of proposed treatment when such risks might affect a patient's decision to forgo treatment constitutes a prima facie violation of a physician's duty to disclose. If a patient can establish that a physician withheld information concerning the inherent and potential hazards of a proposed treatment, consent is abrogated. Consent for a medical procedure may be withdrawn at any time before the act consented to is accomplished.

WRONG SURGICAL PROCEDURE

In *Southwestern Kentucky Baptist Hospital v. Bruce*,[32] a patient admitted for conization of the cervix was taken mistakenly to the operating room for a thyroidectomy. The physician was notified early during surgery that he had the wrong patient on the operating room table. The operation was terminated immediately. The thyroidectomy was not completed, and the incision was sutured. The patient filed an action for malpractice and recovered $10,000 from the physician and $90,000 from the hospital. That the patient mistakenly answered to the name of another patient who had been scheduled for a thyroidectomy did not excuse the failure of the surgeon, the anesthesiologist, and the surgical technician to determine the identity of the patient by examining her identification bracelet. The Kentucky Supreme Court held that the verdict was not excessive in view of the injuries, which consisted of a four-inch incision along the patient's neck, which became infected and required cosmetic surgery.

CORRECT SURGERY: WRONG SITE

The patient in *Holdsworth v. Galler*[33] had a two-centimeter cancerous tumor on the left side of his colon. Unfortunately, the surgeon erroneously performed right-sided colon surgery to remove the tumor. After the surgeon recognized the error, he performed the required left-sided abdominal surgery three days later. At the first surgery on the patient's right side, the surgeon removed the end of the patient's small intestine, his entire right colon, and the majority of his transverse colon; consequently, 40% to 45% of the colon was removed. Three days following the wrong-site surgery, the patient had to undergo left-sided surgery, after which he was left with approximately 20% of his colon. The patient developed complications and died 6 weeks thereafter.

CORRECT PATIENT: WRONG SURGERY

The plaintiff was diagnosed with a herniated disk at L4–L5. His surgeon performed a laminectomy. During a review of the plaintiff's postoperative X-rays, the surgeon noted that he had mistakenly removed the disk at L3–L4. The plaintiff testified that after the surgery his condition progressively worsened.

The plaintiff's expert testified that removal of the healthy disk caused the space between L3–L4 to collapse and the vertebrae to shift and settle. Even the defendant's expert witness testified that the removal of the healthy disk would increase the likelihood that the plaintiff would be more susceptible to future injuries.

The trial court directed a verdict against the defendant based on the defendant's own admission and that of his expert that he was negligent and that his negligence caused at least some injury to the patient. The defendant appealed. The Illinois Appellate Court held the evidence was sufficient to support a determination that the defendant's negligence caused the plaintiff's pain and suffering.[34]

REMOVAL OF THE WRONG KIDNEY: COVER-UP

The physician–petitioner in *In re Muncan*[35] did not review either the patient's CT scan or MRI films prior to surgery. In addition, he did not have the films with him in the operating room on the day of surgery. Had he done so, he would have discovered that the CT scan report erroneously indicated that there was a mass in the patient's left kidney when in fact such mass was located in the patient's right kidney.

During surgery, the physician did not observe any gross abnormalities or deformities in the left kidney and was unable to palpate any masses. Nonetheless, he removed the left kidney. The physician was later advised that he had removed a healthy kidney and that he might have removed the wrong kidney. The physician discharged the patient with a postoperative diagnosis of left renal mass, failing to note that he had in fact removed a tumor-free kidney. In September 1999, another CT scan revealed the presence of a six-centimeter by seven-centimeter mass in the patient's right kidney; the physician deemed this to be a new tumor that was not present on the CT scan conducted four months earlier. The diagnosis, however, appears highly suspect given the medical testimony that this new tumor was in the same location and had the same consistency and appearance as the tumor appearing in the prior CT study. The record also makes clear that it was highly unlikely that a tumor of this dimension could have achieved such size during the relatively brief period of time between the two CT studies.

The Supreme Court of New York, Appellate Division, Third Department held that the evidence was sufficient to support an inference of fraud. The physician knew he removed the wrong kidney and instead of taking steps to rectify the situation, he intentionally concealed his mistake.

NEEDLE FRAGMENT LEFT IN PATIENT

On March 31, 1964, the patient–plaintiff was admitted to the medical center for treatment of metastatic malignant melanoma on her left groin.[36] On April 6, 1964, an unknown resident performed a bone marrow biopsy. The needle broke during the procedure, and a fragment lodged in the patient. The patient was told that the needle would be removed the following day, when surgery was to be performed to remove a melanoma from her groin. The operating surgeons, Dr. Peede and Dr. Kilgore, were informed of the presence of the needle fragment prior to surgery. A notation by Peede stated that the needle fragment had been removed.

The needle fragment, however, had not been removed. The patient remained asymptomatic until she was hospitalized for back pain in September 1985. During her hospitalization, the patient learned that the needle fragment was still in her lower back. The needle fragment was finally removed in October 1985. The physician's discharge report suggested that there was a probable linkage between the needle fragment and recurrent strep infections that the patient had been experiencing. Although the patient's treating physicians had known as early as 1972 that the needle fragment had not been removed, there was no evidence that the patient was aware of this fact.

The defendant–physicians argued that the statute of limitations had tolled under Mississippi Code, thus barring the case from proceeding to trial. The circuit court entered a judgment for the physicians, and the plaintiff appealed.

The Mississippi Supreme Court held that the plaintiff's action was not time barred and was, therefore, remanded for trial. A patient's cause for action begins to accrue and the statute of limitations begins to run when the patient can reasonably be held to have knowledge of the disease or injury. In this instance, the patient began to experience infections and back pain in 1985. Moreover, this is the date she discovered that the needle was causing her problems, never having been informed previously that the needle from the 1964 biopsy procedure remained lodged within her.

IMPROPER PERFORMANCE OF A PROCEDURE

In *Ozment v. Wilkerson*,[37] Mrs. Wilkerson was suffering from Crohn's disease, a chronic ailment that affects the colon and small intestine. Part of the treatment for the disease is to allow the patient's GI system to rest, and this means that the patient cannot eat. The patient is given a concentrated caloric solution intravenously. To deliver the needed nutritional solution, Dr. Ozment needed to place a central venous catheter into Wilkerson's body. Wilkerson's pericardial sac was punctured during the procedure. As a result, a condition known as cardiac tamponade (accumulation of fluids in the pericardial sac) occurred. Wilkerson required emergency surgery to correct this condition and to repair the puncture. The defendants, following a jury verdict favorable to the plaintiffs, filed an appeal.

The Alabama Supreme Court held expert testimony that supported the jury's finding that the catheter was inserted incorrectly. The plaintiff's expert, Dr. Moore, testified that the tip of the catheter should have been placed in the superior vena cava and should not have extended into the heart. Moore also stated that placing the tip of the catheter in the atrium, or against the wall of the atrium, was a deviation from the standard of care ordinarily exercised by a physician in the same line of practice under similar circumstances. Moore stated that the intravenous central line perforated the right atrium and caused the cardiac tamponade. Moore's testimony provided sufficient evidence from which the jury could determine that Ozment inserted the catheter incorrectly and had thereby breached his duty of care to Wilkerson.

FAILURE TO MAINTAIN AN ADEQUATE AIRWAY

In *Ward v. Epting*,[38] the anesthesiologist failed to establish and maintain an adequate airway and resuscitate properly a 22-year-old post-surgical patient, which resulted in the patient's death from lack of oxygen. Expert testimony based on autopsy and blood gas tests showed that the endotracheal tube had been removed too soon after surgery and that the anesthesiologist, in an attempt to revive the patient, reinserted the tube into the esophagus. The record on appeal was found to have contained ample evidence that the anesthesiologist failed to conform to the standard of care and that such deviation was the proximate cause of the patient's death.

PATHOLOGIST MISDIAGNOSES CANCER

On July 1, 1988, the patient, in *Anne Arundel Med. Ctr., Inc. v. Condon*,[39] underwent a routine mammogram ordered by her gynecologist, which revealed suspicious findings in her right breast. Advised by her physician that her breast needed further examination, the patient selected a surgeon to perform a biopsy. The biopsy was ultimately performed on July 19, 1988. Based on the pathology report, the surgeon advised the patient that she did not have cancer but that she should undergo frequent mammograms. On February 7, 1990, the patient returned to her surgeon complaining of an inflammation of her right breast in the same area of her previous biopsy. The surgeon again recommended and performed a biopsy on February 15. Based on the second biopsy, the patient was advised that she was suffering from invasive carcinoma of the breast. On February 23, 1990, she underwent a bilateral modified radical mastectomy. The patient alleged that the first biopsy specimen was incorrectly interpreted by the pathologist and that the pathologist's failure to interpret invasive carcinoma was a departure from the standard of care required and was the proximate cause of her injuries. On the eve of trial, December 9, 1992, counsel for the pathologist settled the claim against his client for $1 million.

AGGRAVATION OF A PREEXISTING CONDITION

Aggravation of a preexisting condition through negligence might cause a physician to be liable for malpractice. If the original injury is aggravated, liability will be imposed only for the aggravation, rather than for both the original injury and its aggravation. In *Nguyen v. County of Los Angeles*,[40] an 8-month-old girl went to the hospital for tests on her hip. She had been injected with air for a hip study and suffered respiratory arrest. She later went into cardiac arrest and was resuscitated, but she suffered brain damage that was aggravated by further poor treatment. The Los Angeles Superior Court jury found evidence of medical malpractice, ordering payments for past and future pain and suffering as well as medical and total care costs that projected to the child's normal life expectancy.

LOSS OF CHANCE TO SURVIVE

In *Boudoin v. Nicholson, Baehr, Calhoun & Lanasa*,[41] expert testimony supported a finding of loss of chance to survive. A diagnostic radiologist's improper reading of a patient's X-ray resulted in a loss of chance to survive a chest-wall cancer. Boudoin had suffered a minor shoulder injury while lifting something at his job as a pipefitter. Because the pain did not subside after a few days, on May 19, he went to see Dr. Nicholson, the family practitioner who had treated him since he was 18. Based upon Boudoin's complaint of pain in the outer chest and a physical examination, Dr. Nicholson took a chest X-ray that, in his opinion, showed nothing remarkable and diagnosed Boudoin's injury as a muscle strain and prescribed accordingly. Nevertheless, he sent the X-ray to be evaluated by a diagnostic radiologist, Hendler. The radiology report returned to Nicholson read in part:

> CHEST: Cardiac, hilar, and mediastinal shadows do not appear unusual. Both lung fields and angles appear clear. A 3.5-cm. broad-based benign osteomatous projection is noted at the level of the vertebral border of the inferior aspect of the left scapula. IMPRESSION: 1—No evidence of active pulmonary or cardiac pathology.

On April 18, 1989, Boudoin returned to Nicholson complaining of night sweats, weight loss, and pain in his left chest. A chest X-ray showed a large abnormal mass.

Dr. Rigby surgically removed the tumor. After recovering from his surgery, Boudoin underwent concurrent radiation and chemotherapy. Boudoin and his family were informed that even with chemotherapy, the prognosis was very poor. Further treatment was restricted to alleviating pain until Boudoin's death on December 18, 1990. Hendler appealed an award of $560,000 based upon a jury's finding that the physician's improper reading of Boudoin's X-ray resulted in a loss of chance to survive a chest-wall cancer. The appeals court affirmed the finding of liability and causation but reduced the amount of the award.

The patient in *Downey v. University Internists of St. Louis, Inc.*[42] entered the hospital for heart-bypass surgery. Two chest X-rays were taken during this hospitalization. The X-rays were interpreted as showing a lesion in the patient's left lung and that a neoplasm could not be completely ruled out. If clinically warranted, CT scanning could be performed. No further tests or evaluations were ordered in response to these reports. A jury found that the now-deceased patient had a material chance of surviving his cancer and that his chance of survival was lost due to the physician's negligence. The jury, however, did not award damages to compensate for the harm suffered. The Missouri Court of Appeals found that the verdict of no-damage award was inconsistent with the evidence and remanded the case for a new trial.

Possibility of Survival Destroyed

On February 5, 1988, Mr. Griffett had been taken to the emergency department with a complaint of abdominal pain.[43] Two emergency department physicians evaluated him and ordered X-rays, including a chest X-ray. Dr. Bridges, a radiologist, reviewed the chest X-ray and noted in his written report that there was an abnormal density present in the upper lobe of Griffett's right lung. Griffett was referred to Dr. Ryan, a gastroenterologist, for follow-up care. Ryan admitted Griffett to the hospital for a 24-hour period and then discharged him without having reviewed the radiology report of the February 5 chest X-ray. On March 1, 1988, Griffett continued to experience intermittent pain. A nurse in Ryan's office suggested that Griffett go to the hospital emergency department if his pain became persistent.

In November 1989, Dr. Baker examined Griffett, who was complaining of pain in his right shoulder. Baker diagnosed Griffett's condition as being cancer of the upper lobe of his right lung. The abnormal density on the February 5, 1988, chest X-ray was a cancerous tumor that had doubled in size from the time it had been first observed. The tumor was surgically removed in February 1990; however, Griffett died in September 1990.

The Virginia Supreme Court held that the plaintiff had sufficiently identified Muller as an expert witness capable of testifying as to the question of causation. Evidence was sufficient to establish that the failure to diagnose lung cancer, in connection with the emergency department visit, was the proximate cause of the patient's death. The duty to review an X-ray contained in a patient's medical record should not vary between an internist and a gastroenterologist. Evidence showed that Ryan's negligence destroyed any substantial possibility of Griffett's survival.

LACK OF DOCUMENTATION

It is imperative that patient records of treatment in the physician's office, as well as in the health care facility, be maintained. A jury could consider lack of documentation as sufficient evidence for finding a physician guilty of negligence.

PREMATURE DISCHARGE

The premature discharge of a patient is risky business. The intent of discharging patients more expeditiously is often due to a need to reduce costs. As pointed out by Dr. Nelson, an obstetrician and board member of the American Medical Association, such decisions "should be based on medical factors and ought not be relegated to bean counters."[44]

FAILURE TO FOLLOW-UP

Failure to provide follow-up care can result in a lawsuit if such failure results in injury to a patient. In *Truan v. Smith*,[45] the Tennessee Supreme Court entered judgment in favor of the plaintiffs, who had brought action against a treating physician for damages alleged to have been the result of malpractice by the physician in the examination, diagnosis, and treatment of breast cancer. In January or February 1974, the patient noticed a change in the size and firmness of her left breast, which she attributed to an implant. She later noticed discoloration and pain on pressure. While being examined by the defendant on March 25, 1974, for another ailment, the patient brought her symptoms to the physician's attention but received no significant response, and the physician made no examination of the breast at that time. The patient brought her symptoms to the attention of her physician for the second time on May 6, 1974. She had been advised by the defendant to observe her left breast for 30 days for a change in symptoms, which at the time of the examination included discomfort, discoloration, numbness, and sharp pain. She was given an appointment for one month later. The patient, on the morning of her appointment, June 3, 1974, called the physician's office and informed the nurse that her symptoms had not changed and that she would like to know if she should keep her appointment. The nurse indicated that she would pass on her message to the physician. The patient assumed she would be called back if it was necessary to see the physician. By late June the symptoms became more acute, and the patient made an appointment to see the defendant physician on July 8, 1974. The patient also was scheduled to see a specialist on July 10, 1974, at which time she was admitted to the hospital and was diagnosed as having a malignant mass. A radical mastectomy was performed. Expert witnesses expressed the opinion that the mass had been palpable 7 months before the removal. When the defendant undertook to give the plaintiff a complete physical examination and embarked on a wait-and-see program as an aid in diagnosis, the physician should have followed up with his patient, who died before the conclusion of the trial. The state supreme court held that the evidence was sufficient to support a finding that the defendant was guilty of malpractice in failing to inform his patient that cancer was a possible cause of her complaints and in failing to make any effort to see his patient at the expiration of the observation period instituted by him.

INFECTIONS

Nosocomial (hospital-acquired) infections are a leading cause of injury and unnecessary deaths. Such infections have been linked to unsanitary conditions in the environment and poor practices (e.g., hand-washing technique). The Centers for Disease Control and Prevention estimates that nearly 2 million patients annually get a hospital-acquired infection. There are estimates that as many as 90,000 of these patients die annually as a result of these infections.[46]

Infections a Recognized Risk

The mere fact that a patient contracted an infection after an operation will not, in and of itself, cause a surgeon to be liable for negligence. The reason for this, according to the Nebraska Supreme Court in *McCall v. St. Joseph Hospital*,[47] is as follows:

> Neither authority nor reason will sustain any proposition that negligence can reasonably be inferred from the fact that an infection originated at the site of a surgical wound. To permit a jury to infer negligence would be to expose every doctor and dentist to the charge of negligence every time an infection originated at the site of a wound. We note the complete absence of any expert testimony or any offer of proof in this record to the effect that a staphylococcus infection would automatically lead to an inference of negligence by the people in control of the operation or the treatment of the patient.[48]

Preventing Spread of Infection

A district court of appeals held in *Gill v. Hartford Accident & Indemnity Co.*[49] that the physician who performed surgery on a patient in the same room as the plaintiff should have known that the patient's infection was highly contagious. The failure of the physician to undertake steps to prevent the spread of the infection to the plaintiff and his failure to warn the plaintiff led the court to find that hospital authorities and the plaintiff's physician caused an unreasonable increase in the risk of injury. As a result, the plaintiff suffered injuries causally related to the negligence of the defendant.

Poor Infection-Control Technique

A jury verdict in the amount of $300,000 was awarded in *Langley v. Michael*[50] for damages arising from the amputation of the plaintiff's thumb. Evidence that the orthopedic surgeon failed to deeply cleanse, irrigate, and debride the injured area of the patient's thumb constituted proof of a departure from that degree of skill and learning ordinarily used by members of the medical profession, and that failure directly contributed to the patient's loss of the distal portion of his thumb.

OBSTETRICS

One of the most vulnerable medical specialties with significant risk exposure to malpractice suits is obstetrics. The following cases illustrate why the risks are high.

C-Section Delay Causes Injury

The plaintiffs' experts in *Northern Trust Co. v. University of Chicago Hospitals and Clinic*[51] supported their contention that an obstetrical nurse's delay in placing a fetal monitor and an additional delay caused by the unavailability of a second operating room for a cesarean section caused an infant's mental retardation. Although there was contrary expert opinion, there was no error in the trial court's denial of the hospital's motion for judgment notwithstanding the verdict.

Failure to Perform C-Section

A medical malpractice action was brought against two obstetricians, a pediatrician, and the hospital in *Ledogar v. Giordano*[52] because of a newborn infant's prenatal and postnatal hypoxia, which allegedly caused brain damage resulting in autism. The record contained sufficient proof of causation to support a verdict in favor of the plaintiff when an expert obstetrician testified that both obstetricians were negligent in failing to perform a cesarean section at an earlier time, that the hospital staff departed from proper medical standards of care by not monitoring the fetal heartbeat at least every 15 minutes, and that, with a reasonable degree of medical certainty, it was probable that the fetus suffered hypoxia during labor.

Failure to Attend Delivery: Fetus Decapitated

The plaintiff in *Lucchesi v. Stimmell*[53] brought an action against a physician for intentional infliction of emotional distress, claiming that the physician failed to be present during unsuccessful attempts to deliver her premature fetus, and that he thereafter failed to disclose to her that the fetus was decapitated during attempts to achieve delivery by pulling on the hip area to free the head. The judge instructed the jury that it could conclude that the physician had been guilty of extreme and outrageous conduct for staying at home and leaving the delivery in the hands of a first-year intern and a third-year resident, neither of whom was experienced in breech deliveries.

The intentional infliction of emotional distress requires that the following four elements be proven: (1) the defendant's conduct was intentional or reckless; (2) the conduct was extreme and outrageous; (3) the conduct caused emotional distress to the plaintiff; and (4) the emotional distress was severe. All of these elements were present in *Lucchesi v. Stimmell*.

Failure to Perform Timely C-Section

The attending physician in *Jackson v. Huang*[54] was negligent in failing to perform a timely cesarean section. The attending physician applied too much traction when he was faced with shoulder dystocia, a situation in which a baby's shoulder hangs under the pubic bone, arresting the progress of the infant through the birth canal. As a result, the infant suffered permanent injury to the brachial plexus nerves of his right shoulder and arm. On appeal of this case, no error was found in the trial court's finding of fact when such finding was supported by testimony of the plaintiff's expert witness. The trial judge accepted the testimony of Dr. Forte, the expert witness, who testified that the defendant possessed the necessary skill and knowledge relevant to the practice of obstetrics and gynecology. The defendant, because of prolonged labor and weight of the baby, should have anticipated the possibility of shoulder dystocia and performed a timely cesarean section.

Wrongful Death of Unborn Fetus

A medical malpractice action was filed against the physician in *Modaber v. Kelley*[55] for personal injuries and mental anguish caused by the stillbirth of a child. The circuit court entered judgment on a jury verdict against the obstetrician, and an appeal was taken. The Virginia Supreme Court held that the evidence was sufficient to support a finding that the obstetrician's conduct during the patient's pregnancy caused direct injury to the patient. Evidence at trial showed that the physician failed to treat the mother's known condition of toxemia, including the development of high blood pressure and the premature separation of the placenta from the uterine wall, and that the physician thereafter failed to respond in a timely fashion when the mother went into premature labor. The court also held that injury to the unborn child constituted injury to the mother and that she could recover for the physical injury and mental anguish associated with the stillbirth. The court found that the award of $750,000 in compensatory damages was not excessive.

PSYCHIATRY

The major risk areas of psychiatry include commitment, electroshock, duty to warn, and suicide. Matters relating to admission, consent, and discharge are governed by statute in most states.

Commitment

The recent emphasis on patient rights has had a major impact on the necessity to perform an appropriate assessment prior to commitment. The various state statutes often provide requirements granting an individual's rights to legal counsel and other procedural safeguards (e.g., patient hotline) governing the admission, retention, and discharge of psychiatric patients.

Most states have enacted administrative procedures that must be followed. The various statutes often require that two physicians certify the need for commitment. Physicians who participate in the commitment of a patient should do so only after first examining the patient and reaching their own conclusions. Reliance on another's examination and recommendation for commitment could give rise to a claim of malpractice. Commitment is generally necessary in those situations in which a person might be in substantial danger of injuring himself or herself or third persons.

Commitment Upheld

Evidence was determined to be legally and factually sufficient to support a trial court's order committing a patient diagnosed with a psychotic disorder to a state hospital inpatient mental health services for a period to exceed 90 days. Two incidents in which the patient altered razors into weapons constituted recent overt acts that tended to confirm the likelihood of serious harm to a patient.[56]

Duty to Warn

In *Tarasoff v. Regents of the University of California*,[57] a former patient allegedly killed a third party after revealing his homicidal plans to his therapist. His therapist made no effort to inform the victim of the patient's intentions. The California Supreme Court held that when a therapist determines or reasonably should determine that a patient poses a serious danger of violence to others, there is a duty to exercise reasonable care to protect the foreseeable victims and to warn them of any impending danger. Discharge of this duty also can include notifying the police or taking whatever steps are reasonably necessary under the circumstances.

Under Nebraska law, the relationship between a psychotherapist and a patient gives rise to an affirmative duty to initiate whatever precautions are reasonably necessary to protect the potential victims of a patient. This duty develops when a therapist knows or should know that a patient's dangerous propensities present an unreasonable risk of harm to others.[58]

Exceptions to Duty to Warn

The Maryland Court of Special Appeals in *Shaw v. Glickman*[59] held that a plaintiff could not recover against a psychiatric team on the theory that they were negligent in failing to warn the plaintiff of the patient's unstable and violent condition. The court held that making such a disclosure would violate statutes pertaining to privilege against disclosure of communications relating to treatment of mental or emotional disorders. The court found that a psychiatrist might have a duty to warn the potential victim of a dangerous mental patient's intent to harm. However, the duty could be imposed only if the psychiatrist knew the identity of the prospective victim.

There was no duty on the part of the hospital or treating psychiatrists in *Sharpe v. South Carolina Department of Mental Health*[60] to warn the general public of the potential danger that might result from a psychiatric patient's release from a state hospital. There was no identifiable threat to a decedent who was shot by the patient approximately 2 months after the patient's release from voluntary commitment under a plan of outpatient care. In addition, there was nothing in the record indicating that the former patient and the decedent had known each other prior to the patient's release.

Suicidal Patients

Organizations have a duty to exercise reasonable care to protect suicidal patients from foreseeable harm. This duty exists whether the patient is voluntarily admitted or involuntarily committed. The District Court in *Abille v. United States*[61] held that evidence supported a finding that the attending physician had not authorized a change in status of a suicidal patient to permit him to leave the ward without an escort. The nursing staff allowed him to leave the ward, and he found a window from which he jumped. This constituted a breach of the standard of due care under the law in Alaska, where the act or omission occurred.

The attendant in *Fernandez v. State*[62] left a patient alone in her room for 5 minutes when the patient appeared to be asleep. During the attendant's absence, the patient injured herself in a repeated suicide attempt. The court found that even if the hospital assumed a duty to observe the patient continually, such a 5-minute absence would not constitute negligence. Therefore, the hospital could not be held liable for the patient's injuries.

However, in a case in which a patient with a 14-year history of mental problems escaped from a hospital and committed suicide by jumping off a roof,[63] the record showed the patient was to be checked every 15 minutes. There was no evidence that such checks had been made.

The New York Supreme Court, Appellate Division, in *Eady v. Alter*[64] held that an intern's notation on the hospital record that the patient tried to jump out the window was sufficient to establish a prima facie case against the hospital. The patient succeeded in committing suicide by jumping out the window approximately 10 minutes after having been seen by the intern. Testimony had been given that the patient was restrained inadequately after the reported attempted suicide.

Failure to Provide Appropriate Evaluation

John Doe was at his father's home seeking help in overcoming a heroin addiction. Doe was acting noticeably withdrawn and began vomiting. The plaintiff–father took his son to a local hospital. Doe tested negative for the presence of drugs in his blood and was discharged with instructions to attend a drug rehab program. The following day the father became aware that his son had attempted suicide. He called the office of a drug rehab program for help and was advised to take Doe to the hospital's crisis center.

The crisis center referred the father and his son to the hospital's emergency department. The father explained to the emergency department nurse that his son had attempted suicide by cutting his wrist. Doe's wrist was bandaged. The father and his son proceeded to the crisis center. Following an interview by a nurse and physician, the physician and nurse advised the father that his son was not suicidal but was "acting out" and looking for attention. Hospitalization was not offered, and the plaintiff was advised to follow up with a drug rehab program. Doe's medical records contain no information regarding voluntary hospitalization being recommended or offered, nor do the records reflect that the son refused any offer of voluntary hospitalization.

They returned home, and Doe went to bed. When the father checked Doe at about 6:00 a.m., he was gone. He telephoned the home of his ex-wife and was relieved to learn that his son was there. The father agreed to pick him up before the mother left for work. A few minutes later, the mother called and told the father that their son had left the house. The father immediately went to look for his son. While searching for his son, he noticed flashing lights on a nearby highway. When he went to see what was happening, he saw paramedics administering cardiopulmonary resuscitation (CPR) to his son. The father was told that his son jumped in front of a dump truck and was killed.

A lawsuit was filed against the defendants. At trial, the physician testified that the deceased declined voluntary admission to the hospital. However, in a deposition prior to trial, he testified that he could not recall whether Doe had declined voluntary admission or not. On cross-examination, the physician conceded that he had never specifically recommended hospitalization to Doe.

The nurse testified that voluntary hospitalization was offered as an option to the plaintiff and his son but was not recommended. That option, if in fact offered, was not recorded in the hospital record.

The plaintiff's medical experts testified that: (1) because of Doe's two suicide attempts, he needed hospitalization; (2) additional steps should have been taken prior to ruling out major depression; (3) in all probability, Doe would not have killed himself had he been hospitalized earlier and put on medications; and (4) Doe's prior suicide attempts should have been taken more seriously. They opined that the failure to hospitalize Doe and keep him under close supervision was a deviation from accepted standards of medical practice. The defendants' expert testified to the contrary but conceded on cross-examination that Doe had at least three high-risk factors for suicide.

The trial largely turned to a contest between the experts. The jury, by its verdict, accepted the opinions of the plaintiff's experts. The court found, after a review of the record, no reason to disturb the jury's verdict. The plaintiff, as administrator of the estate of his late son, recovered a verdict of $425,000 against the defendants for their failure to provide appropriate evaluation and hospitalization of Doe.[65]

ABANDONMENT

The relationship between a physician and a patient, when established, continues until it is ended by the mutual consent of the parties, the patient's dismissal of the physician, the physician's withdrawal from the case, or agreement that the physician's services are no longer required. A physician who decides to withdraw his or her services must provide the patient with reasonable notice so that the services of another physician can be obtained. Premature termination of treatment is often the subject of a legal action for abandonment; the unilateral termination of a physician–patient relationship by the physician without notice to the patient. The following elements should be established for a patient to recover damages for abandonment:

- Medical care was unreasonably discontinued.
- The discontinuance of medical care was against the patient's will.
- Termination of the physician–patient relationship must have been brought about by a unilateral act of the physician. There can be no issue of abandonment if the relationship is terminated by mutual consent or by dismissal of the physician by the patient.
- The physician failed to arrange for care by another physician.

- Foresight indicated that discontinuance might result in physical harm to the patient.
- Actual harm was suffered by the patient.

PHYSICIAN–PATIENT RELATIONSHIP

The following suggestions can help to decrease the probability of malpractice suits:

- Personalize your treatment. A patient is more inclined to sue an impersonal physician than one with whom he or she has developed a good relationship.
- Conduct a thorough assessment/history and physical examination that includes a review of all body systems.
- Develop a problems list and comprehensive treatment plan that addresses the patient's problems.
- Provide sufficient time and care to each patient. Take the time to explain treatment plans and follow-up care to the patient, his or her family, and other professionals who are caring for your patient.
- Request consultations when indicated and refer if necessary.
- Closely monitor the patient's progress and, as necessary, make adjustments to the treatment plan as the patient's condition warrants.
- Maintain timely, legible, complete, and accurate records. Do not make erasures.
- Do not guarantee treatment outcome.
- Provide for cross-coverage during days off.
- Do not overextend your practice.
- Avoid prescribing over the telephone.
- Do not become careless because you know the patient.
- Seek the advice of counsel should you suspect the possibility of a malpractice claim.

Notes

1. 301 N.W.2d 156 (Wis. 1981).
2. 211 N.E.2d 253 (Ill. 1965).
3. 394 N.E.2d 770 (Ill. App. Ct. 1979).
4. 540 P.2d 1398, 1400 (Or. 1975).
5. No. 04AP-72 (Ohio Ct. App. 2004).
6. Warnick v. Natchez Community Hospital, Inc., No. 2003-CA-01513-SCT (Miss. 2004).
7. 218 N.W.2d 492 (Iowa 1928).
8. 520 N.Y.S.2d 751 (N.Y. App. Div. 1987).
9. 737 S.W.2d 455 (Ark. 1987).
10. 85 Conn. App. 854 (Conn. App. 2004).
11. EHCA Dunwoody, L.L.C. v. Daniel, 627 S.E.2d 830 (Ga. App. 2006).
12. 294 F. Supp. 466 (D.S.C. 1968).
13. 865 F. Supp. 433 (N.D. Ohio 1994).
14. 235 A.2d 889 (N.J. 1967).
15. 568 N.W.2d 93 (Mich. App. 1997).
16. 594 A.2d 1309 (N.J. 1991).
17. 530 A.2d 1217 (D.C. 1987).
18. Gomez v. Tri City Community Hosp., 4 S.W.3d 281 (Tex. App. 1999).
19. 531 A.2d 226 (D.C. 1987).
20. Snyder v. George Washington Univ., 890 A.2d 237 (D.C. App. 2006).
21. 653 A.2d 541 (Md. App.1995).
22. Valentine v. Kaiser Found. Hosps., 15 Cal. Rptr. 26 (Cal. Ct. App.1961) (dictum).
23. 402 S.W.2d 855 (Ky. Ct. App. 1966).
24. 33 Cal. Rptr. 673 (Cal. Ct. App. 1963).
25. 209 So. 2d 809 (Miss. 1968).
26. 647 So. 2d 1366 (La. App. 3d Cir. 1994).
27. 542 N.Y.S.2d 328 (N.Y. App. Div. 1989).
28. 523 N.Y.S.2d 645 (N.Y. App. Div. 1988).
29. 489 So. 2d 392 (La. Ct. App. 1986).
30. 582 So. 2d 1272 (La. 1991).
31. 570 N.E.2d 1249 (Ill. App. Ct. 1991).
32. 539 S.W.2d 286 (Ky. 1976).
33. 785 A.2d 25 (2001).
34. Bombagetti v. Amine, 627 N.E.2d 230 (Ill. App. Ct. 1993).
35. 745 N.Y.S.2d 304 (N.Y. App. Div. 2002).
36. Williams v. Kilgore, 618 So. 2d 51 (Miss. 1992).
37. 646 So. 2d 4 (Ala. 1994).
38. 351 S.E.2d 867 (S.C. Ct. App. 1987).

39. 649 A.2d 1189 (1994).
40. No. C538628 (L.A. Co. Cal. Super. Ct.).
41. 698 So. 2d 469 (La. App. 4 Cir. 1997).
42. No. ED83231 (Mo. App. 2004).
43. Griffett v. Ryan, 443 S.E.2d 149 (Va. 1994).
44. Anita Manning, AMA Calls Drive-Thru Birth Risky, USA TODAY, June 21, 1995, at 1.
45. 578 S.W.2d 73 (Tenn. 1979).
46. JP Burke. Infection Control-A Problem for Patient Safety. NEW ENG. J. MED. 2003; 348; 651–656.
47. 165 N.W.2d 85 (Neb. 1969).
48. Id. at 89.
49. 337 So. 2d 420 (Fla. Dist. Ct. App. 1976).
50. 710 S.W.2d 373 (Mo. Ct. App. 1986).
51. No. 1-02-3838 (Ill. App. Ct. Rpt. 2004).
52. 505 N.Y.S.2d 899 (N.Y. App. Div. 1986).
53. 716 P.2d 1013 (Ariz. 1986).
54. 514 So. 2d 727 (La. Ct. App. 1987).
55. 348 S.E.2d 233 (Va. 1986).
56. In re States of Texas for the Best Interest and Protection of L.H., 183 S.W.3d 905 (Tex. App. 2006).
57. 551 P.2d 334 (Cal. 1976).
58. Lipari v. Sears, Roebuck & Co., 497 F. Supp. 185 (D. Neb. 1980).
59. 415 A.2d 625 (Md. Ct. Spec. App. 1980).
60. 354 S.E.2d 778 (S.C. Ct. App. 1987).
61. 482 F. Supp. 703 (N.D. Cal. 1980).
62. 356 N.Y.S.2d 708 (N.Y. App. Div. 1974).
63. Fatuck v. Hillside Hosp., 356 N.Y.S.2d 105 (N.Y. App. Div. 1974).
64. 380 N.Y.S.2d 737 (N.Y. App. Div. 1976).
65. Vasilik v. Federbush, 742 A.2d 591 (N.J. Super. Ct. App. Div. 1999).

9

NURSING AND THE LAW

The role of the nurse continues to expand because of a shortage of primary care physicians in certain rural and inner-city areas, ever-increasing specialization, improved technology, public demand, and expectations within the profession itself. A nurse who exceeds his or her scope of practice as defined by state nurse practice acts can be found to have violated licensure provisions or to have performed tasks that are reserved by statute for another health care professional. Because of increasingly complex nursing and medical procedures, it is sometimes difficult to distinguish the tasks that are clearly reserved for the physician from those that can be performed by the professional nurse. Nurses, however, generally have not encountered lawsuits for exceeding their scope of practice unless negligent conduct is an issue.

NURSE LICENSURE

The common organizational pattern of nurse licensing authority in each state is to establish a separate board, organized and operated within the guidelines of specific legislation, to license all professional and practical nurses. Each board is in turn responsible for the determination of eligibility for initial licensing and relicensing; for the enforcement of licensing statutes, including suspension, revocation, and restoration of licenses; and for the approval and supervision of training institutions. A licensing board has the authority to suspend a license; however, it must do so within existing rules and regulations.

Requirements for Licensure

Formal professional training is necessary for nurse licensure in all states. The course requirements vary, but all courses must be completed at board-approved schools or institutions. Each state requires that an applicant pass a written examination, which is generally administered twice annually. A licensing board can draft examinations, or a professional examination service or national examining board can prepare them. Some states waive their written examination for applicants who present a certificate from a national nursing examination board. Graduate nurses are generally able to practice nursing under supervision while waiting for the results of their examination. The four basic methods by which boards license out-of-state nurses are (1) reciprocity, (2) endorsement, (3) waiver, and (4) examination.

Reciprocity

Reciprocity is a formal or informal agreement between states whereby a nurse licensing board in one state recognizes licensees of another state if the board of that state extends reciprocal recognition to licensees from the first state. To have reciprocity, the initial licensing requirements of the two states must be essentially equivalent.

Endorsement

Although some nurse licensing boards use the term "endorsement" interchangeably with "reciprocity," the two words have different meanings. In licensing by endorsement, boards determine whether out-of-state nurses' qualifications are equivalent to their own state requirements at the time of initial licensure. Many states make it a condition for endorsement that the qualifying examination taken in another state be comparable to their own. As with reciprocity, endorsement becomes much easier when uniform qualification standards are applied by the different states.

Waiver

Licensing out-of-state nurses can be accomplished by waiver and examination. When applicants do not meet all the requirements for licensure but have equivalent qualifications, the specific prerequisites of education, experience, or examination can be waived.

Examination

Some states will not recognize out-of state licensed nurses and make it mandatory that all applicants pass a licensing examination. Most states grant temporary licenses for nurses. These licenses may be issued pending a decision by a licensing board on permanent licensure or may be issued to out-of-state nurses who intend to be in a jurisdiction for a limited, specified time.

Graduates of schools in other countries are required to meet the same qualifications as are nurses trained in the United States. Many state boards have established special training, citizenship, and experience requirements for students who are educated abroad; others insist on additional training in the United States. Nurses who complete their studies in a foreign country are required to pass an English proficiency examination and/or a licensing examination administered in English. A few states have reciprocity or endorsement agreements with some foreign countries.

Suspension and Revocation of License

Nurse licensing boards have the authority to suspend or revoke the license of a nurse who is found to have violated specified norms of conduct. Such violations can include procurement of a license by fraud; unprofessional, dishonorable, immoral, or illegal conduct; performance of specific actions prohibited by statute; and malpractice.

Suspension and revocation procedures are most commonly contained in the licensing act; in some jurisdictions, however, the procedure is left to the discretion of the board or is contained in the general administrative procedure acts. For the most part, suspension and revocation proceedings are administrative, rather than judicial, and do not carry criminal sanctions.

Practicing Without a License

Health care organizations are required to verify that each nurse's license is current. The mere fact that an unlicensed practitioner is hired would not generally in and of itself impose additional liability unless a patient suffered harm as a result of the unlicensed nurse's negligence.

NURSE ANESTHETIST

Administration of anesthesia by a nurse anesthetist requires special training and certification. Nurse-administered anesthesia was the first expanded role for nurses that required certification. Oversight and availability of an anesthesiologist are required by most organizations. The major risks for nurse anesthetists include improper placement of an airway, failure to recognize significant changes in a patient's condition, and the improper use of anesthetics (e.g., wrong anesthetic, wrong dose, wrong route).

Supervision of Nurse Anesthetist Required

Medical supervision of nurse anesthetists is generally required in hospital settings. Failure to properly supervise a nurse anesthetist can lead to a lawsuit, as was the case in *Denton Reg'l Med. Ctr. v. LaCroix*,[1] where Mrs. LaCroix was admitted to the hospital's women's pavilion for the birth of her first child, Lawryn. She was admitted to the hospital under the care of Dr. Dulemba, her obstetrician. Prior to undergoing a cesarean section, LaCroix complained several times of breathing difficulty. When Dr. McGehee, the pediatrician, arrived, he noticed that LaCroix appeared to be in respiratory distress and heard her say, "I can't breathe." Dr. McGehee asked Nurse Blankenship, a certified registered nurse anesthetist (CRNA), if LaCroix was okay. She responded that LaCroix was just nervous. Mr. LaCroix claimed that his wife whispered to him that she could not breathe. Mr. LaCroix then shouted, "She can't breathe. Somebody please help my wife." Blankenship asked that Mr. LaCroix be removed from the operating room because his wife was having what appeared to her to be a seizure.

Blankenship could not establish an airway. She told one of the nurses: "Get one of the anesthesiologists here now!" Dr. Green, who was in his car, was paged. Upon receiving the page, he immediately drove to the women's pavilion, where Dulemba had already started the C-section. When Lawryn was delivered, she was not breathing, and Dr. McGehee had to resuscitate her. Meanwhile, Blankenship worked to establish an airway for LaCroix. The intubation was, however, an esophageal intubation. Dr. Dulemba stated that he thought that the intubation was esophageal. LaCroix's blood pressure and pulse dropped, and she went into cardiac arrest. A physician and nurse from the hospital's emergency department responded to a code for assistance. McGehee testified that the emergency department physician said that he did not know how to resuscitate pregnant women and left without providing any medical care. Dr. Dulemba and a nurse began cardiopulmonary resuscitation on LaCroix. Dr. McGehee, having finished treating Lawryn, took control of the code. LaCroix suffered irreversible brain damage.

Blankenship and Dr. Hafiz, the Denton Anesthesiology Associates (DAA), PA, anesthesiologist on call for the women's pavilion on the day of LaCroix's incident, settled with the LaCroixes by paying \$500,000 and \$750,000, respectively. The trial court entered a judgment against the hospital, awarding the LaCroixes approximately \$8.8 million in damages.

The evidence established that the hospital owed a duty to the plaintiff to have an anesthesiologist provide or supervise all anesthesia care, including having an anesthesiologist personally present or immediately available in the operating suite. The hospital's breach of this duty proximately caused the patient's brain damage.

NURSE PRACTITIONER

Nurse practitioners (NPs) are RNs who have completed the necessary education to engage in primary health care decision making. The NP is trained in the delivery of primary health care and the assessment of psychosocial and physical health problems, such as the performance of routine examinations and the ordering of routine diagnostic tests. A physician may not delegate a task to an NP when regulations specify that the physician must perform it personally or when the delegation is prohibited under state law or by an organization's own policies.

The potential risks of liability for the NP are as real as the risks for any other nurse. The standard of care required most likely will be set by statute. If not, the courts will determine the standard based on the reasonable person doctrine (i.e., what would a reasonably prudent NP do under similar circumstances?). The standard would be established through the use of expert testimony of other NPs in the field. Because of potential liability problems and pressure from physicians, hospitals have been historically reluctant to use NPs to the full extent of their training. Such reluctance has been diminishing as the competency of NPs has been well demonstrated in practice.

Nurse Practitioner's Negligence Imputed to Physician

The negligence of a nurse practitioner can be imputed to a physician if the physician is the employer of the nurse. The plaintiff in *Adams v. Krueger*[2] went to her physician's office for diagnosis and treatment. An NP who was employed by the physician performed her assessment and diagnosed the plaintiff as having genital herpes. The physician prescribed an ointment to help relieve the patient's symptoms. The plaintiff eventually consulted with another physician who advised her that she had a yeast infection, not genital herpes.

The plaintiff and her husband filed an action against the initial treating physician and his NP for their failure to correctly diagnose and treat her condition. The action against the physician was based on his failure to review the NP's diagnosis and treatment plan.

The Idaho Supreme Court held that the negligence of the nurse was properly imputed to the physician. The Idaho Supreme Court held that the physician and NP stood in a master–servant relationship and that the nurse acted within the scope of her employment. Consequently, her negligence was properly attributed to her employer/physician.

CLINICAL NURSE SPECIALIST

A clinical nurse specialist (CNS) is a professional RN with an advanced academic degree, experience, and expertise in a clinical specialty (e.g., obstetrics, pediatrics, psychiatry). Further, the CNS acts as a resource for the management of patients with complex needs and conditions. The CNS participates in staff development activities related to his or her clinical specialty and makes recommendations to establish standards of care for those patients. The CNS functions as a change agent by influencing attitudes, modifying behavior, and introducing new approaches to nursing practice. The CNS collaborates with other members of the health care team in developing and implementing the therapeutic plan of care for patients.

NURSE MIDWIFE

Nurse midwives provide comprehensive prenatal care including delivery for patients who are at low risk for complications. For the most part, they manage normal prenatal, intrapartum, and postpartum care. Provided there are no complications, normal newborns are also cared for by a nurse midwife. Nurse midwives often provide primary care for women's issues from puberty to postmenopause.

NURSE MANAGERS

The chief nursing officer (CNO) is a qualified RN who has administrative authority, responsibility, and accountability for the function, activities, and training of the nursing staff. CNOs are generally responsible for maintaining standards of practice, maintaining current policy and procedure manuals, making recommendations for staffing levels based on need, coordinating and integrating nursing services with other patient care services, selecting nursing staff, and developing orientation and training programs.

A manager who knowingly fails to supervise an employee's performance or assigns a task to an individual whom he or she knows, or should know, is not competent to perform can be held personally liable if injury occurs. The employer will be liable under the doctrine of respondeat superior as the employer of both the manager and the individual who performed the task in a negligent manner. The manager is not relieved of personal liability even though the employer is liable under respondeat superior.

In determining whether a nurse with supervisory responsibilities has been negligent, the nurse is measured against the standard of care of a competent and prudent nurse in the performance of supervisory duties. Those duties include the setting of policies and procedures for the prevention of accidents in the care of patients.

Failure to Supervise

Nursing managers must properly supervise the care rendered to patients by their subordinates. Failure to do so can lead to disciplinary action by a state regulatory agency. This was the case in *Hicks v. New York State Department of Health*[3] in which the court held that evidence was sufficient to support a finding that a practical nurse was guilty of resident neglect for failing to ensure that the resident was properly cared for during her assigned shift. The record demonstrated that the petitioner was responsible for ensuring that the nursing aides' tasks were properly accomplished by conducting a visual check of each resident while making rounds at the end of her shift. The nurse's record indicated that a security guard found a resident lying in the dark, half in his bed and half still restrained in an overturned wheelchair. The nurse's record indicated that the resident was covered in urine and stool. The commissioner of health denied the petitioner's request to expunge the patient neglect report and assessed a penalty of $200, of which the petitioner was required to pay $50.

SPECIAL-DUTY NURSE

A special-duty nurse is a health care professional employed by a patient or patient's family to perform nursing care for the patient. An organization is generally not liable for the negligence of a special-duty nurse unless a master–servant relationship can be determined to exist between the organization and the special-duty nurse. If a master–servant relationship exists between the organization and the special-duty nurse, the doctrine of respondeat superior may be applied to impose liability on the organization for the nurse's negligent acts.

A special-duty nurse might be required to observe certain rules and regulations as a precondition to working in the organization. The observance of organization rules is insufficient, however, to establish a master–servant relationship between the organization and the nurse. Under ordinary circumstances, the patient employs the special-duty nurse, and the organization has no authority to hire or fire the nurse. The organization does, however, have the responsibility to protect the patient from incompetent or unqualified special-duty nurses.

FLOAT NURSE

A float nurse is a health care professional who rotates from unit to unit based on staffing needs. "Floaters" can benefit an understaffed unit, but they also might present a liability as well if they are assigned to work in an area outside their expertise. If a patient is injured because of a floater's negligence, the standard of care required of the floater will be that required of a nurse on the assigned patient care unit.

NURSING ASSISTANT

A nursing assistant is an aide who has been certified and trained to assist patients with activities of daily living. The nursing assistant provides basic nursing care to patients under the direction and supervision of an RN or LPN. The nursing assistant helps with positioning, turning, and lifting and performs a variety of tests and treatments. The nursing assistant establishes and maintains interpersonal relationships with patients and other hospital personnel while ensuring confidentiality of patient information.

Failure to Follow Policy: Patient Scalded

Failure to follow hospital policy can result in a successful lawsuit for the plaintiff, as was the case in *Moon Lake Convalescent Center v. Margolis, Ovitz*,[4] where a 73-year-old resident of a convalescent center died after immersion in a tub of hot water that had been prepared by a nursing assistant. Ovitz had paralysis of his left side and could articulate only the words "yes" and "no." The nursing assistant checked the water with his hand and bathed the resident. Later in the day, a nurse noticed that the resident's leg was bleeding and his skin was sloughing off. The paramedics were contacted, and they transferred the resident to a hospital after determining that the patient had suffered third-degree burns. Dr. Drueck, the surgeon at the hospital, observed that Ovitz had suffered third-degree burns over 40% of his body, primarily on his back, buttocks, both sides, genitals, and lower legs.

Ovitz developed pneumonia during his hospitalization and died. There was testimony from Drueck that the cause of death was due to complications following the burns. The center's daily temperature logs indicated that it knew that the water temperature in the system at times fluctuated above its bathing policy, sometimes exceeding 110 degrees Fahrenheit, yet the center failed to take adequate measures to protect residents from exposure to excessive water temperatures. The center's own written policy was violated when the nursing assistant left the resident unattended in his bath. The appellate court held that revocation of the center's license was warranted in this case.

AGENCY STAFF

Health care organizations are at risk for the negligent conduct of agency staff. Because of this risk, it is important to be sure that agency workers have the necessary skills and competencies to carry out the duties and responsibilities assigned by the organization.

STUDENT NURSES

Student nurses are entrusted with the responsibility of providing nursing care to patients. They are personally liable for their own negligent acts, and the facility is liable for their acts on the basis of respondeat superior. A student nurse is held to the standard of a competent professional nurse when performing nursing duties. The courts, in several decisions, have taken the position that anyone who performs duties customarily performed by professional nurses is held to the standards of professional nurses. Every patient has the right to expect competent nursing services even if students provide the care as part of their clinical training. It would be unfair to deprive a patient of compensation for an injury simply because the nurse was a student.

NURSING DIAGNOSIS

Various states recognize that nurses can render a nursing diagnosis. As was the case in *Cignetti v. Camel*[5] where the defendant physicians ignored a nurse's assessment of a patient's diagnosis, which contributed to a delay in treatment and injury to the patient. The nurse testified that she told the physician that the patient's signs and symptoms were not those associated with indigestion. The defendant physician objected to this testimony, indicating that such a statement constituted a medical diagnosis by a nurse. The trial court permitted the testimony to be entered into evidence. Section 335.01(8) of the Missouri Revised Statutes (1975) authorizes an RN to make an assessment of persons who are ill and to render a nursing diagnosis. On appeal, the Missouri Court of Appeals affirmed the lower court's ruling, holding that evidence of negligence presented by a hospital employee, for which an obstetrician was not responsible, was admissible to show the events that occurred during the patient's hospital stay.

MEDICATION ERRORS

Nurses are required to handle and administer a vast variety of drugs that are prescribed by physicians and dispensed by an organization's pharmacy. Medications might range from aspirin to highly dangerous drugs (e.g., potassium chloride) administered through IV solutions. Medications must be administered in the prescribed manner and dose to prevent serious harm to patients.

The practice of pharmacy includes the ordering, preparation, dispensing, and administration of medications. These activities can be carried out only by a licensed pharmacist or by a person exempted from the provisions of a state's pharmacy statutes. Nurses are exempted from the various pharmacy statutes when administering a medication on the oral or written order of a physician.

Failure to Administer Drugs

In *Kallenberg v. Beth Israel Hospital*,[6] a patient died after her third cerebral hemorrhage because of the failure of the physicians and staff to administer necessary medications. When the patient was admitted to the hospital, her physician determined that she should be given a specific drug to reduce her blood pressure and make her condition operable. For an unexplained reason, the drug was not administered. The patient's blood pressure rose, and after the final hemorrhage, she died. The jury found the hospital and physicians negligent by failing to administer the drug and ruled that the negligence caused the patient's death. On appeal, the appellate court found that the jury had sufficient evidence to decide that the negligent treatment had been the cause of the patient's death.

Failure to Document Drug Wastage

The nurse in *Matthias v. Iowa Board of Nursing*[7] failed to conform to minimum standards of practice by neglecting to document the loss or wastage of controlled substances. The minimum standard of acceptable practice requires nurses to count controlled substances each shift, to document all loss or wastage of controlled substances, and to obtain the signature of a witness to the disposal of controlled substances. Iowa Code section 147.\-55\-(2) allows a professional license to be suspended or revoked when the licensee engages in professional incompetency. Iowa Administrative Code section 655-4.\-19\-(2)\-(c), which regulates the actions of the board, defines professional incompetency as including "[w]illful or repeated departure from or failure to conform to the minimum standards of acceptable and prevailing practice of nursing in the state of Iowa."

Matthias argued that the board erred as a matter of law because it failed to find that she knowingly or willfully failed to conform to the minimum standards of practice regarding documentation of loss or wastage of controlled substances. The Iowa Court of Appeals found that there was substantial evidence supporting the board's finding that Matthias engaged in repeated departures from the minimum standards of nursing. The board, therefore, did not need to find that the departure was also willful.

Administering Unprescribed Drugs

In *People v. Nygren*,[8] evidence was considered sufficient to establish probable cause for charging the director of nursing and a charge nurse with second-degree assault in the administration of unprescribed doses of Thorazine to a resident at a time when the patient was incapable of providing consent. There was probable cause to believe that the defendants committed the offense charged and that it would have been established if the prosecution had been permitted to present its witnesses, two of whom would have testified that the nurses administered the unprescribed doses of the drug. The treating physician told the special investigator from the attorney general's office that Thorazine never had been prescribed for the resident while he was in the nursing facility. The resident was mentally retarded and incapable of consenting to administration of the drug. Medical evidence of the amount of Thorazine in the resident's blood was consistent with stupor and impairment of physical and mental functions.

Failure to Clarify Orders

A nurse is responsible for making an inquiry if there is uncertainty about the accuracy of a physician's medication order in a patient's record. In the Louisiana case of *Norton v. Argonaut Insurance Co.*,[9] the court focused attention on the responsibility of a nurse to obtain clarification of an apparently erroneous order from the patient's physician. The medication order, as entered in the medical record, was incomplete and subject to misinterpretation. Believing the order to be incorrect because of the dosage, the nurse asked two physicians present on the patient care unit whether the medication should be given as ordered. The two physicians did not interpret the order as the nurse did and therefore did not share the same concern. They advised the nurse that the attending physician's instructions did not appear out of line. The nurse did not contact the attending physician but instead administered the misinterpreted dosage of medication. As a result, the patient died from a fatal overdose of the medication.

The court upheld the jury's finding that the nurse had been negligent in failing to verify the order with the attending physician prior to administering the drug. The nurse was held liable, as was the physician who wrote the ambiguous order that led to the fatal dose. The court noted that it is the duty of a nurse to make absolutely certain what the physician intended regarding both dosage and route.

Administering the Wrong Dosage

The nurse in *Harrison v. Axelrod*[10] was charged with patient neglect because she administered the wrong dosage of the drug Haldol to a patient on seven occasions while she was employed at a nursing facility. The patient's physician had prescribed a 0.5 milligram dosage of Haldol. The patient's medication record indicated that the nurse had been administering dosages of 5.0 milligrams, the dosage sent to the patient care unit by the pharmacy. A department of health investigator testified that the nurse admitted that she administered the wrong dosage and that she was aware of the facility's medication administration policy, which she breached by failing to check the dosage supplied by the pharmacy against the dosage ordered by the patient's doctor. The nurse denied that she made these admissions to the investigator. The commissioner of the department of health made a determination that the administration of the wrong dosage of Haldol on seven occasions constituted patient neglect.

On appeal, the New York Supreme Court, Appellate Division, held that the evidence established that the nurse administered the wrong dosage of the prescribed drug Haldol to the patient. This was a breach of the facility's medication administration policy and was sufficient to support the determination of patient neglect.

Administering Drugs by the Wrong Route

The nurse in *Fleming v. Baptist General Convention*[11] negligently injected the patient with a solution of Talwin and Atarax subcutaneously rather than intramuscularly. The patient suffered tissue necrosis as a result of the improper injection. The suit against the hospital was successful. On appeal, the court held that the jury's verdict for the plaintiff found adequate support in the testimony of the plaintiff's expert witness on the issues of negligence and causation.

Failure to Discontinue a Drug

A health care organization will be held liable if a nurse continues to inject a solution into a patient after noticing its ill effects. In the Florida case of *Parrish v. Clark,*[12] the court held that a nurse's continued injection of saline solution into an unconscious patient's breast after the nurse noticed ill effects constituted negligence. After something was observed to be wrong with the administration of the solution, the nurse had a duty to discontinue its use.

Failure to Note an Order Change

In *Larrimore v. Homeopathic Hospital Association,*[13] the physician wrote an instruction on the patient's order sheet changing the method of administration from intramuscular to oral. When a nurse on the patient unit who had been off duty for several days was preparing to medicate the patient by injection, the patient objected and referred the nurse to the physician's new order. The nurse, however, told the patient she was mistaken and administered the medication intramuscularly. The court determined the jury could find the nurse negligent by applying ordinary common sense to establish the applicable standard of care.

NEGLIGENT INJECTION

In *Bernardi v. Community Hospital Association,*[14] a 7-year-old patient was in the hospital after surgery for the drainage of an abscessed appendix. The attending physician left a written postoperative order requiring an injection of tetracycline every 12 hours. During the evening of the first day after surgery, the nurse, employed by the hospital and acting under this order, injected the prescribed dosage of tetracycline in the patient's right gluteal region. It was claimed that the nurse negligently injected the tetracycline into or adjacent to the sciatic nerve, causing the patient to permanently lose the normal use of the right foot. The court did not hold the physician responsible. It concluded that if the plaintiff could prove the nurse's negligence, the hospital would be responsible for the nurse's act under the doctrine of respondeat superior. The physician did not know which nurse administered the injection because he was not present when the injection was given, and he had no opportunity to control its administration. The hospital was found liable under respondeat superior. The hospital was the employer of the nurse. Only it had the right to hire and fire her. Only it could assign the nurse to certain hours, designated areas, and specific patients.

FAILURE TO FOLLOW PHYSICIAN'S ORDERS

Evidence in *Redel v. Capital Reg. Med. Ctr.*[15] noted that nurses failed to follow the treating doctor's orders and established a submissible case of medical negligence against the hospital. It was established that, following bilateral knee replacement surgery, the action of nurses caused permanent drop foot to the patient. They failed to follow the doctor's verbal orders to watch the patient closely and to place him in one continuous passive motion machine at a time during physical therapy.

FAILURE TO RECORD PATIENT'S CARE

The plaintiff in *Pellerin v. Humedicenters, Inc.*[16] went to the emergency department at Lakeland Medical Center complaining of chest pain. An emergency department physician, Dr. Gruner, examined her and ordered a nurse to give her an injection consisting of 50 mg of Demerol and 25 mg of Vistaril. Although the nurse testified that she did not recall giving the injection, she did not deny giving it, and her initials are present in the emergency department record. The nurse admitted that she failed to record the site and mode of injection in the emergency department records. She said she might have written this information in the nurse's notes, but no such notes were admitted into evidence.

The plaintiff testified that she felt pain and a burning sensation in her hip during the injection. The burning persisted afterward and progressively worsened over the next several weeks. The pain spread to an area approximately 10 inches in diameter around the injection site. She could not sleep on her right side, work, perform household chores, or participate in sports without experiencing pain. She also testified that she had a lump around the injection site and that her skin was numb in that area.

The appeals court found that there was sufficient evidence to support a jury finding that the nurse had breached the applicable standard of care in administering an injection of Vistaril into Pellerin's hip. The jury awarded the plaintiff $90,304.68 in total damages. The nurse admitted that she failed to record the site and mode of injection in the emergency department records. According to the testimony of two experts in nursing practice, failing to record this information is below the standard of care for nursing.

FAILURE TO IDENTIFY CORRECT PATIENT

The plaintiff in *Meena v. Wilburn*[17] injured her leg and developed an ulcer because of poor blood circulation. Due to the plaintiff's diabetic condition, the ulcer did not heal. Dr. Maples, a vascular surgeon, performed surgery. Two days following surgery, Dr. Meena was at the hospital covering for one of his partners, Dr. Petro, who had asked him to remove the staples from one of his patients, 65-year-old Slaughter. Slaughter shared a semiprivate room with the plaintiff. Meena testified that he went and picked up Slaughter's chart at the nurse's desk and asked one of the nurses which bed Slaughter was in. Meena claimed that he was led to believe that she was in the bed next to the window. He picked up the chart and asked Greer, a nurse, to accompany him to the plaintiff's room. Shortly thereafter, Meena received an emergency call at the nursing station. He said that he asked Greer to take out the staples because he had to respond to an emergency call at another hospital. Greer conceded during her testimony that, before removing staples from a patient, a nurse should read the chart, be familiar with the chart, look at the patient's wristband, and compare the arm band to the chart—all of which she failed to do. Greer rationalized her failure: "When the doctor I work for is standing at the foot of a patient's bed, I would have no doubt—no reason to doubt what he tells me to do."

Greer began to remove the plaintiff's staples. The plaintiff's skin split open, revealing the layer of fat under the skin. Greer stopped the procedure and left the room to check the medical records maintained at the nursing station. She realized that she had removed staples from the wrong patient. At that point, she encountered Maples and explained to him what had happened. Maples immediately restapled the skin.

Following discharge, the plaintiff's health began to falter and she developed a fever of 101 degrees Fahrenheit. The tissue where the staples had been removed became infected. The plaintiff was ultimately readmitted to the hospital; she remained there for approximately 22 days. Her condition gradually improved and, presumably, she had recovered completely with the exception of some scarring and skin indention.

A complaint was filed against Meena and Greer. After 4 days of trial, the jury returned a verdict against Meena and assessed damages in the amount of $125,000. The jury declined to hold the nurse liable for the plaintiff's injuries. Meena appealed, claiming that the jury's exoneration of the nurse, who removed the surgical staples, was grounds for a new trial on the issue of the physician's liability. Further, Meena argued that the jury was bound to return a verdict against both defendants, inasmuch as the defendants were sued as joint tort-feasors. The Mississippi Supreme Court held that the jury's exoneration of Greer was not grounds for a new trial on the issue of the physician's liability.

This case was settled in 1992. In light of The Joint Commission's present day national patient safety goal requiring two forms of patient identification prior to rendering care or treatment, the patient's injury might have been avoided.

INFECTIONS

Failure to follow proper infection-control procedures (e.g., proper hand-washing techniques) can result in cross-contamination between patients, staff, and visitors. Staff members who administer to patients, moving from one patient to another, must wash their hands after changing dressings and carrying out routine procedures.

Cross-Contamination

The patient in *Helmann v. Sacred Heart Hospital*[18] was returned to his room following hip surgery. The patient's roommate complained of a boil under his right arm. A culture was taken of drainage from the wound and was identified as *Staphylococcus aureus*. The infected roommate was transferred immediately to an isolation room. Until this time, hospital employees administered to both patients regularly, moving from one patient to another without washing their hands as they changed dressings and carried out routine procedures. On the day the roommate was placed in isolation, the plaintiff's wound erupted, discharging a large amount of purulent drainage. A culture of the drainage showed it to have been caused by the presence of *Staphylococcus aureus*. The infection penetrated into the patient's hip socket, destroying tissue and requiring a second operation. The court ruled that there was sufficient circumstantial evidence from which the jury could have found that the patients were infected with the same *Staphylococcus aureus* strain and that the infection was caused by the hospital's employees' failure to follow sterile techniques in ministering to its two patients.

Failure to Notify Physician

The failure of nurses to follow adequate nursing procedures in treating decubitus ulcers was found to be a factor leading to the death of a nursing facility resident in *Montgomery Health Care v. Ballard*.[19] Two nurses testified that they did not know that decubitus ulcers could be life threatening. One nurse testified that she did not know that the patient's physician should be called if there were symptoms of infection. Such allegations would indicate that there was a lack of training and supervision of the nurses who were treating the patient. The seriousness of such failure was driven home when the court allowed $2 million in punitive damages.

INAPPROPRIATE CARE

The plaintiffs in *Morris v. Children's Hospital Medical Center*[20] alleged in their complaint that, while hospitalized at Children's Hospital Medical Center, the patient suffered a laceration to her arm as a result of treatment administered by the defendants and their agents that fell below the accepted standard of care. Morris alleged from personal observation that the laceration to her daughter's arm was caused by the jagged edges of a plastic cup that had been split and placed on her arm to guard an IV site. A nurse, in her affidavit, who stated her qualifications as an expert, expressed her opinion that the practice of placing a split plastic cup over an IV site as a guard constituted a breach of the standard of nursing care.

FAILURE TO FOLLOW INSTRUCTIONS

Failure of a staff nurse to follow the instructions of a supervising nurse to wait for her assistance before performing a procedure led to the revocation of the nurse's license in *Cafiero v. North Carolina Board of Nursing.*[21] The nurse had failed to heed instructions to wait for assistance before connecting a heart monitor to an infant. The heart monitor was connected incorrectly and resulted in an electrical shock to the infant. The board of nursing, under the nursing practice act, revoked the nurse's license. The board had the authority to revoke the nurse's license even though her work before and after the incident had been exemplary. The dangers of electric cords are within the realm of common knowledge. The record showed that the nurse failed to exercise ordinary care in connecting the infant to the monitor.

FAILURE TO REPORT PHYSICIAN NEGLIGENCE

An organization can be liable for failure of nursing personnel to take appropriate action when a patient's personal physician is unavailable, unwilling, or unable to cope with a situation that threatens the life or health of the patient. In a California case, *Goff v. Doctors General Hospital,*[22] a patient was bleeding seriously after childbirth because the physician failed to suture her properly. The nurses testified that they were aware of the patient's dangerous condition and that the physician was not present in the hospital. Both nurses knew the patient would die if nothing was done, but neither contacted anyone except the physician. The hospital was liable for the nurses' negligence in failing to notify their supervisors of the serious condition that caused the patient's death. Evidence was sufficient to sustain the finding that the nurses who attended the patient and who were aware of the excessive bleeding were negligent and that their negligence was a contributing cause of the patient's death. The measure of duty of the hospital toward its patients is the exercise of that degree of care used by hospitals generally. The court held that nurses who knew that a woman they were attending was bleeding excessively were negligent in failing to report the circumstances so that prompt and adequate measures could be taken to safeguard her life.

FAILURE TO QUESTION DISCHARGE

A nurse has a duty to question the discharge of a patient if he or she has reason to believe that such discharge could be injurious to the health of the patient. Jury issues were raised in *Koeniguer v. Eckrich*[23] by expert testimony that the nurses had a duty to attempt to delay the patient's discharge if her condition warranted continued hospitalization. By permissible inferences from the evidence, the delay in treatment that resulted from the premature discharge contributed to the patient's death. Summary dismissal of this case against the hospital by a trial court was found to have been improper.

Swollen Beyond Recognition: Failure to Act

Failure to take appropriate and timely action can lead to serious lawsuits. As was the case in *NKC Hosps., Inc. v. Anthony,*[24] Mrs. Anthony was in her first pregnancy under the primary care of Dr. Hawkins, her personal physician. Mrs. Anthony was in good health, 26 years of age, employed, and about 30 weeks along in her pregnancy. On September 5, 1989, Mrs. Anthony's husband took her to the emergency department of Norton Hospital. She was experiencing nausea, vomiting, and abdominal pain. Because of her pregnancy, she was referred to the hospital's obstetrical unit. In the obstetrical unit, Mrs. Anthony came under the immediate care of Moore, a nurse, who performed an assessment.

Dr. Hawkins was called and she issued several orders, including an IV start, blood work, urinalysis, and an antinausea prescription. Later that night, a second call was made to Dr. Hawkins, giving her the test results and informing her that the patient was in extreme pain. Believing that Mrs. Anthony had a urinary tract infection, antibiotics were ordered along with an order for her discharge from the hospital.

That same night a third call was made to Dr. Hawkins because of the pain Mrs. Anthony was experiencing, as observed by Nurse Moore. Mr. Anthony also talked with Dr. Hawkins about his wife's pain. Nurse Moore became concerned about Hawkins's discharge order. Although aware of Nurse Moore's evaluation, Dr. Hawkins prescribed morphine sulfate but was unrelenting in her order of discharge.

Dr. Love, the resident physician on duty, did not see or examine the patient, although a prescription for morphine was ordered and administered pursuant to the telephoned directions of Dr. Hawkins. At approximately 2:00 a.m., the morphine was administered to Mrs. Anthony. She rested comfortably for several hours but awakened in pain again. At 6:00 a.m., the patient was discharged in pain.

During trial testimony, Hale, a nursing supervisor, admitted that it was a deviation from the standard of nursing care to discharge a patient in significant pain. Nurse Moore, who was always concerned with the patient's pain, had grave reservations about her discharge. She suggested that Dr. Love examine Mrs. Anthony. She even consulted her supervisor, Nurse Hale.

At approximately 10:00 a.m., Mrs. Anthony was readmitted to the hospital. Upon readmission, Dr. Hawkins began personal supervision of her patient. It was determined that Mrs. Anthony had a serious respiratory problem. The next day the patient was transferred to the hospital's intensive care unit (ICU).

The following day, the baby was delivered by cesarean section. It was belatedly determined at that time that Mrs. Anthony's condition was caused by a perforation of the appendix at the large bowel, a condition not detected by anyone at the hospital during her first admission. Almost three weeks later, while still in Norton Hospital, Mrs. Anthony died of acute adult respiratory distress syndrome, a complication resulting from the delay in the diagnosis and treatment of her appendicitis.

Judgment was brought against the hospital. At trial, Dr. Fields, an expert witness for the estate of Mrs. Anthony, testified that the hospital deviated from the standard of care. Every patient who presents himself or herself to the labor and delivery area, the emergency department, or any area of the hospital should be seen by a physician before anything is undertaken, and certainly before he or she is allowed to leave the institution. Further, to provide the patient with medication in the form of a prescription without the physician ever seeing the patient was below any standard of care with which Dr. Fields was acquainted. An award of more than $2 million was returned, with the apportionment of causation attributable to Dr. Hawkins as 65% and to the hospital as 35%. The hospital argued that the trial court erred in failing to grant its motions for directed verdict and for judgment notwithstanding the verdict because of the lack of substantial causation in linking the negligence of the hospital to Mrs. Anthony's death.

The Kentucky Court of Appeals found that the hospital failed to have Mrs. Anthony examined by a physician and by discharging her in pain. The hospital should have foreseen the injury to Mrs. Anthony because its own staff was questioning the judgments of Dr. Hawkins while at the same time failing to follow through with the standard of care required of it. The defense that the hospital's nurses were only following a "chain of command" by doing what Hawkins ordered is not persuasive. The nurses were not the agents of Dr. Hawkins. All involved had their independent duty to Anthony.

The evidence presented a woman conscious of her last days on earth, swollen beyond recognition, tubes exiting almost every orifice of her body, in severe pain, and who deteriorated to the point where she could not verbally communicate with loved ones. The trial court, when confronted with a motion for a new trial on excessive damages, must evaluate the award mirrored against the facts. No question, the award was monumental, but so was the injury.

FAILURE TO NOTE CHANGES IN PATIENT'S CONDITION

Nurses have the responsibility to observe the condition of patients under their care and report any pertinent findings to the attending physician. Failure to note changes in a patient's condition can lead to liability on the part of the nurse and the organization.

Failure to Recognize That the Patient Stopped Breathing

The recovery room nurse in *Eyoma v. Falco*,[25] who had been assigned to monitor a postsurgical patient, left the patient and failed to recognize that the patient stopped breathing. Nurse Falco had been assigned to monitor the patient in the recovery room. She delegated that duty to another nurse and failed to verify that the nurse accepted that responsibility.

Nurse Falco admitted she never got a verbal response from the other nurse, and when she returned there was no one near the decedent. She acknowledged that Dr. Brotherton told her to watch the decedent's breathing, but she claimed she was not told that decedent had been given narcotics. She maintained that upon her return she checked the decedent and observed his respirations to be eight per minute.

Thereafter, Brotherton returned and inquired about the decedent's condition. Falco informed the doctor that the patient was fine. However, upon his personal observation, Brotherton realized that the decedent had stopped breathing.

The decedent, because of oxygen deprivation, entered a comatose state and remained unconscious for over a year until his death.[26]

The jury held the nurse to be 100% liable for the patient's injuries. The court held that there was sufficient evidence to support the verdict.

FAILURE TO REPORT DETERIORATING CONDITION

An organization's policies and procedures should prescribe the guidelines for staff members to follow when confronted with a physician or other health care professional whose action or inaction jeopardizes the well-being of a patient. Guidelines that are in place, but not followed, are of no value, as the following cases illustrate. Such was the case in *Utter v. United Hospital Center, Inc.*[27] where the patient suffered an amputation that the jury determined resulted from the failure of the nursing staff to properly report the patient's deteriorating condition. The nursing staff, according to written procedures in the nursing manual, was responsible for reporting such changes. It was determined that deviation from hospital policy constituted negligence.

FAILURE TO REPORT PATIENT SYMPTOMS

In *Citizens Hospital Association v. Schoulin*,[28] an accident victim sued the hospital and the attending physician for their negligence in failing to discover and properly treat his injuries. The court held that there was sufficient evidence to sustain a jury verdict that the hospital's nurse was negligent in failing to inform the physician of all the patient's symptoms, to conduct a proper examination of the plaintiff, and to follow the directions of the physician. Thus, because the nurse was the employee of the hospital, the hospital was liable under the doctrine of respondeat superior.

In another case arising from the death of a hospital patient following hernia surgery, evidence supported findings that both the patient's treating physician and hospital deviated from applicable standards of care, and deviations were the cause of the patient's death. The applicable standard of care required the nurse to notify the physician if the patient complained of restlessness and had a heart rate fluctuating between 120 and 136. If the cardiologist had been called, it was probable that the patient could have been successfully treated. Hospital personnel had deviated from the standard of care when they observed bleeding from the patient and did not inform the physician, and that the physician deviated from the standard of care when he failed to call a cardiac consult for the patient. In addition, a nursing expert testified that the nurse had deviated from the standard of care when he failed to call the physician when the patient pulled off his oxygen mask and complained of difficulty breathing.[29]

TIMELY REPORTING OF PATIENT'S SYMPTOMS

In *Hiatt v. Grace*,[30] on appeal by the hospital and the nurse, the Kansas Supreme Court held that there was sufficient evidence to authorize the jury to find that the nurse was negligent in failing to timely notify the physician that delivery of the plaintiff's child was imminent. This delay resulted in an unattended childbirth with consequent injuries. The trial court awarded the plaintiff $15,000.

FAILURE TO REPORT DEFECTIVE EQUIPMENT

Failure to report defective equipment can cause a nurse to be held liable for negligence if the failure to report is the proximate cause of a patient's injuries. The defect must be known and not hidden from sight.

FAILURE TO CORRECTLY TRANSCRIBE TELEPHONE ORDERS

Failure to take correct telephone orders can be just as serious as failure to follow, understand, and/or interpret a physician's order(s). Nurses must be alert in transcribing orders because there are periodic contradictions between what physicians claim they ordered and what nurses allege they ordered. Orders should be read back after they are transcribed for verification purposes. Verification of an order by another nurse on a second telephone is helpful, especially if an order is questionable. Any questionable orders must be verified with the physician who initiated the order. Physicians must authenticate their verbal order(s) by signing the written order in the medical record. Nurses who disagree with a physician's order should not carry out an obvious erroneous order. In addition, they should confirm the order with the prescribing physician and report to the supervisor any concerns they might have with a particular order.

MISIDENTIFYING INFANTS

The inadvertent or negligent switching of infants can lead to liability for damages. Damages in the amount of $110,000 were awarded for the inadvertent switching of two babies born at the same time in *De Leon Lopez v. Corporacion Insular de Seguros*.[31]

RESTRAINTS

Standards for the application of both physical and chemical restraints have been evolving over the past decade, and they are becoming more stringent. Because of patient rights issues, injuries, and the improper and indiscreet use of restraints, organizations are attempting to develop restraint-free environments.

Failure to Follow Policy

The plaintiffs in *Estate of Hendrickson v. Genesis Health Venture, Inc.*[32] filed an action for negligence, breach of contract, and negligent infliction of emotional distress against Genesis ElderCare Network Services, Inc. (GENS), among others.

Hendrickson suffered a massive stroke while she was a patient at a hospital in the summer of 1996. The stroke left her totally dependent on others for her daily care. During one of her admissions to Salisbury Center, a nursing home, operated by the defendant GENS, Ferguson went into Hendrickson's room while making rounds and found Hendrickson dead, her head wedged between the mattress and the adjacent bed rail.

A jury found that Hendrickson's death was caused by negligence. On appeal, GENS argued that the plaintiff failed to show that it knew or should have known of the risk of injury to Hendrickson from the side rails. The North Carolina Court of Appeals disagreed, finding there was evidence tending to show that nursing assistants employed by GENS were aware that Hendrickson, on several occasions before her death on October 30, had slid to the edge of the bed and became caught between the edge of the mattress and the bed rail. Plaintiffs offered evidence showing that GENS had a restraint policy in effect that required a restraint assessment form for any resident for whom the use of restraints was required. The nursing staff was required to document the effectiveness of less restrictive measures. The assessment was required to be reviewed by a restraint alternative team/committee. Evidence was offered showing that no restraint assessment form had been completed for Hendrickson. In addition, her medical records contained no nursing notes documenting the use of less restrictive measures than the bed rails. The defendant argued that the bed rails were required for positioning and safety and were not restraints, so that no restraint assessment was required. While the evidence was conflicting as to whether the bed rails were used as a restraint or as a safety measure, evidence indicated that the rails should have been considered a restraint in connection with Hendrickson's care, as per organization policy.

The court of appeals concluded that the plaintiffs offered sufficient evidence to sustain a finding by the jury that defendant GENS was negligent in failing to conform to its own policies with respect to the use of physical restraints and that such negligence was the proximate cause of Hendrickson's death.

FAILURE TO TAKE VITAL SIGNS

Bradshaw, in *Brandon HMA, Inc. v. Bradshaw*,[33] had been admitted to Rankin Medical Center (RMC) under the care of Dr. Bobo for treatment of bacterial pneumonia. She was prescribed oxygen and various medications. A general surgeon inserted a chest tube in Bradshaw's left side to drain some fluid that accumulated. Due to the pain and discomfort associated with a chest tube, Extra Strength Tylenol and Lorcet Plus were prescribed for pain. Bobo also prescribed Ativan to relieve anxiety. During the afternoon and evening following insertion of the chest tube, two nurses periodically checked Bradshaw, took her vital signs, and noted that she exhibited "no distress." Around 11:00 p.m., Lewis, an LPN, was assigned by Nail, the floor's charge nurse, to provide care to Bradshaw. Before checking on Bradshaw, Lewis reviewed the notes and a tape left by the previous nurse that detailed Bradshaw's condition. Around midnight, Lewis made his first visit to Bradshaw's room, took her vital signs, and noted she was experiencing some pain on her left side. Sometime before 1:00 a.m., a respiratory therapist checked on Bradshaw and did not notice any problems, but did note that Bradshaw was restless. Shortly after 1:00 a.m., Lewis made his second visit to Bradshaw's room. She continued to complain of pain in her chest. Lewis, however, did not take her vital signs. He gave her an Extra Strength Tylenol and made a note indicating that the patient was complaining of pain on the left side and appeared to be in distress. At 2:00 a.m. during Lewis's next visit, Bradshaw again complained that she could not sleep and that the pain had increased. Despite her complaints, Lewis again failed to take her vital signs. Instead, he consulted Nail and administered an injection of Ativan to relieve Bradshaw's anxiety and restlessness. Forty minutes later, Bradshaw again complained of increased pain. Lewis noticed that she was sitting up in bed and her respiration had become short and rapid. Feeling that the earlier Lorcet Plus was wearing off, Lewis administered another dose. Lewis again failed to check Bradshaw's vital signs.

Nail, while in Bradshaw's room at 3:00 a.m., did not note any problems. When Lewis returned to Bradshaw's room at 3:30 a.m., her condition had significantly worsened. She was nauseous, disoriented, covered in sweat, and did not follow verbal commands. Lewis checked her vital signs and found her temperature had fallen to 95.8 degrees. Realizing the seriousness of Bradshaw's condition, Lewis left the room to find Nail. At this point, testimony among RMC's employees varies. Lewis and Washington, a nurses' aide, testified that Lewis found Nail and Washington conversing in the hallway. According to the two testimonies, Nail and Lewis discussed Bradshaw's condition and returned to the room at 3:40 a.m.

When Lewis and Nail returned to the room, they found Bradshaw was cyanotic, had stopped breathing, and had no pulse. Nail called a "code" and started cardiopulmonary resuscitation (CPR). The code team arrived and revived Bradshaw by administering epinephrine. Bradshaw was transferred to ICU where she remained comatose for 2 weeks. She was eventually transferred to a rehabilitation center for treatment. While in treatment, MRIs of Bradshaw's brain were ordered and showed evidence of brain damage due to lack of oxygen. Bradshaw's present condition as a result of the cardiopulmonary arrest and hypoxic brain damage is permanent and severe. She has significant difficulty in moving due to rigidity in her muscles and is prone to bouts of spasms. Bradshaw cannot walk without assistance and often falls due to a lack of stability. She is unable to perform many daily activities without the aid of her mother or someone else, including dressing, brushing her teeth, driving a car, and going to the bathroom.

Bradshaw filed suit against Brandon HMA, Inc., for negligent nursing care. Bradshaw alleged that nursing personnel failed to properly monitor her, report vital information to her physician, and allowed her condition to deteriorate to a critical stage before providing urgently needed care and implementing life support. The jury found in favor of Bradshaw and awarded $9 million in damages. The judge entered a final judgment on the jury verdict, and Brandon filed an appeal.

On appeal, the Supreme Court of Mississippi upheld the judgment of the circuit court. *Nine million did not seem excessive. Bradshaw will live out her years with both emotional and physical pain, and her present existence will not remotely resemble her former life.*

SURGERY: FOREIGN OBJECTS LEFT IN PATIENTS

Romero v. Bellina[34] describes how both nurses and surgeons are responsible for sponge counts. Bellina performed laser surgery on Romero at the hospital. During surgery, Bellina was assisted by Markey and Toups, surgical nurses employed by the hospital. Before the final suturing of the incision, the nurses erroneously informed Bellina that all the lap pads had been accounted for.

The day after the procedure, Romero complained of severe abdominal pain. A few months later, she discovered a mass in her abdomen near the area where the surgery was performed. She visited her treating physician, Dr. Blue, who determined through an X-ray that the mass in her abdomen was a lap sponge from the surgery with Bellina. Romero underwent corrective surgery with a different physician to remove the sponge.

The plaintiffs settled their claims with the hospital, and the case proceeded to trial against Bellina. After a bench trial, the trial court rendered judgment in favor of the plaintiffs for $170,966.41, and Bellina filed an appeal.

In ruling against Bellina, the trial court held that a surgeon's duty to remove foreign objects placed in a patient's body is an independent, nondelegable duty. The trial court found that Bellina was 70% at fault and the nurses employed by the hospital were 30% at fault. On appeal, Bellina argued that the trial judge erred in concluding that, in Louisiana, a surgeon cannot rely on surgical nurses to count sponges to make sure none are left inside a patient. Prevailing case law in Louisiana, however, holds that a surgeon has a nondelegable duty to remove all sponges placed in a patient's body.

The Louisiana Court of Appeals held that although nurses have an independent duty, apart from the surgeon's duty, to account for the sponges, and that they can be concurrently at fault with the surgeon for leaving a sponge in the patient's body, the nurses' count is a remedial measure that cannot relieve the surgeon of his or her nondelegable duty to remove the sponge in the first instance. Bellina had an independent, nondelegable duty to remove from the patient's body the foreign substance that he had placed into her.

Current jurisprudence more accurately reflects the modern team approach to surgery, whereby the nurses' count is a remedial measure that does not discharge the surgeon's independent duty to ensure that all sponges are removed before an incision is closed.

NEGLIGENT PROCEDURE: AMPUTATING INFANT'S FINGER

A nurse employed by the defendant in *Ahmed v. Children's Hospital of Buffalo*[35] amputated nearly one-third of a 1-month-old infant's index finger while cutting an IV tube with a pair of scissors. Surgery to reattach the amputated portion of the finger was unsuccessful. The plaintiffs were awarded $87,000 for past pain and suffering and $50,000 for future damages. The defendant moved to set aside the verdict and sought a new trial, claiming that damages were excessive. The trial court rejected much of the testimony presented by the plaintiffs.

An appeals court determined that it was the jury's function to assess the credibility of witnesses and to evaluate the testimony regarding the child's pain, suffering, and disability. The trial court was found to have improperly invaded the jury's province to evaluate the nature and extent of the injury. The appellate court found that the jury's award of damages did not deviate materially from what would be reasonable compensation. The jury's verdict was reinstated.

MONITOR ALARM DISCONTINUED

In *Odom v. State Department of Health and Hospitals*,[36] the appeals court held that the decedent's cause of death was directly related to the absence of being placed under the watch of a heart monitor. Jojo was born 12 weeks prematurely at the HPL Medical Center. Jojo remained in a premature infant's nursery and was eventually placed into two different foster homes prior to his admission to Pinecrest Foster Home. While Jojo was a Pinecrest resident, Mr. and Mrs. Odom adopted Jojo. He was unable to feed himself and was nourished via a gastrostomy tube. Because he suffered from obstructive apnea, he became dependent on a trach tube.

At Pinecrest, Jojo was assigned to Home 501. While making patient rounds, Ms. Means found Jojo with his trach out of the stoma. She called for help, and Ms. Wiley, amongst others, responded. Wiley immediately took the CPR efforts under her control. She noticed that Jojo was breathless and immediately reinserted the trach. She then noticed that Jojo was still hooked to a monitor.

No one had heard the heart monitor's alarm sound. Means asserts that the monitor was on because she saw that the monitor's red lights were blinking, indicating the heart rate and breathing rate. She stated that she took the monitor's leads off of Jojo to put the monitor out of the way, but the alarm did not sound. CPR efforts continued while Jojo was placed on a stretcher and sent by ambulance to HPL. Jojo was pronounced dead at HPL's emergency department at 7:02 p.m.

The Odoms filed a petition against Pinecrest, alleging that Jojo's death was caused by the negligence and fault of Pinecrest, its servants, and employees. Judgment was for the plaintiffs. The trial court's reason for judgment was enlightening because it stated that the monitor should have been on but was, however, disconnected by the staff and this was the cause, in fact, of Jojo's injury. The appeals court found that the record supported the trial court's findings. There was overwhelming evidence upon which the trial court relied to find that the monitor had been turned off, in breach of the various physicians' orders with which the nurses should have complied. The monitor was supposed to be on Jojo to warn the nurses of any respiratory distress episodes that he might experience. A forensic pathologist's report showed the cause of Jojo's death to be hypoxia, secondary to respiratory insufficiency, secondary to apnea episodes. Thus, Jojo's cause of death was directly related to the absence of being placed under the watch of a heart monitor.

CHANCE OF SURIVIVAL DIMINISHED

Mr. Ard, in *Ard v. East Jefferson Gen. Hosp.*,[37] began feeling nauseous. He was in pain and had shortness of breath. Although his wife rang the call bell several times, it was not until sometime later that evening that someone responded and administered medication for his nausea. The nausea continued to worsen. Mrs. Ard then noticed that her husband was having difficulty breathing. Believing that her husband was dying, she continued to call for help. She estimated that she rang the call bell for 1 1/4 hours before anyone responded. A code was eventually called. Unfortunately, Mr. Ard did not survive the code. There was no documentation in the medical records between 5:30 p.m. and 6:45 p.m. that would indicate any nurse or physician checked on Ard's condition. This finding collaborated Mrs. Ard's testimony regarding this time period.

A wrongful death action was filed against the hospital, and the district court granted judgment for Mrs. Ard. The hospital appealed.

Ms. Krebs, an expert in general nursing, stated that it should have been obvious to the nurses from the physicians' progress notes that the patient was a high risk for aspiration. This problem was never addressed in the nurses' care plan or in the nurses' notes.

On May 20, Ard's assigned nurse was Ms. Florscheim. Krebs stated that Florscheim did not perform a full assessment of the patient's respiratory and lung status. There was nothing in the record indicating that she completed such an evaluation after he vomited. Krebs also testified that a nurse did not conduct a swallowing assessment at any time. Although Florscheim testified that she checked on the patient around 6:00 p.m., there was no documentation in the medical record.

Ms. Farris, an expert in intensive care nursing, testified for the defense. She disagreed with Krebs that there was a breach of the standard of care. However, on cross-examination, she admitted that if a patient was in the type of distress described by Mrs. Ard and no nurse checked on him for 1 1/4 hours, that would fall below the expected standard of care. An appeals court concluded there was ample evidence to support the trial judge's conclusion that the nursing staff breached the standard of care. Ard would have had a much better chance of survival if he had been transferred to the intensive care unit. The court raised the general damages award from $50,000 to $150,000.

Notes

1. 947 S.W.2d 941 (Tex. Ct. App. 1997).
2. 856 P.2d 864 (Idaho 1993).
3. 570 N.Y.S.2d 395 (N.Y. App. Div. 1991).
4. 535 N.E.2d 956 (Ill. App. Ct. 1989).
5. 692 S.W.2d 329 (Mo. Ct. App. 1985).
6. 357 N.Y.S.2d 508 (N.Y. App. Div. 1974).
7. No. 2-153/01-1019 (Iowa Ct. of App. 2002).
8. 696 P.2d 270 (Colo. 1985).
9. 144 So. 2d 249 (La. Ct. App. 1962).
10. 599 N.Y.S.2d 96 (N.Y. App. Div. 1993).
11. 742 P.2d 1087 (Okla. 1987).
12. 145 So. 2d 848 (Fla. 1933).
13. 181 A.2d 573 (Del. 1962).
14. 443 P.2d 708 (Colo. 1968).
15. 165 S.W.3d 168 (Mo. App. 2005).
16. 696 So. 2d 590 (La. App. 1997).
17. 603 So.2d 866 (1992).
18. 381 P.2d 605 (Wash. 1963).
19. 565 So. 2d 221 (Ala. 1990).
20. 597 N.E.2d 1110 (Ohio Ct. App. 1991).
21. 403 S.E.2d 582 (N.C. Ct. App. 1991).
22. 333 P.2d 29 (Cal. Ct. App. 1958).
23. 422 N.W.2d 600 (S.D. 1988).
24. 849 S.W.2d 564 (Ky. Ct. App. 1993).
25. 589 A.2d 653 (N.J. Super. App. Div. 1991).
26. Id. at 655.
27. 236 S.E.2d 213 (W. Va. 1977).
28. 262 So. 2d 303 (Ala. 1972).
29. Leblanc v. Walsh, 922 So.2d 1248 (La. App. 2006).

30. 523 P.2d 320 (Kan. 1974).
31. 931 F.2d 116 (1st Cir. 1991).
32. 151 N.C. App. 139, 565 S.E.2d 254 (2002).
33. 809 So. 2d 611 (2001).
34. 798 So. 2d 279 (2001).
35. 661 N.Y.S.2d 164 (N.Y. App. Div. 1997).
36. 733 So. 2d 91 (La. App. 3 Cir. 1999).
37. 636 So. 2d 1042 (La. Ct. App. 1994).

10

Liability by Departments and Health Care Professionals

Dying at the Hospital's Door: A Child Lost, Troubling Questions*

While communications were breaking down among a child's parent, a 9-1-1 dispatcher, and hospital personnel, the child's condition was quickly deteriorating. Twelve hours later, the three-year-old girl was brain dead, and she expired three days later. Although there are several central issues involved in this story, the frustrating dialogue that took place is particularly important.

The 9-1-1 dispatcher answers the phone.

DISPATCHER: 9-1-1; is this an emergency?

PARENT: Yes, it's an emergency. I need an ambulance. I have a 3-year-old daughter that's passed out on me.

DISPATCHER: OK. Where do you need the ambulance?

PARENT: I'm right in front of the emergency exit in . . . Hospital.

DISPATCHER: You're right in front of the emergency exit?

PARENT: Yes, that's exactly where I am. And they won't do a . . . thing in this place.

The dispatcher phones the hospital emergency department:

DISPATCHER: There's a guy that says he's right outside your emergency exit. And he needs an ambulance. He says his 3-year-old daughter is passed out.

HOSPITAL: This is a guy who wants to be seen quicker. We're busy—so he figured if he called 9-1-1 he'd be seen quicker.

DISPATCHER: Well, he's saying he needs an ambulance right away. Is somebody going to go out there, or not?

HOSPITAL: There's nothing we can do.[1]

The parents were offered an out-of-court settlement totaling $200,000. This tragedy might have been prevented if the patient had been screened and triaged by a person competent to determine the patient's need for immediate care. Failure to assign triage responsibility to a competent individual can lead to lawsuits that involve not only the hospital, but also the supervisor who assigns responsibilities to unqualified staff members.

This chapter presents an overview of selected departments and health care professions. Health care professionals are held to the prevailing standard of care required in their profession, which includes proper assessments, reassessments, diagnosis, treatment, and follow-up care. The following legal cases have application to all health care professionals.

CHIROPRACTOR

A chiropractor is required to exercise the same degree of care, judgment, and skill exercised by other reasonable chiropractors under like or similar circumstances. He or she has a duty to determine whether a patient is treatable through chiropractic means and to refrain from chiropractic treatment when a reasonable chiropractor would or should be aware that a patient's condition will not respond to chiropractic treatment. Failure to conform to the standard of care can result in liability for any injuries suffered.

DENTISTRY

Dental malpractice cases are generally related to patients who suffer from complications of a dental procedure. They can involve the improper treatment of dental infections or complications from the improper administration of anesthesia. Complications can also include damage to the nerves of the lower jaw, face, chin, lips, and tongue. Injuries can involve high-speed drills damaging the tongue and result in permanent loss of sensation or taste.

Drill Bit Left in Tooth

The patient in *Mazor v. Isaacman*[2] visited the defendant–dentist in August 1997 for routine root canal surgery. After the surgery, the patient began experiencing constant pain in the tooth in which the root canal was performed. The dentist told the patient that such pain was ordinarily felt after root canal surgery. In February 1999, the patient visited another dentist who discovered that a piece of a drill bit had been left inside the patient's tooth during the previous root canal. The patient filed a lawsuit against the defendant–dentist for dental malpractice. The defendant–dentist filed a motion to dismiss, arguing that the patient did not bring the claim within the 1-year statute of limitations. The Tennessee Court of Appeals held that the patient had 1 year from the time she discovered or should have discovered the foreign object in which to file her lawsuit.

EMERGENCY DEPARTMENT

Emergency departments are high-risk areas that tend to be a main source of lawsuits for hospitals. The courts recognize a general duty to care for all patients presenting themselves to hospital emergency departments. Not only must hospitals accept, treat, and transfer emergency department patients if such is necessary for the patients' well-being, but they must adhere to the standards of care they have set for themselves, as well as to national standards.

Hospitals under the Emergency Medical Treatment and Active Labor Act (EMTALA) discussed on page 156 are required to provide either stabilizing treatment or appropriate transfer for patients with emergency medical conditions.

Objectives of Emergency Care

The objectives of emergency care are the same regardless of severity. No matter how seemingly trivial the complaint, each patient must be examined. Treatment must begin as rapidly as possible, function is to be maintained or restored, scarring and deformity are to be minimized. Every patient must be treated regardless of ability to pay.

> As the Sixth Circuit points out, there are many reasons other than indigence that might lead a hospital to give less than standard attention to a person who arrives at the emergency room doors. These might include: prejudice against the race, sex, or ethnic group of the patient; distaste

> for the patient's condition (e.g., acquired immune deficiency syndrome [AIDS] patients); personal dislike or antagonism between medical personnel and the patient; disapproval of the patient's occupation; or political or cultural opposition. If a hospital refuses treatment to persons for any of these reasons, or gives cursory treatment, the evil inflicted would be quite akin to that discussed by Congress in the legislative history, and the patient would fall squarely in the statutory language.[3]

No Duty to Patient Who Left

The patient and her sister became upset with the care offered and left the hospital and went home without proper discharge. The patient died 2 days later at home. The county coroner's office initiated a postmortem examination and determined that the patient died from meningoencephalitis. The patient made a conscious decision to leave the hospital on her own accord without the knowledge or permission of the hospital. She did not tell the doctors, nurses, or anyone else that she was leaving the emergency room; she just left the emergency room without informing anyone.

In a wrongful death medical malpractice action alleging negligence, the trial court properly granted summary judgment because under Ohio law, an emergency room nurse had no duty to interfere with an individual who left the emergency room without telling anyone and who refused treatment.[4]

Failure to Admit

Roy went to the emergency department complaining of chest pains. The attending physician, Dr. Gupta, upon examination, performed an electrocardiogram that showed ischemic changes indicating a lack of oxygen to the heart tissue. He applied a transdermal nitroglycerin patch and gave Roy a prescription for nitroglycerin. After monitoring her progress, he sent her home. Several hours later, she returned to the emergency department, experiencing more chest pains. Three days later, Roy died of a massive myocardial infarction.

Gupta was found negligent in failing to hospitalize Roy. The trial court found that had Roy been hospitalized on her first visit, her chances of survival would have been increased. On appeal, the Louisiana Court of Appeal held that Gupta was negligent by failing to advise Roy that she should be hospitalized for chest pains. All of the medical expert witnesses, except Dr. Kilpatrick, a defense witness, testified that Roy should have been admitted. Kilpatrick testified that such a decision varied greatly among physicians. The trial court disregarded his testimony because of his hostile responses to questioning.

The trial judge was not convinced by Gupta's explanation of why Roy was not hospitalized. He focused on Gupta's failure to have X-rays taken during the first visit, which might have allowed him to determine whether the ischemic changes were due to her hypertension medication or indicated the beginning of a heart attack. The relative simplicity of the technique and its obvious availability lent credence to the trial judge's belief that the requisite attention was not paid to Roy's complaints. The law does not require proof that proper treatment would have been the difference between Roy's living or dying. It requires only proof that proper treatment would have increased her chances of survival.[5]

Documentation Sparse and Contradictory

An ambulance team found 26-year-old Feeney intoxicated, sitting on a street corner in South Boston. Feeney admitted to alcohol abuse but denied that he used drugs. His condition interfered with conducting an examination, and he was transported by ambulance to the hospital.

Documentation at the hospital between 10:45 p.m. and 11:30 p.m. was sparse and contradictory. The minimum standard for nursing care required monitoring the patient's respiratory rate every 15 minutes. It was doubtful that this occurred. This monitoring would have more likely permitted the nursing staff to observe changes in the patient's breathing patterns and/or the onset of respiratory arrest. The emergency department physician failed to evaluate the patient and to initiate care within the first few minutes of Feeney's entry into the emergency facility. The emergency physician had an obligation to determine who was waiting for physician care and how critical the need was for that care. Had the standards been maintained, respiratory arrest might have been averted. According to the autopsy report, respiratory arrest was the sole cause of death.

The failure to provide adequate care rationally could be attributed to the staff nurse assigned to the area in which the patient lay, as well as to the physicians in charge. The hospital was implicated on the basis of the acts or omission of its staff.[6]

Emergency Medical Treatment Under EMTALA

In 1986, Congress passed the Emergency Medical Treatment and Active Labor Act (EMTALA) that forbids Medicare-participating hospitals from "dumping" patients out of emergency departments. The act provides that:

> [i]n the case of a hospital that has a hospital emergency department, if any individual . . . comes to the emergency department and a request is made on the individual's behalf for examination or treatment for a medical condition, the hospital must provide for an appropriate medical screening examination within the capability of the hospital emergency department, including ancillary services routinely available to the emergency department, to determine whether or not an emergency medical condition . . . exists.[7]

Under EMTALA, hospital emergency rooms are subject to two principal obligations, commonly referred to as (1) the appropriate medical screening requirement and (2) the stabilization requirement. The appropriate medical screening requirement obligates hospital emergency rooms to provide an appropriate medical screening to any individual seeking treatment to determine whether the individual has an emergency medical condition. If an emergency medical condition exists, the hospital is required to provide stabilization treatment before transferring the individual.

Stabilizing the Patient

Patients can be transferred only after they have been medically screened by a physician, stabilized, and cleared for transfer by the receiving institution. Stabilized means "with respect to an emergency medical condition . . . to provide such medical treatment of the condition as may be necessary to assure, within reasonable medical probability, that no material deterioration of the condition is likely to result from or to occur during the transfer of the individual from a facility."[8]

Transfer Prior to Stabilizing Patient

The plaintiff in *Huckaby v. East Ala. Med. Ctr.*[9] brought an action against the hospital alleging that the patient was transferred from the hospital's emergency department before her condition was stabilized. The patient went to the hospital, suffering from a stroke. The complaint alleged that the patient's condition was critical and materially deteriorating. The attending emergency department physician, Dr. Wheat, informed the patient's family that she needed the services of a neurosurgeon but that the hospital had problems in getting neurosurgeons to accept patients. Upon the recommendation of Wheat, the patient was transferred to another hospital where she expired soon after arrival. The plaintiff alleged that Wheat did not inform the family regarding the risks of transfer and that the transfer of the patient in an unstable condition was the proximate cause of her death. The US District Court held that the plaintiff stated a cause of action under EMTALA for which monetary relief could be granted.

Inappropriate Transfer

In *Burditt v. U.S. Department of Health and Human Services*,[10] EMTALA was violated by Dr. Burditt, a physician, when he ordered a woman with dangerously high blood pressure (210/130) and in active labor with ruptured membranes to be transferred from the emergency department of one hospital to another hospital 170 miles away. The physician was assessed a penalty of $20,000. Dr. Louis Sullivan, secretary of the Department of Health and Human Services at that time, issued this statement:

> This decision sends a message to physicians everywhere that they need to provide quality care to everyone in need of emergency treatment who comes to a hospital. This is a significant opinion and we are pleased with the result.[11]

The American Public Health Association, in filing an amicus curiae, advised the appeals court that if Burditt wants to ensure that he will never be asked to treat a patient not of his choosing, then he ought to vote with his feet by affiliating only with hospitals that do not accept Medicare funds or do not have an emergency department.

Wrong Record—Fatal Mistake

Dr. McManus had not realized that he had made a grave and fatal mistake. Dr. McManus had looked at the wrong chart . . . .

Terry Trahan, in *Trahan v. McManus*,[12] was taken to the hospital after being injured in an automobile accident. Terry's parents were informed about the accident and asked to come to the hospital. Mrs. Trahan drove to the hospital and consulted with Dr. McManus, the emergency department physician who treated Terry. Dr. McManus assured Mrs. Trahan that it would be all right to take her son home because there was nothing more that could be done for him at the hospital.

Upon ordering discharge, however, Dr. McManus had not realized that he had made a grave and fatal mistake. Dr. McManus had looked at the wrong chart in determining Terry's status. Dr. McManus had looked at a chart that indicated that the patient's vital signs were normal. In fact, the correct chart showed that Terry had three broken ribs as a result of the accident. His blood pressure was 90/60 when he was admitted to the emergency department. Forty-five minutes after being admitted, Terry's blood pressure had dropped to 80/50, and his respiration rate had doubled. Terry's vital signs clearly indicated that he was suffering from internal hemorrhaging.

In the 7 hours following his discharge, Terry's condition continued to worsen. Terry complained to his parents about severe pain. He could not turn from his back to his side without the aid of his father. Several hours after being brought home from the hospital, Mr. Trahan noticed that Terry's abdomen was swelling. Mrs. Trahan immediately called the hospital. Mr. Trahan asked Terry if he wanted to sit up. Terry replied, "Well, we can try." Those were Terry's final words. Terry slumped in his father's arms and his head fell forward. When Mr. Trahan attempted to lift Terry's head, Terry's face was white. Mr. Trahan immediately laid his son down on the bed, realizing for the first time that his son was not breathing and had no pulse. He attempted CPR as Mrs. Trahan called for an ambulance. Mr. Trahan continued CPR until the ambulance arrived a few minutes later. Terry was pronounced dead on arrival at the hospital.

Subsequently, during a medical review panel proceeding in which the Trahans participated, Dr. McManus admitted liability by tendering his $100,000 limit of liability, pursuant to the Medical Malpractice Act.

A jury returned a verdict absolving Dr. McManus of any liability, finding that Terry's injuries would have occurred despite the physician's failure to use reasonable care in his treatment of Terry. The Trahans appealed. On appeal, the jury's determination was found to be clearly erroneous when it concluded that the physician's actions were not the cause-in-fact of Terry's death. The record is replete with testimony, including Dr. McManus's own admissions, that he acted negligently when he discharged Terry, that his actions led to Terry's death, and that there was treatment available that could have made a difference.

Duty to Contact On-Call Physician

Hospitals are expected to notify specialty on-call physicians when their particular skills are required in the emergency department. A physician who is on call and fails to respond to a request to attend a patient can be liable for injuries suffered by the patient because of his or her failure to respond.

Timely Response Required

Hospitals are not only required to care for emergency patients, but they also are required to do so in a timely fashion. In *Marks v. Mandel*,[13] a Florida trial court was found to have erred in directing a verdict against the plaintiff. It was decided that the relevant inquiry in this case was whether the hospital and the supervisor should bear ultimate responsibility for failure of the specialty on-call system to function properly. Jury issues had been raised by evidence that the standard for on-call systems was to have a specialist attending the patient within a reasonable time period of being called.

Failure to Contact On-Call Physician

In *Thomas v. Corso*,[14] a patient had been brought to the hospital emergency department after he was struck by a car. A physician did not attend to him even though he had dangerously low blood pressure and was in shock. There was some telephone contact between the nurse in the emergency department and the physician who was providing on-call coverage. The physician did not act upon the hospital's call for assistance until the patient was close to death. Expert testimony was not necessary to establish what common sense made evident: the patient who was struck by a car may have suffered internal injuries and should have been evaluated and treated by a physician. Lack of attention in such cases is not reasonable care by any standard. The concurrent negligence of the nurse, who failed to contact the on-call physician after the patient's condition worsened, did not relieve the physician of liability for his failure to respond to his on-call duty. Because of the nurse's negligence, the hospital is liable under the doctrine of respondeat superior.

Failure to Respond to Call

Treatment rendered by hospitals is expected to be commensurate with that available in the same or similar communities or in hospitals generally. In *Fjerstad v. Knutson*,[15] the South Dakota Supreme Court found that a hospital could be held liable for the failure of an on-call physician to respond to a call from the emergency department. An intern who attempted to contact the on-call physician and was unable to do so for 3½ hours treated and discharged the patient. The hospital was responsible for assigning on-call physicians and ensuring that they would be available when called. The patient died during the night in a motel room as a result of asphyxia resulting from a swelling of the larynx, tonsils, and epiglottis that blocked the trachea. Testimony indicated that the emergency department's on-call physician was to be available for consultation and was assigned that duty by the hospital. Expert testimony also was offered that someone with the decedent's symptoms should have been hospitalized and that such care could have saved the decedent's life. The jury believed that an experienced physician would have taken the necessary steps to save the decedent's life.

Notice of Inability to Respond to Call

In *Millard v. Corrado*,[16] the Missouri Appellate Court found that on-call physicians owe a duty to provide reasonable notice when they will be unavailable to respond to calls. Physicians who cannot fulfill their on-call responsibilities must provide notice as soon as practicable when they learn of the circumstances that will render them unavailable. Imposing a duty on on-call physicians to notify hospital staff of their unavailability does not place an unreasonable burden. In this case, a mere telephone call would have significantly reduced the 4-hour time period between an accident and life-saving surgery. Whatever slight inconvenience may be associated with notifying the hospital of the on-call physician's availability is trivial when compared to the substantial risk to patients.

Telephone Medicine Costly

The diagnosis and treatment of patients by telephone can be costly. As noted in *Futch v. Attwood*,[17] the record shows that on the morning of February 28, 1990, Lauren, a 4-year-old diabetic child, awoke her mother, Wanda. She had vomited two or three times and her glucose reading was high. Wanda administered Lauren's morning insulin and intended to feed her a light breakfast before bringing her to see Dr. Attwood, a pediatrician, at about 9:45 a.m. According to the plaintiff, Attwood did not check Lauren's blood sugar level or her urine to determine whether ketones were present. If Attwood had done so, Lauren's condition could have been quickly corrected by the simple administration of insulin. Instead of administering insulin, however, Attwood prescribed the use of Phenergan suppositories to address Lauren's symptoms. Lauren's symptoms of nausea continued, and she was taken to the hospital emergency department. The hospital personnel contacted Attwood. Attwood returned the call and again prescribed a Phenergan injection. Attwood did not go to the hospital and had not been given Lauren's vital signs when he suggested such an injection, and he further failed to order any blood or urine tests.

Wanda returned home with Lauren at approximately 8:00 p.m. and put her to bed, waking her around midnight to administer the prescribed medication. Lauren woke but went back to sleep. Early the next morning, Wanda awoke and found Lauren with labored breathing. While attempting to wake up the 4-year-old, the only responses, according to plaintiff's brief, were "huh" followed by moaning. Wanda telephoned Attwood and informed him of her daughter's far-worsened condition. Attwood admitted Lauren to the hospital at 6:30 a.m. that morning.

Hospital records revealed that Lauren's glucose level was 507 at the time of admission with her blood acid revealing diabetic ketoacidosis. At approximately 9:13 a.m., Lauren went into respiratory arrest as a result of her brain swelling with rupturing into the opening at the base of her neck. Lauren was immediately transported by helicopter to Children's Hospital in New Orleans and diagnosed with ketoacidotic coma, cerebral edema, and bilateral pulmonary edema. She was pronounced dead at 5:07 p.m. on March 2, 1990.

The mother witnessed her daughter's decline in health, and her protracted wait was punctuated only by various traumatic episodes: Lauren's respiratory intubation; her respiratory failure and consequent code blue; numerous medical staff scurrying in and out to see Lauren behind doors closed to Wanda; and, finally, Wanda's being asked to consider whether she would prefer to "pull the plug" on her daughter or to watch her linger indefinitely. Wanda decided to let her go and did. For Wanda, the period following Lauren's death has been marked by the inevitable sense of loss of a daughter and by the guilt of a mother whose unrelenting loss compels her to ask what she might have done differently to save her child's life.

Prevention of Lawsuits in the Emergency Department

Emergency department lawsuits can be reduced by implementing and enforcing some fundamental commonsense policies, procedures, and programs by:

- treating each patient courteously and promptly
- treating all patients regardless of ability to pay
- triaging and treating seriously ill patients first
- establishing an on-call list for specialists
- requiring consultations when determined necessary
- communicating with the patient and the patient's family to ensure that a complete and accurate picture of the patient's symptoms and complaints is obtained
- ensuring all caregivers are effectively communicating with one another
- providing continuing education programs for all staff members
- not taking lightly any patient's complaint (this may well be the single most fatal mistake in emergency departments)
- accepting the concept that all patients, regardless of ailment, must receive care
- requiring that hospitals determine what types of patients and levels of care they can safely address
- knowing when to admit or transfer a patient

Emergency Rooms Vital to Public Safety

McBride, in *Simmons v. Tuomey Regional Medical Center*,[18] was involved in an accident while driving his moped. Upon learning of the accident, Simmons, McBride's daughter, rushed to the scene, where she found emergency service personnel attending to an injury to the back of her father's head. McBride was taken to Tuomey where Simmons signed an admission form for her father. The admission form contained the following provision:

> The Physicians Practicing in this Emergency Room are not Employees of the Tuomey Regional Medical Center. They are Independent Physicians, as are All Physicians Practicing in this Hospital.

While in Tuomey's emergency department, Drs. Cooper and Anderson examined McBride. Despite McBride's confused state, the physicians decided to treat his contusions and release him from the hospital. The physicians, apparently attributing McBride's confusion to intoxication, did not treat his head injury.

The next day, McBride returned to Tuomey where his head injury was diagnosed as a subdural hematoma. Ultimately, McBride was transported to Richland Memorial Hospital. Approximately 6 weeks later, McBride died of complications from the hematoma.

When Simmons brought suit, Tuomey moved for summary judgment by alleging that it was not liable because the physicians were independent contractors. Tuomey relied on its June 1987 contract with Coastal Physicians Services, which set forth the procedures by which Coastal would provide emergency department physicians to Tuomey. The carefully worded contract referred numerous times to physicians as independent contractors and stated that Tuomey agreed not to exercise any control over the means, manner, or methods by which any Physician supplied by Coastal carries out his duties. The trial court accorded great weight to the Coastal–Tuomey contract when it granted Tuomey's motion for summary judgment. Simmons appealed, arguing that the trial court erred in granting summary judgment on the issues of actual agency, apparent agency, and nondelegable duty.

Few things are more comforting in today's society than knowing that immediate medical care is available around the clock at any hospital. As the Texas Court of Appeals astutely observed:

> Emergency rooms are aptly named and vital to public safety. There ex-

ists no other place to find immediate medical care. The dynamics that drive paying patients to a hospital's emergency rooms are known well. Either a sudden injury occurs, a child breaks his arm or an individual suffers a heart attack, or an existing medical condition worsens, a diabetic lapses into a coma, demanding immediate medical attention at the nearest emergency room. The catch phrase in legal nomenclature, "time is of the essence," takes on real meaning. Generally, one cannot choose to pass by the nearest emergency room, and after arrival, it would be improvident to depart in hope of finding one that provides services through employees rather than independent contractors.[19]

The public not only relies on the medical care rendered by emergency departments, but it also considers the hospital as a single entity providing all of its medical services. A set of commentators observed:

> [T]he hospital itself has come to be perceived as the provider of medical services. According to this view, patients come to the hospital to be cured, and the doctors who practice there are the hospital's instrumentalities, regardless of the nature of the private arrangements between the hospital and the physician. Whether or not this perception is accurate seemingly matters little when weighed against the momentum of changing public perception and attendant public policy.[20]

Public reliance and public perceptions, as well as the regulations imposed on hospitals, have created an absolute duty for hospitals to provide competent medical care in their emergency departments. Hospitals contributed to the shift in public perception through commercial advertisements. By actively soliciting business, hospitals effectively removed themselves from the sterile world of altruistic agencies. The Alaska Supreme Court, the first American court to recognize a nondelegable duty in the hospital context, wrote:

> Not only is [finding a nondelegable duty] consonant with the public perception of the hospital as a multifaceted health care facility responsible for the quality of medical care and treatment rendered, it also treats tort liability in the medical arena in a manner that is consistent with the commercialization of American medicine.[21]

Given the cumulative public policies surrounding the operation of emergency departments and the legal requirement that hospitals provide emergency services, hospitals must be accountable in tort for the actions of caregivers who work in their emergency departments. The court in this case agreed with a New York court, which wrote:

> In this Court's opinion it is public policy, and not traditional rules of the law of agency or the law of torts, which should underlie the decision to hold hospitals liable for malpractice which occurs in their emergency rooms. In this regard the observation of former U.S. Supreme Court Justice Oliver Wendell Holmes is apt: "The true grounds of decision are consideration of policy and of social advantage, and it is vain to suppose that solutions can be attained merely by logic and the general propositions of law which nobody disputes. Propositions as to public policy rarely are unanimously accepted, and still more rarely, if ever, are capable of unanswerable proof."[22]

The appeals court in Tuomey held that hospitals have a nondelegable duty to render competent service to the patients of their emergency departments.

LABORATORY

An organization must provide for clinical laboratory services to meet the needs of its patients. Each health care organization is responsible for the quality and timeliness of the services provided. Because it is often necessary to contract out certain tests, the organization should be sure that it is contracting for services with a reputable licensed laboratory.

An organization's laboratory provides data that are vital to a patient's treatment. Among its many functions, the laboratory monitors therapeutic ranges, measures blood levels for toxicity, places and monitors instrumentation on patient units, provides education for the nursing staff (e.g., glucose monitoring), provides valuable data utilized in research studies, provides data on the most effective and economical antibiotic for treating patients, serves in a consultation role, and provides valuable data as to the nutritional needs of patients.

Failure to Follow Recommended Transfusion Protocol

Fowler, in *Fowler v. Bossano*,[23] gave birth to twins on March 26, 1996. Due to premature birth, the twins were transferred to LCMH and were cared for by Bossano, a neonatologist. The infants experienced complications and problems associated with premature birth, including respiratory and feeding difficulties. The twins' treatment included blood transfusions. Bossano stated that the twins proceeded through these difficulties and began to make progress, but then Ryan (one of the twins) took a turn for the worse. According to Bossano, Ryan's condition generally continued to deteriorate until he died on May 25. Bossano stated that the most likely cause of death was a viral infection. At his urging, an autopsy was performed, and the pathologist found the presence of cytomegalovirus inclusion (CMV) disease. Bossano stated that he learned that the lab at the hospital did not, at that time, screen for the presence of the virus in the blood used for transfusions.

The Fowlers filed suit naming both Bossano and the hospital as defendants. They sought damages associated with a survival action and those for wrongful death.

The jury found for the plaintiffs. LCMH breached the applicable standard of care by failing to test the blood used for this transfusion for CMV. The evidence presented was sufficient to support the jury's determination that the hospital's breach of the standard of care was the cause of Ryan's death.

Mismatched Blood

A laboratory technician in *Barnes Hospital v. Missouri Commission on Human Rights*[24] had been discharged because of inferior work performance. On three occasions, the employee allegedly mismatched blood. The employee filed a complaint with the Commission on Human Rights, alleging racial discrimination as a reason for his discharge by the hospital. The hospital appealed, and the circuit court reversed the commission's order. The technician appealed to the Missouri Supreme Court, which held that the evidence did not support the ruling of racial discrimination by the Missouri Commission on Human Rights.

Lost Chance of Survival: Changes in Pap Smear

The patient had several gynecological examinations, including Pap smears, in 1977, 1978, 1980, 1984, 1986, and 1987. The patient's physician performed the examinations. Specimens for the Pap test were submitted to a laboratory for evaluation. The laboratory procedure included a clerk who assigned each specimen a number when it was received. A cytotechnologist would then screen the specimen. If the specimen was determined to be abnormal, it would be marked for review by a pathologist. Out of the Pap tests that were determined to be normal, only 1 in 10 was actually viewed by a pathologist. The pathologist made recommendations based on the classification of the Pap tests. A biopsy would be recommended if the Pap test was determined to be Class IV.

Except for the Pap test in 1987, which showed premalignant cellular changes, all of the patient's other Pap tests were determined to be negative. In 1986, the laboratory made a notation to the patient's physician that "moderate inflammation" was present. The patient's physician, who was treating her with antibiotics for a foot inflammation, thought that the medication would also treat the other inflammation. In September 1987, the patient returned to her physician complaining of pain, erratic periods, and tiredness. After completing a physical, her physician took a Pap test, which he sent to the laboratory. He also referred her to a gynecologist. The pathologist recommended a biopsy. Biopsies and further physical examinations revealed squamous cell carcinoma that had spread to her pelvic bones. Her Pap tests were reexamined by the laboratory, which reported that the 1986 smear showed that malignancy was highly likely. The patient was referred to the University of Minnesota to determine whether she was a viable candidate for radiation treatment. The cancer, however, had spread, and the patient was not considered a candidate for radiation treatment because she had no chance of survival. When the university reviewed all of the available slides, they found cellular changes back to 1984.

The patient sued in 1988, alleging that the laboratory failed to detect and report cellular changes in her Pap tests in time to prevent the spread of the cancer. Before trial, the patient died. Her husband and sister were substituted as plaintiffs, and the complaint was amended to include a wrongful death action. After trial, a jury awarded $3.7 million in damages, which were reduced to $1 million by the circuit court. The jury found against the laboratory, and the laboratory appealed.

The South Dakota Supreme Court upheld the jury verdict and restored the $3.7 million damage award. The court determined that evidence relating to negligence claims pertaining to Pap tests taken more than 2 years before filing the action were admissible because the patient had a continuing relationship with the clinical laboratory as a result of her physician submitting her Pap tests to the laboratory over a period of time.[25]

MEDICAL ASSISTANT

The medical assistant is an unlicensed person who provides administrative, clerical, and/or technical support to a licensed practitioner. A licensed practitioner is generally required to be physically present in the treatment facility, medical office, or ambulatory facility when a medical assistant is performing procedures. Employment of medical assistants is expected to grow much faster than the average for all occupations as the health services industry expands. This growth is due in part to technological advances in medicine and a growing and aging population. Increasing use of medical assistants in the rapidly growing health care industry will most likely result in continuing employment growth for the occupation.

Medical assistants work in physicians' offices, clinics, nursing homes, and ambulatory care settings. The duties of medical assistants vary from office to office, depending on the location and size of the practice and the practitioner's specialty. In small practices, medical assistants usually are generalists, handling both administrative and clinical duties. Those in large practices tend to specialize in a particular area, under supervision. Administrative duties often include answering telephones, greeting patients, updating and filing patients' medical records, filling out insurance forms, handling correspondence, scheduling appointments, arranging for hospital admission and laboratory services, and handling billing and bookkeeping. Clinical duties vary according to state law and include assisting in taking medical histories, recording vital signs, explaining treatment procedures to patients, preparing patients for examination, and assisting the practitioner during examinations.

Poor Communications

In 1987, the patient–plaintiff in *Follett v. Davis*[26] had her first office visit with Dr. Davis. In the spring of 1988, the plaintiff discovered a lump in her right breast and made an appointment to see Davis; however, the clinic had no record of her appointment. The clinic's employees directed her to radiology for a mammogram. The plaintiff was not offered an examination by Davis or any other physician at the clinic, and she was not scheduled for an examination as a follow-up to the mammogram. A technician examined the plaintiff's breast and confirmed the presence of a lump in her right breast. After the mammogram, clinic employees told her that she would hear from Davis if there were any problems with her mammogram.

The radiologist explained in his deposition that the mammogram was not normal. Davis reviewed the mammogram report and considered it to be negative for malignancy. He was unaware about the lump in the patient's breast, and there was no evidence that clinic employees informed him about it. The clinic, including Davis, never contacted the plaintiff about her lump or the mammogram. On April 6, 1990, the plaintiff called the clinic and was told that there was nothing to worry about unless she heard from Davis. On September 24, 1990, the plaintiff returned to the clinic after she had developed pain associated with the lump. A mammogram performed on that day gave results consistent with cancer. Three days later, Davis made an appointment for the plaintiff with a clinic surgeon for a biopsy and treatment. Davis subsequently transferred her care to other physicians. In October 1990, the biopsy confirmed the diagnosis of cancer. In August 1992, the plaintiff filed her complaint.

NUTRITIONAL SERVICES

Health care organizations are expected to provide patients with diets that meet their individual needs. Failure to do so can lead to negligence suits. The daughter of the deceased in *Lambert v. Beverly Enterprises, Inc.*[27] filed an action claiming that her father had been mistreated. The deceased allegedly suffered malnutrition as a direct result of the acts or omissions of personnel, and that the plaintiff's father suffered actual damages that included substantial medical expenses and mental anguish due to the injuries he sustained. A motion to dismiss the case was denied.

PARAMEDIC

Many states have enacted legislation that provides civil immunity to paramedics who render emergency lifesaving services. In *Riffe v. Vereb Ambulance Service, Inc.*,[28] a wrongful death action was filed by appellants against Vereb Ambulance Service, St. Francis Hospital, and Custozzo. The complaint alleged that, while responding to an emergency call, defendant Custozzo, an emergency medical technician employed by Vereb, began administering lidocaine to Anderson as ordered over the telephone by the medical command physician at the defendant hospital. While en route to the hospital, Anderson was administered lidocaine 44 times the normal dosage. Consequently, normal heart function was not restored, and Anderson was pronounced dead at the hospital shortly thereafter.

The superior court held that the liability of medical technicians could not be imputed to the hospital. The court noted the practical impossibility of the hospital carrying ultimate responsibility for the quality of care and treatment given patients by emergency medical services (EMS).

The deceased's parents in *Lemann v. Essen Lane Daiquiris*[29] filed a wrongful death action after paramedics failed to transport their son to the hospital for evaluation after they had treated him following a fight in the parking lot of a bar. It was determined that the parents failed to establish that the paramedics breached their duty to care when they did not transport their son to the hospital. Police officers at the scene testified that the deceased was intoxicated and had slurred speech and erratic behavior. Paramedics testified that they found him to be alert and oriented. In addition he twice refused to be transported to the hospital and signed a waiver form that acknowledged his refusal to the paramedics to transport him to the hospital.

PHARMACY

Because of the immense variety and complexity of medications now available, it is practically impossible for nurses or doctors to keep up with the information required for safe medication use. The pharmacist has become an essential resource in modern hospital practice.[30]

Among the nonoperative adverse events, medication errors are considered to be a leading cause of medical injury in the United States. Antibiotics, chemotherapeutic drugs, and anticoagulants are the three categories of drugs responsible for many drug-related adverse events. The prevention of medication errors requires recognition of common causes and the development of practices to help reduce the incidence of errors. With thousands of drugs, many of which look alike and sound alike, it is understandable why medication errors are so common. The following listing describes some of the more common types of medication errors:

- prescription errors include: wrong patient; wrong drug; wrong dose; wrong route; wrong frequency; transcription errors (often due to illegible handwriting and improper use of abbreviations); and inadequate review of medication for appropriateness
- dispensing errors include: improper preparation of medication; failure to properly formulate medications; dispensing expired medications; mislabeling containers; delivering the wrong dosages to floor stock; and misinterpretation of the physician's order
- administration errors include: wrong patient; wrong route; double dosing (drug administered more than once); failure to administer medications; wrong frequency; administering discontinued drugs; administering drugs without an authorized order; wrong dose (e.g., IV rate); documentation errors; transcription errors (often due to illegible handwriting and improper use of abbreviations); inaccurate transcription to medication administration record (MAR); charted but not administered; administered but not documented on the MAR; discontinued order not noted on the MAR; and medication wasted and not recorded

The practice of pharmacy essentially includes preparing, compounding, dispensing, and retailing medications. These activities may be carried out only by a pharmacist with a state license or by a person who is exempted from the provisions of a state's pharmacy statutes. The entire stock of drugs in a pharmacy is subject to strict government regulation and control. The pharmacist is responsible for developing, coordinating, and supervising all pharmacy activities and reviewing the drug regimens of each patient.

Controlled Substances Act

The Comprehensive Drug Abuse Prevention and Control Act of 1970, commonly known as the Controlled Substances Act (CSA), replaced virtually all preexisting federal laws dealing with narcotics, depressants, and stimulants.

> The CSA places all substances that are regulated under existing federal law into one of five schedules. This place-

ment is based upon the substance's medicinal value, harmfulness, and potential for abuse or addiction. Schedule I is reserved for the most dangerous drugs that have no recognized medical use, while Schedule V is the classification used for the least dangerous drugs. The act also provides a mechanism for substances to be controlled, added to a schedule, decontrolled, removed from control, rescheduled, or transferred from one schedule to another.[31]

Federal Food, Drug and Cosmetic Act

The Federal Food, Drug and Cosmetic Act (FDCA) applies to drugs and devices carried in interstate commerce and to goods produced and distributed in federal territory. The act's requirements apply to almost every drug that would be dispensed from a pharmacy because nearly all drugs and devices, or their components, are eventually carried in interstate commerce.

Section 502 of the act sets forth the information that must appear on the labels or the labeling of drugs and devices. The label must contain, among other special information: (1) the name and place of business of the manufacturer, packer, or distributor; (2) the quantity of contents; (3) the name and quantity of any ingredient found to be habit forming, along with the statement "Warning—may be habit-forming"; (4) the established name of the drug or its ingredients; (5) adequate directions for use; (6) adequate warnings and cautions concerning conditions of use; and (7) special precautions for packaging.

The regulation implementing the labeling requirements of Section 502 exempts prescription drugs from the requirement that the label bear "adequate directions for use for laymen" if the drug is in the possession of a pharmacy or under the custody of a practitioner licensed by law to administer or prescribe legend drugs.[32] This particular exemption applies only to prescription drugs meeting the other requirements. Ordinary household remedies in the custody or possession of a practitioner or pharmacist would not fall under the labeling exemption.

If the drug container is too small to bear a label with all the required information, the label may contain only the quantity or proportion of each active ingredient and the lot or control number. The prescription legend may appear on the outer container of such drug units. The lot or control number may appear on the crimp of a dispensing tube, and the remainder of the required label information may appear on other labeling within the package.

Besides the label itself, each legend drug must be accompanied by labeling, on or within the sealed package from which the drug is to be dispensed, bearing full prescribing information including indications; dosage; routes, methods, and frequency of administration; contraindications; side effects; precautions; and any other information concerning the intended use of the drug necessary for the prescriber to use the drug safely. This information usually is contained in what is known in the trade as the package insert.

State Regulations

Besides federal laws affecting the manufacture, use, and handling of drugs, the different states have controlling legislation. All states regulate the practice of pharmacy, as well as the operation of pharmacies. State regulations generally provide that: (1) each health care organization must ensure the availability of pharmaceutical services to meet the needs of patients; (2) pharmaceutical services must be provided in accordance with all applicable federal and state laws and regulations; (3) pharmaceutical services must be provided under the supervision of a pharmacist; (4) space and equipment must be provided within the organization for the proper storage, safeguarding, preparation, dispensing, and administration of drugs; (5) each organization must develop and implement written policies and procedures regarding accountability, distribution, and assurance of quality of all drugs; and (6) each organization must develop and follow current written procedures for the safe prescription and administration of drugs.

State laws require that pharmacies be licensed and that they be under the supervision of a person licensed to practice pharmacy. The pharmacist usually can be either an employee of the organization or a consultant. The authority of an organization to operate a pharmacy is conditioned on compliance with licensing requirements affecting the pharmacy premises and its personnel. The statutes applying to pharmacies usually empower regulatory agencies, such as the state pharmacy board, to issue rules and regulations as necessary.

Dispensing and Administration of Drugs

The *dispensing of medications* is the processing of a drug for delivery or for administration to a patient pursuant to the order of an appropriately licensed health care practitioner. It consists of checking the directions on the label with the directions on the prescription to determine accuracy; selecting the drug from stock to fill the order; counting, measuring, compounding, or preparing the drug; placing the drug in the proper container; and adding to a written prescription any required notations.

The *administration of a medication* is an act in which a single dose of a prescribed drug is given to a patient by an authorized person in accordance with federal and state laws and regulations. The complete act of administration includes removing an individual dose from a previously dispensed, properly labeled container (including a unit-dose container), verifying it with the physician's order, giving the individual dose to the proper patient, and recording the time and dose given.

Each dose of a drug administered must be recorded on the patient's clinical records. A separate record of narcotic drugs must be maintained. In the event that an emergency arises requiring the immediate administration of a particular drug, the patient's record should be documented properly, showing the necessity for administration of the drug on an emergency basis. Procedures should be in place for handling emergency situations.

Storage of Drugs

Drugs must be stored in their original containers and must be labeled properly. The label should indicate the patient's full name, physician, prescription number, strength of the drug, expiration date of all time-dated drugs, and the address and telephone number of the pharmacy dispensing the drug. The medication containers must be stored in a locked cabinet at the nurses' station. Medications containing narcotics or other dangerous drugs must be stored under double lock (e.g., a locked box within the medicine cabinet). The keys to the medicine cabinet and narcotics box must be in the possession of authorized personnel. Medications for external use only must be marked clearly and kept separate from medications for internal use. Medications that are to be taken out of use must be disposed of according to federal and state laws and regulations.

Hospital Formulary

Health care organizations use a formulary system, whereby physicians and pharmacists create a formulary listing of drugs used in the institution. The formulary contains the brand names and generic names of drugs. Under the formulary system, a physician agrees that his or her prescription, which calls for a brand-name drug, may be filled with the generic equivalent of that drug (i.e., a drug that contains the same active ingredients in the same proportions).

Expanding Role of the Pharmacist

Historically, the role of the pharmacist was centered on the management of the pharmacy and the accurate dispensing of drugs. The duties and responsibilities of pharmacists have moved well beyond the concept of filling prescriptions and dispensing drugs. Schools of pharmacy have recognized the ever-expanding role of the pharmacist into the clinical aspects of patient care—so much so that educational requirements are getting more stringent, with emphasis on clinical education and application.

Duty to Monitor Patient's Medications

In *Baker v. Arbor Drugs, Inc.*,[33] a Michigan court imposed a duty on a pharmacist to monitor a patient's medications. Three different prescriptions were prescribed by the same physician and filled at the same pharmacy. The pharmacy maintained a computer system that detected drug–drug interactions. The pharmacy advertised to consumers that it could, through the use of a computer-monitoring system, provide a medication profile for its customers that would alert its pharmacists to potential drug–drug interactions. Because the pharmacy advertised and used the computer system to monitor the medications of its customers, the pharmacist voluntarily assumed a duty of care to detect the harmful drug–drug interaction that occurred in this case.

Warning Patients About Potential for Overdose

A Pennsylvania court held that a pharmacist failed to warn the patient about the maximum dosage of a drug the patient could take.[34] This failure resulted in an overdose, causing permanent injuries. Expert testimony focused on the fact that a pharmacist who receives inadequate instructions as to the maximum recommended dosage has a duty to ascertain whether the patient is aware of the limitations concerning the use of the drug. The pharmacist should have contacted the prescribing physician to clarify the prescription.

Refusal to Honor a Questionable Prescription

In *Hooks v. McLaughlin*,[35] the Indiana Supreme Court held that a pharmacist had a duty to refuse to refill prescriptions at an unreasonably faster rate than prescribed pending directions from the prescribing physician. The Indiana code provides that a pharmacist is immune from civil prosecution or civil liability if he or she, in good faith, refuses to honor a prescription because, in his or her professional judgment, the honoring of the prescription would aid or abet an addiction or habit.[36]

PHYSICAL THERAPY

Physical therapy is the art and science of preventing and treating neuromuscular or musculoskeletal disabilities through the evaluation of an individual's disability and rehabilitation potential; the use of physical agents (heat, cold, ultrasound, electricity, water, and light); and neuromuscular procedures that, through their physiologic effect, improve or maintain the patient's optimum functional level. Because of different physical disabilities brought on by various injuries and medical problems, physical therapy is an extremely important component of a patient's total health care.

Incorrectly Interpreting Physician's Orders

Pontiff, in *Pontiff v. Pecot & Assoc.*[37] filed a petition for damages against Pecot and Associates and Morris. Pontiff alleged Pecot and Associates had been negligent in failing to properly train, supervise, and monitor its employees, including Morris, and that Pecot and Associates was otherwise negligent. Pontiff alleged that employee Morris failed to exercise the degree of care and skill ordinarily exercised by physical therapists, failed to heed his protests that he could not perform the physical therapy treatments she was supervising, and failed to stop performing physical therapy treatments after he began to complain that he was in pain. Pontiff claimed he felt a muscle tear while he was exercising on the butterfly machine, a resistive exercise machine.

Pontiff's expert, Boulet, a licensed practicing physical therapist, testified that Pecot deviated from the standard of care of physical therapists by introducing a type of exercise that, according to her, was not prescribed by Dr. deAraujo, the treating physician. She stated that Pecot added resistive or strengthening exercises to Pontiff's therapy and that these were not a part of the physician's prescription. Pecot argued that resistive exercises were implicitly part of the prescription, even if her interpretation of the prescription was not reasonable.

Legally, under Louisiana law, a physical therapist may not treat a patient without a written physical therapy prescription. Ethically, the Physical Therapists' Code of Ethics, Principle 3.4, states that any alteration of a program or extension of services beyond the program should be undertaken in consultation with the referring practitioner. Because resistive exercises were not set forth in the original prescription, Boulet stated that consultation with the physician was necessary before Pontiff could be advanced to that level. Only in the case where a physician has indicated on the prescription that the therapist is to evaluate and treat would the therapist have such discretion. There was no such indication on the prescription written by deAraujo.

Davis, a physical therapist in private practice and Pecot's expert witness, testified that the program that Pecot designed for Pontiff was consistent with how she interpreted the prescription for therapy that the physician wrote. Davis, however, did not at any time state that Pecot's interpretation was a reasonable one. In fact, Davis herself would not have interpreted the prescription in the manner that Pecot did. Davis testified only that Pecot's introduction of resistive exercises was reasonable based on her interpretation of the prescription.

It is clear that Pecot, as a licensed physical therapist, owed a duty to Pontiff, her client. Pecot's duty is defined by the standard of care of similar physical therapists and the Association of Physical Therapists of America. If Pecot found the prescription to be ambiguous, she had a duty to contact the prescribing physician for clarification. The appeals court found that the trial court was correct in its determination that Pontiff presented sufficient evidence to show that this duty was breached and that Pecot's care fell below the standard of other physical therapists.

PHYSICIAN'S ASSISTANT

One of the solutions to the shortage of physicians in certain rural and inner-city areas has been to train allied health professionals, such as a physician's assistant (PA), to perform the more routine and repetitive medical procedures. A physician may delegate to a PA such tasks as suturing minor wounds, administering injections, and performing routine history and physical examinations. A physician may not delegate a task to a PA in those instances where regulations specify that the physician must perform it or when the delegation is prohibited under state law or by the facility's own policies.

PAs are responsible for their own negligent acts. The employer of a PA can be held liable for the PA's negligent acts on the basis of respondeat superior. To limit the potential risk of liability for a PA's negligent acts, PAs should be monitored and supervised by a physician. Guidelines and procedures also should be established to provide a standard mechanism for reviewing a PA's performance.

PODIATRIST

The legal concerns of podiatrists, similar to those of surgeons, include misdiagnosis and negligent surgery. The podiatrist, for example, in *Strauss v. Biggs*[38] was found to have failed to meet the standard of care required of a podiatrist and that failure resulted in injury to the patient. The podiatrist, by his own admission, stated that his initial incision in the patient's foot had been misplaced. The trial court was found not to have erred in permitting the jury to consider additional claims that the podiatrist acted improperly by failing to refer the patient, stop the procedure after the first incision, inform the patient of possible nerve injury, and provide proper postoperative treatment. Testimony of the patient's experts was adequate to show that such alleged omissions violated the standard of care required of podiatrists.

RESPIRATORY THERAPIST

Respiratory therapy is the allied health profession responsible for the treatment, management, diagnostic testing, and control of patients with cardiopulmonary deficits. A respiratory therapist is a person employed in the practice of respiratory care who has the knowledge and skill necessary to administer respiratory care.

Respiratory therapists are responsible for their negligent acts. A respiratory therapist's employer is responsible for the negligent acts of the therapist under the legal doctrine of respondeat superior.

Failure to Remove Endotracheal Tube

The court in *Poor Sisters of St. Francis v. Catron*[39] held that the failure of nurses and a respiratory therapist to report to the supervisor that an endotracheal tube had been left in the plaintiff longer than the customary period of 3 or 4 days was sufficient to allow the jury to reach a finding of negligence. The patient experienced difficulty speaking and underwent several operations to remove scar tissue and open her voice box. At the time of trial, she could not speak above a whisper and breathed partially through a hole in her throat created by a tracheotomy. The hospital was found liable for the negligent acts of its employees and the resulting injuries to the plaintiff.

Multiple Use of Same Syringe

The respiratory therapist in *State University v. Young*[40] was suspended for using the same syringe for drawing blood from a number of critically ill patients. The therapist had been warned several times of the dangers of that practice and that it violated the state's policy of providing quality patient care.

Restocking the Code Cart

Dixon had been admitted to the hospital and was diagnosed with pneumonia in her right lung. Dixon's condition began to deteriorate and she was moved to the intensive care unit (ICU). A code blue was eventually called signifying that her cardiac and respiratory functions were believed to have ceased. During the code, a decision was made to intubate, which is to insert an endotracheal tube into Dixon so that she could be given respiratory support by a mechanical ventilator. As Dixon's condition stabilized, Dr. Taylor, Dixon's physician at that time, ordered that she gradually be weaned from the respirator. Blackham, a respiratory therapist employed by the hospital, extubated Dixon at 10:15 p.m. Taylor left Dixon's room to advise her family that she had been extubated. Blackham decided an oxygen mask would provide better oxygen to Dixon but could not locate a mask in the ICU, so he left ICU and went across the hall to the critical care unit (CCU). When Blackham returned to Dixon's room with the oxygen mask and placed it on Dixon, he realized that she was not breathing properly. Blackham realized that she would have to be reintubated as quickly as possible.

A second code was called. Shackleford, a nurse in the cardiac CCU, responded to the code. Shackleford recorded on the code sheet that she arrived in Dixon's room at 10:30 p.m. She testified that Blackham said he needed a medium Number 4 MacIntosh laryngoscope blade, which was not on the code cart. The code cart is a cart that is equipped with all the medicines, supplies, and instruments needed for a code emergency. The code cart in the ICU had not been restocked after the first code that morning, so Shackleford was sent to obtain the needed blade from the CCU across the hall. When Shackleford returned to the ICU, the blade was passed to Taylor, who had responded to the code and was attempting to reintubate Dixon. Upon receiving the blade, Taylor was able to quickly intubate Dixon. Dixon was placed on a ventilator, but she never regained consciousness. After the family was informed there was no hope that Dixon would recover the use of her brain, the family requested that no extraordinary measure be taken to prolong her life.

A medical negligence claim was filed against Taylor and the hospital. The jury found that Taylor was not negligent. Evidence presented at trial established that the hospital's breach of duty in not having the code cart properly restocked resulted in a 3-minute delay in the intubation of Dixon. Reasonable minds could accept from the testimony at trial that the hospital's breach of duty was a cause of Dixon's brain death, without which the injury would not have occurred. Foreseeability on the part of the hospital could be established from the evidence introduced by the plaintiff that the written standards for the hospital require every code cart be stocked with a Number 4 MacIntosh blade. This evidence permits a reasonable inference that the hospital should have foreseen that the failure to have the code cart stocked with the blade could lead to critical delays in intubating a patient. Accordingly, there was substantial evidence that failure to have the code cart stocked with the proper blade was a proximate cause of Dixon's injuries.[41]

SEXUAL IMPROPRIETIES

A significant number of cases address health care professionals who have been involved in sexual relationships with their patients. Such cases are being litigated, in many instances, in both civil and criminal arenas. Health care professionals finding themselves in such unprofessional relationships must seek help for themselves as well as refer their patients to other appropriate professionals. Besides being subject to civil and criminal litigation, health care professionals also are subject to having their licenses revoked for sexual improprieties.

Dentist

Revocation of a dentist's license on charges of professional misconduct was properly ordered in *Melone v. State Education Department*[42] on the basis of substantial evidence that while acting in his professional capacity, the dentist engaged in physical and sexual contact with five different male patients within a 3-year period. Considering the dentist's responsible position, the extended time period during which the sexual contacts occurred, the age and impressionable nature of the victims (7 to 15 years of age), and the possibility of lasting effects on the victims, the penalty was not shocking to the court's sense of fairness.

Physician

A hospital technologist in *Copithorne v. Framingham Union Hospital*[43] alleged that a staff physician raped her during the course of a house call. The technologist's claim against the hospital was summarily dismissed for lack of proximate causation. On appeal, the dismissal was found to be improper when the record indicated that the hospital had received notice of allegations that the physician assaulted patients on and off the hospital's premises. The hospital had instructed the physician to have another individual present when visiting female patients and had instructed nurses to keep an eye on him. The physician's sexual assault was foreseeable. There was evidentiary support for the proposition that failure to withdraw the physician's privileges caused the rape when the technologist asserted that it was the physician's good reputation in the hospital that led her to seek his services.

Psychiatrist

The sexual relationship a psychiatrist had with the spouse of a patient was found to be improper in *Richard v. Larry*.[44] California Civil Code Section 43.5, abolishing causes of action for alienation of affection, criminal conversation, and seduction of a patient over the age of consent, did not bar damages for emotional distress caused by the alleged professional negligence of the psychiatrist who had sexual relations with the plaintiff's wife. The psychiatrist owed a special duty to use due care for his patient's health. The statute was not intended to lower the standard of care that psychiatrists owed their patients. Besides an action against the psychiatrist, allegations that the psychiatrist was an agent of the hospital stated a cause of action against the hospital.

SURGERY

Operating rooms, hidden behind closed doors, are often the scenes of negligent acts. A Wyoming man was awarded $1.175 million after doctors removed the wrong cervical disc during spinal surgery.[45] The following cases illustrate a variety of medical errors that have occurred during the course of surgery.

Improper Positioning of Arm

The plaintiff in *Wick v. Henderson*[46] experienced pain in her left arm upon awakening from surgery; an anesthesiologist told her that her arm was stressed during surgery. According to the plaintiff, she sustained an injury to the ulnar nerve in her left upper arm. A malpractice action was filed against the hospital and the anesthesiologist. The plaintiff sought recovery on theory of res ipsa loquitur. There was testimony that the main cause of the injury was the mechanical compression of the nerve by improper positioning of the arm during surgery. The trial court granted the defendants a directed verdict, resulting in dismissal of the case.

On appeal, the Iowa Supreme Court held that the res ipsa loquitur doctrine applied. The plaintiff must prove two foundational facts to invoke the doctrine of res ipsa loquitur. First, she must prove that the defendants had exclusive control and management of the instrument that caused her injury, and second, that it was the type of injury that ordinarily would not occur if reasonable care had been used. As to control, the plaintiff can show an injury resulting from an external force applied while she lay unconscious in the hospital. It is within common knowledge and experience of a layperson that an individual does not enter the hospital for gallbladder surgery and leave with ulnar nerve injury.

CERTIFICATION OF HEALTH CARE PROFESSIONALS

The certification of health care professionals is the recognition by a governmental or professional association that an individual's expertise meets the standards of that group. Some professional groups establish their own minimum standards for certification in those professions that are not licensed by a particular state. Certification by an association or group is a self-regulation credentialing process.

LICENSING HEALTH CARE PROFESSIONALS

Licensure can be defined as the process by which some competent authority grants permission to a qualified individual or entity to perform certain specified activities that would be illegal without a license. As it applies to health care personnel, licensure refers to the process by which licensing boards, agencies, or departments of the several states grant to individuals who meet certain predetermined standards the legal right to practice in a health care profession and to use a specified health care practitioner's title. The commonly stated objectives of licensing laws are to limit and control admission to the different health care occupations and to protect the public from unqualified practitioners by promulgating and enforcing standards of practice within the professions.

The authority of states to license health care practitioners is found in their regulating power. Implicit in the power to license is the authority to collect license fees, establish standards of practice, require certain minimum qualifications and competency levels of applicants, and impose on applicants other requirements necessary to protect the general public welfare. This authority, which is vested in the legislature, may be delegated to political subdivisions or to state boards, agencies, and departments. In some instances, the scope of the delegated power is made specific in the legislation; in others, the licensing authority may have wide discretion in performing its functions. In either case, however, the authority granted by the legislature may not be exceeded.

SUSPENSION AND REVOCATION OF LICENSE

Licensing boards have the authority to suspend or revoke the license of a health care professional who is found to have violated specified norms of conduct. Such violations may include procurement of a license by fraud; unprofessional, dishonorable, immoral, or illegal conduct; performance of specific actions prohibited by statute; and malpractice. Suspension and revocation procedures are most commonly contained in a state's licensing act.

HELPFUL ADVICE FOR CAREGIVERS

- Abide by the ethical code of one's profession.
- Do not criticize the professional skills of others.
- Maintain complete and adequate medical records.
- Seek the aid of professional medical consultants when indicated.
- Inform the patient of the risks, benefits, and alternatives to proposed procedures.
- Practice the specialty in which you have been trained.
- Participate in continuing education programs.
- Keep patient information confidential.
- Check patient equipment regularly, and monitor it for safe use.
- When terminating a professional relationship with a patient, provide adequate notice to the patient.
- Authenticate all telephone orders.
- Obtain a qualified substitute when you will be absent from your practice.
- Be a good listener, and allow each patient sufficient time to express fears and anxieties.
- Safely administer patient medications.
- Closely monitor each patient's response to treatment.
- Provide education and teaching to patients.
- Foster a sense of trust and feeling of significance.
- Communicate with the patient and other caregivers.

Notes

1. RONNIE GREEN, Dying at the Hospital's Door: A Child Lost, Troubling Questions, THE MIAMI HERALD, Apr. 16, 1995, at 14A.
2. No. W2000-01485-COA-R3-CV (Tenn. App. 2002).
3. Cleland v. Bronson Health Care Group, 917 F.2d 266, 272 (6th Cir. 1990).
4. Griffith v. University Hospitals of Cleveland, No. 84314 (Ohio Ct. of App. 2004).
5. Roy v. Gupta, 606 So.2d 940 (La. Ct. App. 1992).
6. Feeney v. New England Medical Center, Inc., 615 N.E.2d 585 (Mass. App. Ct. 1993).
7. 42 U.S.C.A. § 1395dd(a) (1992).
8. 42 U.S.C.A. § 1395dd(3)(A) (1992).
9. 830 F. Supp. 1399 (M.D. Ala. 1993).
10. 934 F.2d 1362 (5th Cir. Tex. 1991).
11. Courts Uphold Law, Regulations against Patient Dumping, NATION'S HEALTH, Aug. 1991, at 1.
12. 689 So. 2d 696 (La. App. 1997).
13. 477 So. 2d 1036 (Fla. Dist. Ct. App. 1985).
14. 288 A.2d 379 (Md. 1972).
15. 271 N.W.2d 8 (S.D. 1978).
16. 14 S.W.3d 42 (Mo. App. 1999).
17. 698 So. 2d 958 (La. App. 1997).
18. 498 S.E.2d 408 (1998).
19. Baptist Mem'l Hosp. Sys. v. Sampson, 969 S.W.2d 945, 947 (Tex. 1998).
20. MARTIN C. MCWILLIAMS, JR. & HAMILTON E. RUSSELL, III, Hospital Liability for Torts of Independent Contractor.
21. Jackson v. Powei, 743 P.2d 1376, 1385 (Alaska 1987).
22. Martell v. St Charles Hosp., 523 N.Y.S.2d 342, 352 (N.Y. Sup. Ct. 1987).
23. 797 So. 2d 160 (2001).
24. 661 S.W.2d 534 (Mo. 1983).
25. Sander v. Geib, Elston, Frost Prof'l Ass'n, 506 N.W.2d 107 (S.D. 1993).
26. 636 N.E.2d 1282 (Ind. Ct. App. 1994).
27. 753 F. Supp. 267 (W.D. Ark. 1990).
28. 650 A.2d 1076 (Pa. Super. 1994).
29. 933 S.2d 627 (La. 2006).
30. INSTITUTE OF MEDICINE, To Err Is Human: Building a Safer Health System, supra note 1, at 194.
31. www.usdoj.gov/dea/agency/csa.htm.
32. 21 C.F.R. § 1.106.
33. 544 N.W.2d 727 (Mich. Ct. App. 1996).
34. Riff v. Morgan Pharmacy, 508 A.2d 1247 (Pa. Super. Ct.1986).
35. 642 N.E.2d 514 (Ind. 1994).
36. IND. CODE § 25-26-13-16(b)(3) (1993).
37. 780 So.2d 478 (2001).
38. 525 A.2d 992 (Del. 1987).
39. 435 N.E.2d 305 (Ind. Ct. App. 1982).
40. 566 N.Y.S.2d 79 (N.Y. App. Div. 1991).
41. Dixon v. Taylor, No. 9224SC760 (Filed 20 July 1993).
42. 495 N.Y.S.2d 808 (N.Y. App. Div. 1985).
43. 520 N.E.2d 139 (Mass. 1988).
44. 243 Cal. Rptr. 807 (Cal. Ct. App. 1988).
45. Baldwin, Medical News Summary: $1.175 million awarded in a medical malpractice case, Casper Star Tribune, 485 N.W.2d 645 (Iowa 1992).
46. 485 N.W.2d 645 (Iowa 1992).

11

Information Management and Health Care Records

To significantly reduce the tens of thousands of deaths and injuries caused by medical errors every year, health care organizations must adopt information technology systems that are capable of collecting and sharing essential health information on patients and their care . . . . These systems should operate seamlessly as part of a national network of health information that is accessible by all health care organizations and that includes electronic records of patients' care, secure platforms for the exchange of information among providers and patients, and data standards that will make health information uniform and understandable to all . . . .

News: Institute of Medicine,
November 20, 2003

The effective and efficient delivery of patient care requires that an organization determine its information needs. Organizations that do not centralize their information needs will often suffer scattered databases, which may result in such problems as duplication of data gathering, inconsistent reports, and inefficiencies in the use of economic resources.

As the principal means of communication between health care professionals in matters relating to patient care, the medical record primarily provides documentation of a patient's illness, symptoms, diagnosis, and treatment, and it is used as a planning tool for patient care. Practitioners also use medical records to document communication; assist in protecting the legal interests of the patient, the organization, and the practitioner; provide a database for use in statistical reporting, continuing education, and research; and provide information necessary for third-party billing and regulatory agencies. Health care organizations are required to maintain a medical record for each patient in accordance with accepted professional standards and practices.

Nurses tend to access the medical record more often than other health care professionals, simply because of the greater amount of time spent caring for patients. Because of the job description, the nurse monitors the patient's illness, response to medication, display of pain and discomfort, and general condition. The patient's care, as well as the nurse's observations, should be recorded on a regular basis. A nurse who has doubt as to the appropriateness of a particular order should verify with the physician the intent of the prescribed order.

Licensure rules and regulations contained in state statutes generally describe the requirements and standards for the maintenance, handling, signing, filing, and retention of medical records. Failure to maintain a complete and accurate medical record reflecting the treatment rendered may affect the ability of an organization and/or physician to obtain third-party reimbursement (e.g., from Medicare, Medicaid, or private insurance carriers). Under federal and state laws, the medical record must reflect accurately the treatment for which the organization or physician seeks payment. Thus, the medical record is important to the organization for medical, legal, and financial reasons.

MANAGING INFORMATION

All organizations, regardless of mission or size, develop and maintain information management systems, which often include financial, medical, and human resource data. Information management is a process intended to facilitate the flow of information within and between departments and caregivers. An information management plan should: determine customer needs, both internal and external (e.g., third-party payers); set goals and establish priorities (e.g., the development of an integrated patient care record); improve accuracy of data collection; provide uniformity of data collection and definitions; limit duplication of entries; deliver timely and accurate information; provide easy access to information; maintain security and confidentiality of information; improve collaboration across the organization through information sharing; establish disaster plans for the recovery of information; orient and train staff on the information management system; and provide an annual review of the plan.

CONTENTS OF THE MEDICAL RECORD

Because the medical record fulfills many crucial roles within a health care organization, practitioners must strive to fulfill all requirements to maintain the integrity and accuracy of records. The inpatient medical record includes: the admission record, which describes pertinent demographic information; consent and authorization for treatment forms; advance directives; medical history and physical examination, including diagnosis and findings that support the diagnosis; patient screenings and assessments (e.g., nursing, functional, nutritional, social, and discharge planning); treatment plans; physicians' orders; progress notes; nursing notes; diagnostic reports; consultation reports; vital signs charts; anesthesia assessment; operative reports; medication administration records; discharge planning documentation; patient education; and discharge summaries.

OWNERSHIP AND RELEASE OF MEDICAL RECORDS

Health care providers who handle medical records must fully understand the related issues of ownership and privacy. Medical records are the property of the provider of care and are maintained for the benefit of the patient. Ownership resides with the organization or professional who renders treatment. Although medical records typically have been protected from public scrutiny by a general practice of nondisclosure, this practice has been waived under a limited number of specifically controlled situations. Some jurisdictions recognize that individuals have a right to privacy and to be protected from the mass dissemination of information pertaining to their personal or private affairs. The right of privacy generally includes the right to be kept out of the public spotlight. The Privacy Act of 1974 was enacted to safeguard individual privacy from the misuse of federal records and to give individuals access to records concerning themselves that are maintained by federal agencies.

Requests by Patients

Patients have a legally enforceable interest in the information contained in their medical records and, therefore, have a right to access their records. Patients may have access to review and obtain copies of their records, including diagnostic tests. Access to information includes that maintained or possessed by a health care organization or a health care practitioner who has treated or is treating a patient. Organizations and physicians can withhold records if the information could reasonably be expected to cause substantial and identifiable harm to the patient (e.g., patients in psychiatric hospitals, institutions for the mentally disabled, and substance abuse treatment programs).

Failure to release a patient's record can lead to legal action. The patient in *Pierce v. Penman*[1] brought a lawsuit seeking damages for severe emotional distress when physicians repeatedly refused to turn over her medical records. The defendants had rendered different professional services to the plaintiff for approximately 11 years. The patient moved and found a new physician, Dr. Hochman. She signed a release authorizing Hochman to obtain her records from the defendant physicians. Hochman wrote a letter for her records but never received a response. The defendants claimed that they never received the request. The patient changed physicians again and continued in her efforts to obtain a copy of the records. Eventually the defendants' offices were burglarized, and the plaintiff's records were allegedly taken. The detective in charge of investigating the burglary stated that he was never notified that any records were taken. The patient was awarded $2500 in compensatory damages and $10,000 in punitive damages.

Requests by Third Parties

The medical record is a peculiar type of property because there is a variety of third-party interest in the information contained in medical records. Health care organizations may not generally disclose information without patient consent. Policies regarding the release of information should be formulated to address the rights of third parties, such as insurance carriers processing claims, physicians, medical researchers, educators, and governmental agencies.

Criminal Investigations

A restriction on disclosing information obtained in a confidential relationship may occur when a patient is the victim of a crime. The hospital in *In re Brink*[2] sought to quash a grand jury request for the medical records pertaining to blood tests administered to a person under investigation. The court of common pleas held that physician–patient privilege did not extend to medical records subpoenaed pursuant to a grand jury investigation. A proceeding before a grand jury is considered secret in nature, inherently preserving the confidentiality of a patient's records.

Medicaid Fraud

Patient records may also be obtained during investigations into such alleged criminal actions as Medicaid fraud. The grand jury in *People v. Ekong*[3] was permitted to obtain certain patient files and records that were in the possession of the physician who was under investigation for Medicaid fraud.

RETENTION OF RECORDS

The length of time medical records must be retained varies from state to state. A California court revoked the license of a nursing facility for failure to keep *adequate* records.

Failure to Preserve X-rays

The plaintiff in *Rodgers v. St. Mary's Hosp. of Decatur*[4] filed a complaint for damages against a hospital, alleging that the hospital breached its statutory duty to preserve for 5 years all of the X-rays taken of his wife. He alleged that the hospital's failure to preserve one of the X-rays was a breach of its duty arising from the state's X-ray retention act and from the hospital's internal regulations. The plaintiff asserted that because the hospital failed to preserve the X-ray, he was unable to prove his case in a lawsuit. The circuit court entered judgment in favor of the hospital, and the plaintiff appealed.

The Illinois Supreme Court held that a private cause of action existed under the X-ray retention act and that the plaintiff stated a claim under the act. The act provides that hospitals must retain X-rays and other such photographs or films as part of their regularly maintained records for a period of 5 years.

The hospital also argued that the loss of one X-ray out of a series of six should not be considered a violation of the statute. The court disagreed, finding that the statute requires that all X-rays be preserved, not just some of them.

COMPUTERIZED RECORDS

Retaining all patient records for 5 years may seem unwieldy, but computers make the task feasible, while also increasing efficiency for many other information management processes. Health care organizations undergoing computerization must determine user needs, design an effective system, select appropriate hardware and software, develop user training programs, develop a disaster recovery plan (e.g., provide for emergency power systems and backup files), and provide for data security. Solid planning and design can lead to great achievements.

Advantages

Computers have become an economic necessity and play an important role in assisting health care providers to improve the quality of health care. In the health care community, computers: retrieve demographic information and consultants' reports, as well as laboratory, radiology, and other test results; improve productivity and quality; reduce costs; support clinical research; play an ever-increasing role in the education process; allow for interactive computer-assisted diagnosis and treatment; generate reminders for follow-up testing; assist in standardizing treatment protocols; assist in the identification of drug–drug and food–drug interactions; and assist in providing telecommunications around the world, transporting picture graphics (e.g., computed tomography scans) between nations.

Disadvantages

With the advent of electronic medical records, organizations, for the most part, have failed to achieve a paperless electronic system. Instead, organizations find themselves with a hybrid system with various elements of a patient's care recorded in both paper and electronic format. Further, computerization has proven to be costly.

MEDICAL RECORD BATTLEGROUND

The contents of a medical record must not be tampered with after an entry has been made; therefore, it should be used wisely. Although the record should be complete and accurate, it should not be used as an instrument for registering complaints about another individual or the organization. Its purpose is to record the patient's course of care. Those individuals who choose to make derogatory remarks in a patient's record about others could find themselves in a courtroom trying to defend such notations in the record. Always consider that comments written during a time of anger may have been based on inaccurate information, which, in turn, could be damaging to one's credibility and future statements.

PATIENT OBJECTS TO RECORD NOTATIONS

As noted in *Dodds v. Johnstone*,[5] during a physical exam the appellee indicated in her progress notes that she believed the appellant had been using cocaine prior to her last office visit. Appellee's notes read: "I believe by physical exam the patient was using cocaine on Friday before her office visit." The appellant filed a complaint in which she alleged that the appellee was negligent in her diagnosis of the appellant and that as a result she incurred a loss of compensation for her automobile accident claim and suffered severe emotional distress. The court reviewed the record of proceedings before the trial court and found that there was no genuine issue of material fact as to negligent infliction of severe emotional distress, loss of employment opportunities, or a decreased insurance settlement as a result of the notation in the patient's medical records.

FALSIFICATION OF RECORDS

When handling medical records, professionals must recognize that intentional alteration, falsification, or destruction to avoid liability for medical negligence is generally sufficient to show actual malice. Punitive damages may be awarded whether or not the act of altering, falsifying, or destroying records directly causes compensable harm. The evidence in *Dimora v. Cleveland Clinic Foundation*[6] showed that the patient had fallen and broken five or six ribs; yet, upon examination, the physician stated in the progress notes that the patient was smiling and laughing pleasantly, exhibiting no pain upon deep palpation of the area. Other testimony indicated that she was in pain and crying. The discrepancy between the written progress notes and the testimony of the witnesses who observed the patient was sufficient to raise a question of fact. The court then considered the possible falsification of documents by the physician in an effort to hide the possible negligence of hospital personnel. The testimony of the witnesses, if believed, would have been sufficient to show that the physician falsified the record or intentionally reported the incident inaccurately to avoid liability for the negligent care of the patient.

The intentional alteration or destruction of medical records to avoid liability for medical negligence is sufficient to show actual malice, and punitive damages may be awarded whether the act of altering, falsifying, or destroying records directly causes compensable harm.[7]

TAMPERING WITH RECORDS

Closely related to falsification, tampering with records sends the wrong signal to jurors and can shatter one's credibility. Altered records can create a presumption of negligence. The court in *Matter of Jascalevich*[8] held:

> We are persuaded that a physician's duty to a patient cannot but encompass his affirmative obligation to maintain the integrity, accuracy, truth and reliability of the patient's medical record. His obligation in this regard is no less compelling than his duties respecting diagnosis and treatment of the patient since the medical community must, of necessity, be able to rely on those records in the continuing and future care of that patient. Obviously, the rendering of that care is prejudiced by anything in those records which is false, misleading or inaccurate. We hold, therefore, that a deliberate falsification by a physician of his patient's medical record, particularly when the reason therefore is to protect his own interests at the expense of his patient's, must be regarded as gross malpractice endangering the health or life of his patient.[9]

Dr. McCroskey faced a lawsuit for tampering with documents. The state board of medical examiners, in a disciplinary hearing in *State Board of Medical Examiners v. McCroskey*,[10] issued a letter of admonition to Dr. McCroskey based upon a series of incidents arising out of the care of a patient's stab wound. Although the patient's condition was initially thought to be stable, he bled to death several hours after his admission to the hospital. McCroskey was the attending surgeon on the date of the incident and, therefore, responsible for the accurate completion of the patient's medical record. McCroskey declined to accept the letter of admonition and a formal disciplinary hearing was held.

McCroskey erased and wrote over a preoperative note made by another physician concerning the patient's estimated blood loss. Specifically, the original record entry was completed by a surgical resident on the date of the patient's death and stated that the patient's blood loss just prior to surgery was "now greater than 3000 cc." Sometime after the autopsy, McCroskey changed the record to read that the patient's blood loss was "now greater than 2000 cc."[11]

The Colorado Supreme Court held that the findings of the board were supported by substantial evidence. Because of the expertise of the board, it was in a position to determine the seriousness of the physician's conduct by placing the events in their proper factual context.

All three of the inquiry panel's witnesses testified that the generally accepted standard of practice requires that a medical record entry be dated with the date it is made. Even one of McCroskey's witnesses acknowledged that misdating the medical record was "certainly something that should not have been done." McCroskey did not simply backdate a trivial note in a patient's medical record. Instead McCroskey's actions took place in the context of a patient's death, which resulted in a coroner's autopsy, peer review activities, publicity, and several legal actions. McCroskey was the attending physician responsible for the accuracy of the patient's medical record, and yet he engaged in conduct that cast doubt upon the medical record's integrity. Under these circumstances, the Board was justified in considering McCroskey's conduct to violate the standard of care.[12]

REWRITING AND REPLACING NOTES

Another temptation of health care professionals is the desire to clarify and explain one's activities in the care of a patient. In a well-publicized case that involved the death of a child, the nurse replaced her original notes with a second set of notes that were much more detailed and indicated that she had seen the patient more frequently than was reported in her original notes.[13] Rewriting one's notes in a patient's medical record casts doubt as to the accuracy of other entries in the record. It is easier to explain why one did not chart all activities than it is to explain why a new entry was recorded and an original note was replaced.

ILLEGIBLE ENTRIES

Illegible handwriting is as ancient as the first stylus. Unfortunately, poor penmanship can cause injury to patients. Medical errors because of poor handwriting can lead to extended length of hospital stays and, in some cases, the death of patients.

Fatal Handwriting Mix-Up

Forty-two-year-old Vasquez died as a result of a handwriting mix-up on the medication prescribed for his heart. Vasquez had been given a prescription for 20 mg of Isordil to be taken four times per day. The pharmacist misread the physician's handwriting and filled the prescription with Plendil, a drug for high blood pressure, which is usually taken at no more than 10 mg per day. As a result, Vasquez was given the wrong medication at eight times the recommended dosage. He died 2 weeks later from an apparent heart attack. The family filed a lawsuit. A West Texas jury ordered the physician, drugstore, and pharmacist to pay

$225,000 to the family. The likelihood of similar occurrences is a growing danger as the number and variety of medications increase with similar names and look-alikes.[14]

FRAUDULENT RECORD KEEPING

Maintaining records, of course, does little good when the records are flawed with errors. In one such case, *Tulier-Pastewski v. State Board for Professional Medical Conduct*,[15] two hospital administrators testified and showed undisputed proof that the physician had recorded a patient was alert during the purported examination when the patient was actually sedated and asleep. Evidence also indicated the physician failed to properly document medical histories and current physical status. Although the physician asserted that evidence of failure to document did not support findings of negligence because there was no expert testimony that her omissions actually caused or created a risk of harm to a patient, an expert witness testified that the missing information as to certain patients was needed for proper assessment of the patient's condition and choice of treatment. This testimony, together with the obvious importance of cardiac information when treating patients with chest pain, provided a rational basis for the conclusion by the administrative review board for professional medical conduct that the physician's deficient medical record keeping could have affected patient care. The physician was found to be practicing medicine negligently on more than one occasion, and fraudulent practice was supported by the record.

INCOMPLETE RECORDS: SUSPENSION OF PRIVILEGES

Not only must the chart be accurate, but health care professionals must promptly complete records after patients are discharged. Persistent failure to conform to a medical staff rule requiring physicians to complete records promptly can be the basis for suspension of medical staff privileges, as was the case in *Board of Trustees Memorial Hospital v. Pratt*.[16]

LEGAL PROCEEDINGS AND THE MEDICAL RECORD

The ever-increasing frequency of personal injury suits mandates that health care organizations maintain complete, accurate, and timely medical records. The integrity and completeness of the medical record are important in reconstructing the events surrounding an alleged negligence in the care of a patient. Medical records aid police investigations, provide information for determining the cause of death, and indicate the extent of injury in workers' compensation or personal injury proceedings.

When health care professionals are called as witnesses in a proceeding, they are permitted to refresh their recollections of the facts and circumstances of a particular case by referring to the medical record. Courts recognize that it is impossible for a medical witness to remember the details of every patient's treatment. The record therefore may be used as an aid in relating the facts of a patient's course of treatment.

If a medical record is admitted into evidence in a legal proceeding, the court must be assured the information is accurate, was recorded at the time the event took place, and was not recorded in anticipation of a specific legal proceeding. When a medical record is introduced into evidence, its custodian must testify as to the manner in which the record was produced and the way in which it is protected from unauthorized handling and change. If a record can be shown to be inaccurate or incomplete or that it was made long after the event it purports to record, its credibility as evidence will be diminished.

CONFIDENTIAL AND PRIVILEGED COMMUNICATIONS

The duty of an organization's employees and staff to maintain confidentiality encompasses both verbal and written communications and applies to consultants, contracted individuals, students, and volunteers. Information about a patient, regardless of the method in which it is acquired, is confidential and should not be disclosed without the patient's permission. All health care professionals who have access to medical records have a legal, ethical, and moral obligation to protect the confidentiality of the information in the records, as well as verbal communications between physicians and patients.

Breach of Physician–Patient Confidentiality

Patients enter the physician–patient relationship assuming that information acquired by physicians will not be disclosed, unless the patient consents or the law requires disclosure. Mutual trust and confidence are essential to the physician–patient relationship. A breach of physician–patient confidentiality is analogous to invasion of privacy, and plaintiffs are entitled to recover damages, including emotional damages, for the harm caused by the physician's unauthorized disclosure.

Ordinary Business Documents

Privileged communications statutes do not protect from discovery the records maintained in the ordinary course of doing business and rendering inpatient care. Such documents often can be subpoenaed after showing cause.

Attorney–Client Privilege

Attorney–client privilege generally will preclude discovery of memorandums written to an organization's general counsel by the organization's risk management director. In *Mlynarski v. Rush Presbyterian–St. Luke's Medical Center*,[17] a memorandum written by the risk management coordinator to the hospital's general counsel was barred from discovery. There was undisputed evidence that the risk management coordinator had consulted with and assisted counsel in determining the legal action to pursue and the advisability of settling a claim that she had been assigned to investigate. Information contained in the memorandum was available from witnesses whose names and addresses were made available to the plaintiff. If the hospital later at trial decided to attempt to impeach those witnesses based on the coordinator's testimony, privilege would be waived, and the hospital would be required to produce the relevant reports.

HEALTH INSURANCE PORTABILITY AND ACCOUNTABILITY ACT

The Health Insurance Portability and Accountability Act (HIPAA) was enacted by Congress in 1996. According to the Centers for Medicare and Medicaid Services, Title I of HIPAA protects health insurance coverage for workers and their families when they change or lose their jobs. Title II of HIPAA, the administrative simplification (AS) provisions, requires the establishment of national standards for electronic health care transactions and national identifiers for providers, health insurance plans, and employers. The AS provisions also address the security and privacy of health information. The standards are meant to improve the efficiency and effectiveness of the nation's health care system by encouraging the widespread use of electronic data interchange in health care.

The HIPAA privacy provision took effect on April 14, 2003. Key privacy provisions include:

- Patients must be able to access their record and request correction of errors.
- Patients must be informed of how their personal information will be used.
- Patient information cannot be used for marketing purposes without the explicit consent of the involved patients.
- Patients can ask their health insurers and providers to take reasonable steps to ensure that their communications with the patient are confidential. For example, a patient can ask to be called at his or her work phone number instead of home or cell phone number.

- Patients can file formal privacy-related complaints with the US Department of Health and Human Services (DHHS) Office for Civil Rights.
- Health insurers or providers must document their privacy procedures, but they have discretion on what to include in their privacy procedure.
- Health insurers or providers must designate a privacy officer and train their employees.
- Providers may use patient information without patient consent for the purposes of providing treatment, obtaining payment for services, and performing the nontreatment operational tasks of the provider's business.

CHARTING—SOME HELPFUL ADVICE

The medical record is the most important document in a negligence action. Both the plaintiff and defendant use it as a basis for their action and defense in a lawsuit. The following suggestions on documentation should prove to be helpful when charting in a patient's record.

- The medical record describes the care rendered to each patient. It should be sufficiently complete to allow those not treating a patient to review the record and assume continuing care when necessary.
- Medical record entries should be timely, legible, clear, and meaningful to a patient's course of treatment. Illegible medical records not only damage one's ability to defend oneself but also can have an adverse effect on the credibility of other health care professionals who read the record and act on what they read.
- The medical record should be complete. This is often a problem with progress notes when there is little new information to report. Progress notes should describe the symptoms or condition being addressed, the treatment rendered, the patient response, and the patient's status at the time treatment is discontinued.
- Long, defensive, or derogatory notes should not be written. Only the facts should be related. Criticism, complaints, emotional comments, and extraneous remarks have no place in the medical record. Such remarks can precipitate a malpractice suit.
- Erasures and correction fluid should not be used to cover up entries. Do not tamper with the chart in any form. A single line should be drawn through a mistaken entry, the correct information entered, and the correction signed and dated.
- Charts related to pending legal action should be placed in a separate file under lock and key. Legal counsel should be notified immediately of any potential lawsuit.
- A medical record has many authors. Entries made by others must not be ignored. Good patient care is a collaborative interdisciplinary team effort. Entries made by health care professionals provide valuable information in treating the patient.

Notes

1. 515 A.2d 948 (Pa. Super. Ct. 1986).
2. 536 N.E.2d 1202 (Ohio Com. Pl. 1988).
3. 582 N.E.2d 233 (Ill. App. Ct. 1991).
4. 597 N.E.2d 616 (Ill. 1992).
5. No. L-03-1303 (Ohio App. 2004).
6. 683 N.E.2d 1175 (Ohio App. 1996).
7. Moskovitz v. Mount Sinai Med. Ctr., 635 N.E.2d 331 (Ohio 1994).
8. 442 A.2d 635 (N.J. Super. Ct. 1982).
9. In re Jascalevich, 182 N.J. Super. 445, 442 A.2d 635, 644–45 (1982).
10. 880 P.2d 1188 (Colo. 1994).

11. Id. at 1192.
12. Id. at 1196.
13. RONNIE GREENE, Examiner: Treatment "Appropriate," THE MIAMI HERALD, April 16, 1995, at 14A.
14. Doctor Held Liable for Fatal Handwriting Mix-up, USA TODAY, Oct. 21, 1999.
15. No. 94969 (Supreme Court of N.Y. App. Div. 2004).
16. 262 P.2d 682 (Wyo. 1953).
17. 572 N.E.2d 1025 (Ill. App. Ct. 1991).

12

PATIENT CONSENT

". . . no right is held more sacred, or is more carefully guarded, by the common law, than the right of every individual to the possession and control of his own person."

Union Pacific Ry. Co. v. Botsford[1]

Consent, in the health care setting, is the voluntary agreement by a person who possesses sufficient mental capacity to make an intelligent choice to allow a medical procedure and/or treatment proposed by another to be performed on himself or herself. Consent changes a touching that otherwise would be nonconsensual to one that is consensual. Consent can be either express or implied.

Express consent can take the form of a *verbal* agreement, or it can be accomplished through the execution of a *written* document authorizing medical care.

Implied consent is determined by some act or silence, which raises a presumption that consent has been authorized.

Consent must be obtained from the patient, or from a person authorized to consent on the patient's behalf, before any medical procedure can be performed. Every individual has a right to refuse to authorize a touching. Touching of another without authorization to do so could be considered a battery. Consent is not required for the normal, routine, everyday touching and bumping that occurs in life. In the process of caring for patients, it is inevitable that they will be touched and handled. Most touching in the health care setting is considered to be routine. Typical routine touching includes bathing, administering medications, dressing changes, and so forth. This chapter reviews the many issues surrounding consent in the health care setting.

INFORMED CONSENT

Whose Decision Is It?

At the end of the day and as recognized by the courts, it is the patient's right to accept or refuse treatment based on the alternatives available. Each patient must be "informed" by his or her treating "physician" as to what the alternatives are. The operation, for example, one gets often depends on where you live. Some patients undergo a mastectomy only to learn that a less-destructive alternative procedure is available. The procedure, a lumpectomy, is argued to have the same survival rate as a mastectomy. In one case a patient claimed the surgeon never "informed" her as to the alternative. In the final analysis, the patient decides!

Informed consent is a legal doctrine that provides that a patient has the right to know the potential risks, benefits, and alternatives of a proposed procedure. Where there are two or more medically acceptable treatment options, the patient has the absolute right to know about and select from the available treatment options after being informed of the alternatives, risks, and benefits of each.

Informed consent is predicated on the duty of the physician to disclose to the patient sufficient information to enable the patient to evaluate a proposed medical or surgical procedure before submitting to it. Informed consent requires that a patient have a full understanding of that to which he or she has consented. The informed consent doctrine provides that a physician has a legal, ethical, and moral duty to respect patient autonomy and to provide only such medical care as authorized by the patient. An authorization from a patient who does not understand to what he or she is consenting is not effective consent.

The right to be free from unwanted medical treatment has long been recognized by the courts. The right to control the integrity of one's own body spawned the doctrine of informed consent.[2] The US Supreme Court, in *Cruzan v. Director, Missouri Dep't of Health*,[3] held that a competent adult patient has the right to decline any and all forms of medical intervention, including lifesaving or life-prolonging treatment.

A physician is not under a duty to elucidate all the possible risks but only those of a serious nature. Expert testimony is often required to establish whether a reasonable physician in the community would make the pertinent disclosures under the same or similar circumstances.

Hospitals generally do not have an independent duty to obtain informed consent or to warn patients of the risks of a procedure to be performed by a physician who is not an agent of the hospital. It is the treating physician who has the education, expertise, skill, and training necessary to treat a patient and determine what information a patient should have to give informed consent. Nurses and other nonphysician hospital employees do not normally possess the knowledge of a particular patient's medical history, diagnosis, or other circumstances that would enable the employee to fully disclose pertinent information to the patient.

ASSESSING DECISION-MAKING CAPACITY

A patient is considered to be competent to make medical decisions regarding his or her care, unless a court determines otherwise. The clinical assessment of decision-making capacity should include the patient's ability to:

- understand the risks, benefits, and alternatives of a proposed test or procedure
- evaluate the information provided by the physician
- express his or her treatment preferences
- voluntarily make decisions regarding his or her treatment plan without undue influence by family, friends, or medical personnel

NURSES AND INFORMED CONSENT

In general, a nurse has no duty to advise a patient as to a particular procedure to be employed; advise the patient as to the risks, benefits, and alternatives to the recommended procedure; or obtain a patient's informed consent to a procedure merely because the physician directed a nurse to have the patient sign a consent form.

PHYSICIANS AND INFORMED CONSENT

Physicians are expected to disclose to their patients the risks, benefits, and alternatives of recommended procedures. Disclosure should include what a reasonable person would consider material to his or her decision of whether or not to undergo treatment.

The Pennsylvania Superior Court held in *Stover v. Surgeons*[4] that the physicians had to discuss alternative prostheses with the patient, where it represented medically recognized alternatives. Evidence that the heart valve actually implanted was no longer in general use at the time of operation was relevant and material to the issue of informed consent.

Although the physicians argued that the choice of prosthesis should belong to them, the court held that if there are other recognized, medically sound alternatives, the patient must be informed about the risks and benefits of them to make a sound judgment regarding treatment, including the desire to execute a waiver of consent. The agreement between the physician and the patient is contractual. Therefore, for valid consent to occur, there must be a finding that both parties understood the nature of the procedure, including what any possible as well as expected results would be. The consent is not valid if the patient did not understand the operation to be performed, its seriousness, the disease or incapacity, and possible results. In the instant case, the physicians failed to inform the patient about the recognized risks of the valve that was implanted.

Finally, the court reasoned that there were alternative valves available that were never discussed with the patient. To arrive at an informed decision concerning her treatment, it was material for her to have been told about the alternatives, risks, and benefits of the different valves available for use.

Physician's Duty to Advise

The duty to inform rests with the physician and requires the exercise of delicate medical judgment. It is the physician—not the hospital—who has the duty of obtaining informed consent. The physician, not the hospital, has the education, training, and experience necessary to advise each patient of risks associated with a proposed procedure. The physician is in the best position to know the patient's medical history and to evaluate and explain the risks of a particular operation in light of the particular medical history.[5]

COURSE OF TREATMENT: PATIENT'S DECISION

The plaintiff–patient in *Matthies v. Mastromonaco*,[6] an elderly woman living alone in a senior citizens' residence, fell and fractured her hip and was taken to the hospital. An orthopedic surgeon, the defendant, reviewed the patient's history, condition, and X-rays, and decided that, rather than utilizing a pinning procedure for her hip involving the insertion of four steel screws, it would be better to adopt a conservative course of treatment, bed rest.

Prior to her injury, the plaintiff maintained an independent style of living. She did her own grocery shopping and other household duties and had been able to climb steps unassisted.

Expert testimony at trial indicated that bed rest was an inappropriate treatment. The defendant was of the opinion that given the frail condition of the patient and her age, she would be best treated in a nursing home and, therefore, opted for a more conservative treatment. At the heart of the informed consent issue was the plaintiff's assertion that she would not have consented to bed rest if she had been informed of the probable effect on the quality of her life.

The New Jersey Supreme Court held that it is necessary to advise a patient when considering alternative courses of treatment. The physician should have explained medically reasonable invasive and noninvasive alternatives, including the risks and likely outcomes of those alternatives, even when the chosen course is noninvasive.

In an informed consent analysis, the decisive factor is not whether a treatment alternative is invasive or noninvasive, but whether the physician adequately presents the material facts so that the patient can make an informed decision. That conclusion does not imply that a physician must explain in detail all treatment options in every case.

If the patient's choice is not consistent with the physician's recommendation, the physician has the option of withdrawing from the case. The patient then has the option to seek another physician who is comfortable with the alternative treatment preferred by the patient.

Mother Asks Children, "Why Did You Let Them Do That to Me?"

Four children, in *Riser v. American Medican Intern, Inc.*,[7] brought a medical malpractice action against Lang, a physician who performed a femoral arteriogram on their 69-year-old mother. Her physician, Dr. Sottiurai, ordered bilateral arteriograms to determine the cause of the patient's impaired circulation. Because De La Ronde Hospital could not accommodate Sottiurai's request, Riser was transferred to Dr. Lang, a radiologist at St. Jude Hospital. Lang performed a femoral arteriogram, not the bilateral brachial arteriogram ordered by Sottiurai. The procedure seemed to go well, and the patient was prepared for transfer back to De La Ronde Hospital. However, shortly after the ambulance departed the hospital, the patient suffered a seizure in the ambulance and was returned to St. Jude. Riser's condition deteriorated, and she died 11 days later. The plaintiffs claimed in their lawsuit that Riser was a poor risk for the procedure.

The district court ruled for the plaintiffs, awarding damages in the amount of $50,000 for Riser's pain and suffering and $100,000 to each child. Lang appealed.

The Louisiana Court of Appeal held that Lang breached the standard of care by subjecting the patient to a procedure that would have no practical benefit to the patient. Further, Lang failed to obtain informed consent from the patient.

Testimony revealed that Lang breached the standard of care by performing a procedure that he knew or should have known would have had no practical benefit to the patient or her referring physician. The defendant himself, as well as the expert witnesses in this case, testified that it is a breach of the standard of care for any physician to subject a patient to a particular test or procedure that has any risk of injury, however small, associated with it if that physician knows or reasonably should know that the procedure will be of no benefit to the patient.

The consent form itself did not contain express authorization for Lang to perform the femoral arteriogram. Sottiurai ordered a brachial arteriogram, not a femoral arteriogram. Riser was under the impression that she was about to undergo a brachial arteriogram, not a femoral arteriogram. Two consent forms were signed; neither form authorized the performance of a femoral arteriogram. O'Neil, one of Riser's daughters, claimed that her mother said following the arteriogram, "Why did you let them do that to me?"[8] Although Lang claims that he explained the procedure to Riser and O'Neil, the trial court, faced with this conflicting testimony, chose to believe the plaintiffs.

INFORMATION TO BE DISCLOSED

A physician should provide as much information about treatment options as is necessary based on a patient's personal understanding of the physician's explanation of the risks of treatment and the probable consequences of the treatment. The needs of each patient can vary depending on age, maturity, and mental status.

Some courts have recognized that the condition of the patient may be taken into account to determine whether the patient has received sufficient information to give consent. The individual responsible for obtaining consent must weigh the importance of giving full disclosure to the patient against the likelihood that such disclosure will seriously and adversely affect the condition of the patient.

The courts generally utilize an "objective test" or "subjective test" to determine whether a patient would have refused treatment if the physician had provided adequate information as to the risks, benefits, and alternatives of the procedure. In the *objective test*, the plaintiff must prove that a "reasonable person" would not have undergone the procedure if he or she had been properly informed. Under the *subjective test theory*, the court examines whether the "individual patient" would have chosen the procedure if he or she had been fully informed. As described in the following cases, the courts favor the objective test.

Objective Standard

When applying the objective standard, the finder of fact may take into account the characteristics of the plaintiff, including the plaintiff's idiosyncrasies, fears, age, medical condition, and religious beliefs. Accordingly, the objective standard affords the ease of applying a uniform standard and yet maintains the flexibility of allowing the finder of fact to make appropriate adjustments to accommodate the individual characteristics and idiosyncrasies of an individual patient. The standard to be applied in informed consent cases is whether a reasonable person in the patient's position would have consented to the procedure or treatment in question if adequately informed of all significant perils. Under the objective analysis, the plaintiff's testimony is only one factor when determining the issue of informed consent. The issue is not whether a particular patient would have chosen a different course of treatment. The issue is whether a reasonable patient would have chosen a different course of treatment.

Subjective Standard

The subjective standard relies solely on the patient's testimony. Patients must testify and prove that they would not have consented to the procedure(s) had they been advised of the particular risk in question. Proponents of the subjective standard argue that a patient should have the right to make medical decisions regarding his or her care regardless of whether the determination is rational or reasonable. The subjective standard, however, potentially places the physician in jeopardy of the patient's hindsight and bitterness. The subjective standard is premised on the credibility of a patient's testimony.

HOSPITAL'S ROLE IN INFORMED CONSENT

Although hospitals are not generally responsible for informing patients as to the risks, benefits, and alternatives to specific procedures, there are some cases in which hospitals have a duty to provide patients with informed consent. The patient–plaintiff, in *Keel v. St. Elizabeth Medical Center, Ky.*,[9] filed a medical malpractice action alleging that the hospital failed to provide him with informed consent when he went there for a CT scan. The scan involved the injection of a contrast dye material. Prior to the test, Keel was given no information concerning any risks attendant to the procedure. The dye was injected, and the scan was conducted. However, the plaintiff developed a thrombophlebitis at the site of the injection.

The plaintiff argued that expert medical testimony was not required to prove the absence of informed consent. The hospital argued that the question of informed consent, like the question of negligence, must be determined against the standard of practice among members of the medical profession.

The Kentucky Supreme Court held that expert testimony was not required to establish lack of informed consent and that the hospital had a duty to inform the patient of the risks associated with the procedure. Responsibility did not lie solely with the patient's personal physician.

In view of the special circumstances of this case, the court found it significant that the hospital offered the plaintiff no information whatsoever concerning any possible hazards of this particular procedure, while at the same time the hospital admits that it routinely questions every patient about to undergo a dye injection as to whether he or she has had any previous reactions to contrast materials. Failure to adequately inform the patient need not be established by expert testimony if the failure is so apparent that laypersons may easily recognize it or infer it from evidence within the realm of common knowledge. A juror might reasonably infer from the nontechnical evidence that the hospital's utter silence as to the risks amounted to an assurance that there were none. The hospital's own questions to patients regarding reactions to the CT scan procedure demonstrated that the hospital recognized the substantial possibility of complications.

ADEQUACY OF CONSENT

When questions arise as to whether adequate consent has been given, some courts take into consideration the information that is ordinarily provided by other physicians. A physician must reveal to his or her patient such information as a skilled practitioner of good standing would provide under similar circumstances. A physician must disclose to the patient the potential of death, serious harm, and other complications associated with a proposed procedure. The scope of a physician's duty to disclose, as noted in *Wooley v. Henderson*,[10] is to be measured by those communications that a reasonable medical practitioner in that branch of medicine would make under the same or similar circumstances.

The plaintiff in *Ramos v. Pyati*[11] brought a medical malpractice action, alleging that the physician performed surgery on his hand outside the scope of surgery to which he consented. The plaintiff had injured his thumb while at work. He was referred to the defendant after seeing three other physicians. The plaintiff was diagnosed as having a ruptured thumb tendon. The plaintiff consented to a surgical repair of the thumb. During surgery, the defendant discovered that scar tissue had formed, causing the ends of the tendons in the thumb to retract. As a result, the surgeon decided to use a donor tendon to make the necessary repairs to the thumb. He chose a tendon from the ring finger. On discovering additional disability from the surgery, the plaintiff filed a suit alleging that his hand was rendered unusable for his employment as a mechanic and that the defendant had breached his duty by not advising him of the serious nature of the operation, by not exercising the proper degree of care in performing the operation, and by failing to discontinue surgery when he knew or should have known that the required surgery would most likely cause a greater disability than the already injured condition of the thumb. The plaintiff testified that although he signed a written consent form authorizing surgery on his thumb, he did not consent to a graft of his ring finger tendon or any other tendon. The plaintiff's expert witness testified that the ring finger is the last choice of four other tendons that could have been selected for the surgery. The circuit court entered a judgment for the plaintiff, and the defendant appealed. The appellate court upheld the judgment for the plaintiff, finding that the plaintiff had not consented to use of the ring finger tendon for repair of the thumb tendon.

VERBAL CONSENT

Verbal consent, if proved, is as binding as written consent, for there is, in general, no legal requirement that a patient's consent be in writing. However, oral consent is more difficult to corroborate.

Verbal Consent to Surgery Sufficient

The plaintiff in *Siliezar v. East Jefferson General Hospital*[12] argued that the defendants breached the standard of care by failing to obtain written consent for a surgical procedure. The trial judge found that the plaintiff failed to sustain her burden of proof that the defendants were liable to her for damages. On appeal, the appellees admitted that they breached hospital policy by failing to obtain written consent prior to surgery. The physician testified that he explained the surgical procedure, as well as the risks of the procedure. He testified that after he explained the procedure and its risks, he left a written consent for the patient to sign. He explained that while it is the policy of the clinic to obtain a written consent prior to performing surgery, the patient did not sign the consent form. The surgeon testified that he did not know why the form was not signed but that the patient did not refuse to sign the form.

At trial, a nurse testified that she placed the patient in an operating room and prepared her for surgery. Although she was not in the room when the surgeon discussed the surgical procedure with the plaintiff, she testified that she was in the next room and was able to hear the physician explain the procedure to the plaintiff. The nurse also had no explanation as to why the consent was not signed. She did state that the patient never said she did not want surgery nor did she ask the physician to stop the procedure. The nurse testified that as the physician performed the surgery, he explained to the patient what he was doing.

Louisiana statutes do not require that a patient's consent be written. Verbal consent was sufficient. The verbal consent included the information required by statute, and the patient was given an opportunity to ask questions and those questions were answered. The plaintiff claimed that she was told that surgery would not be performed. The trial judge did not find her testimony to be credible. The appellate court found that the defendants did not commit malpractice by failing to obtain written consent prior to surgery.

WRITTEN CONSENT

Written consent is preferred over oral consent. It provides evidence of a patient's wishes. Because the function of a written consent form is to preserve evidence of informed consent, the nature of the treatment, the risks, the benefits, and the consequences involved should be incorporated into the consent form. States have taken the view that consent, to be effective, must be informed consent. An informed consent form should include the following elements:

- the nature of the patient's illness or injury
- the procedure or treatment consented to
- the purpose of the proposed treatment
- the risks and probable consequences of the proposed treatment
- the probability that the proposed treatment will be successful
- any alternative methods of treatment and their associated risks and benefits
- the risks and prognosis if no treatment is rendered
- an indication that the patient understands the nature of any proposed treatment, the alternatives, the risks involved, and the probable consequences of the proposed treatment
- the signatures of the patient, physician, and witnesses
- the date the consent is signed

Health care professionals have an important role in the realm of informed consent. They can be instrumental in averting lawsuits by being observant as to a patient's doubts, changes of mind, confusion, or misunderstandings expressed regarding any proposed procedures he or she is about to undergo.

CONSENT FOR ROUTINE PROCEDURES

Many physicians and health care organizations have relied on consent forms worded in such general terms that they permit the physician to perform almost any medical or surgical procedure believed to be in the patient's best interests. There is little difference between a surgical patient who signs no authorization and one who signs a form consenting to whatever procedure the physician deems advisable.

Consent forms signed at the time of admission generally record the patient's consent to routine services, general diagnostic procedures, medical treatment, and the everyday routine touchings of the patient. The danger from its use arises from the potential of unwarranted reliance on it for specific, potentially high-risk procedures or treatments.

CONSENT FOR SPECIFIC PROCEDURES

There are a variety of consent forms found in the health care setting designed to more specifically describe the risks, benefits, and alternatives of particular invasive and noninvasive procedures. Such forms include consent for: anesthesia; cardiac catheterization; surgery; radiation therapy; administration of blood and blood byproducts; chemotherapy; CT and MRI scans; endoscopies; and colonoscopies.

LIMITED POWER OF ATTORNEY

A *limited power of attorney* authorizes, for example, school officials, teachers, and camp counselors to act on the parent's/parents' or legal guardian's behalf when seeking emergency care for injured students or campers. Such consent for treatment provides limited protection in the care of a particular child. Temporary consent indicates a parent's or guardian's intent to have a school official, teacher, or counselor seek emergency treatment when necessary.

IMPLIED CONSENT

Although the law requires consent for the intentional touching that stems from medical or surgical procedures, exceptions do exist with respect to emergency situations. *Implied consent* will generally be presumed when immediate action is required to prevent death or permanent impairment of a patient's health. If it is impossible in an emergency to obtain the consent of the patient or someone legally authorized to consent, the required procedure may be undertaken without liability for failure to procure consent.

Unconscious patients are presumed under law to approve treatment that appears to be necessary. It is assumed that such patients would have consented if they were conscious and competent. However, if a conscious patient expressly refuses to consent to certain treatment, such treatment may not be instituted after the patient becomes unconscious. Similarly, conscious patients suffering from emergency conditions retain the right to refuse consent.

If a procedure is necessary to protect one's life or health, every effort must be made to document the medical necessity for proceeding with medical treatment without consent. It must be shown that the emergency situation constituted an immediate threat to life or health.

In *Luka v. Lowrie*,[13] a case involving a 15-year-old boy whose left foot had been run over and crushed by a train, consultation by the treating physician with other physicians was an important factor in determining the outcome of the case. On the boy's arrival at the hospital, the defending physician and four house surgeons decided it was necessary to amputate the foot. The court said it was inconceivable that, had the parents been present, they would have refused consent in the face of a determination by five physicians that amputation would save the boy's life. Thus, despite testimony at the trial that the amputation might not have been necessary, professional consultation before the operation supported the assertion that a genuine emergency existed and could be implied consent.

STATUTORY CONSENT

Many states have adopted legislation concerning emergency care. An emergency in most states eliminates the need for consent. When a patient is clinically unable to give consent to a lifesaving emergency treatment, the law implies consent on the presumption that a reasonable person would consent to lifesaving medical intervention.

When an emergency situation does arise, there may be little opportunity to contact the attending physician, much less a consultant. The patient's records, therefore, must be complete with respect to the description of his or her illness and condition, the attempts made to contact the physician as well as relatives, and the emergency measures taken and procedures performed. If time does not permit a court order to be obtained, a second medical opinion, when practicable, is advisable.

JUDICIAL CONSENT

Judicial consent may be necessary in those instances where there is concern as to the absence or legality of consent. Judicial intervention is periodically necessary to grant consent on an emergency basis when a court is not in session. A judge should be contacted only after alternative methods have been exhausted and the matter cannot wait for a determination during the normal working hours of the court. Some courts (e.g., Massachusetts trial courts) require an attorney to initiate the call to the justice and to certify that there are no alternatives, other than a judicial response, available in the matter.

WHO MAY CONSENT

Consent of the patient ordinarily is required before treatment. However, when the patient is either physically unable or legally incompetent to consent and no emergency exists, consent must be obtained from a person who is empowered to consent on the patient's behalf. The person who authorizes treatment of another must have sufficient information to make an intelligent judgment on behalf of the patient.

Competent Patients

A competent adult patient's wishes concerning his or her person may not be disregarded. The court in *In re Melideo*[14] held that every human being of adult years has a right to determine what shall be done with his or her own body and cannot be subjected to medical treatment without his or her consent. When there is no compelling state interest that justifies overriding an adult patient's decision, that decision should be respected.

In *Fosmire v. Nicoleau*,[15] the New York Court of Appeals, New York's highest court, stated that the citizens of the state have long had the right to make their own medical care choices without regard to their medical condition or status as parents. The court of appeals held that a competent adult has both a common-law and statutory right under public health law to refuse lifesaving treatment. Citing the state's authority to compel vaccination to protect the public from the spread of disease, to order treatment for persons who are incapable of making medical decisions, and to prohibit medical procedures that pose a substantial risk to the patient alone, the court of appeals did note that the right to choose is not absolute. However, if there is no compelling state interest to justify overriding a patient's refusal to consent to a medical procedure because of religious beliefs, states are reluctant to override such a decision.

Guardianship

A *guardian* is an individual who by law is vested with the power and charged with the duty of taking care of a patient by protecting the patient's rights and managing the patient's estate. Guardianship is often necessary in those instances in which a patient is incapable of managing or administering his or her private affairs because of physical and/or mental disabilities or because he or she is under the age of majority.

Temporary guardianship can be granted by the courts if it is determined that such is necessary for the well-being of the patient. Temporary guardianship was granted by the court in *In re Estate of Dorone*,[16] where the physician and administrator petitioned the court on two occasions for authority to administer blood to a 22-year-old male patient brought to the hospital center by helicopter after an automobile accident was diagnosed as suffering from an acute subdural hematoma. It was determined that the patient would die unless he underwent a cranial operation. The operation required the administration of blood to which the parents would not consent because of their religious beliefs. After a hearing by telephone, the court of common pleas appointed the hospital's administrator as temporary guardian, authorizing him to consent to the performance of blood transfusions during emergency surgery. A more formal hearing did not take place because of the emergency situation that existed. Surgery was required a second time to remove a blood clot, and the court once again granted the administrator authority to authorize administration of blood. The superior court affirmed the orders, and the parents appealed.

The Pennsylvania Supreme Court held that the judge's failure to obtain direct testimony from the patient's parents and others concerning the patient's religious beliefs was not in error when death was likely to result from withholding blood. The judge's decisions granting guardianship and the authority to consent to the administration of blood were considered absolutely necessary in the light of the facts of this case. Nothing less than a fully conscious contemporary decision by the patient himself would have been sufficient to override the evidence of medical necessity.

Consent for Minors

When a medical or surgical procedure is to be performed on a minor, the question arises as to whether the minor's consent alone is sufficient and, if not, from whom consent should be obtained. The courts have held, as a general proposition, that the consent of a minor to medical or surgical treatment is ineffective and that the physician must secure the consent of the minor's parent or someone standing in loco parentis; otherwise, he or she will risk liability. Although parental consent should be obtained before treating a minor, treatment should not be delayed to the detriment of the child.

Parental consent is not necessary when the minor is married or otherwise emancipated. Most states have enacted statutes making it valid for married and emancipated minors to provide effective consent. Several courts have held the consent of a minor to be sufficient authorization for treatment in certain situations. In any specific case, a court's determination that the consent of a minor is effective and that parental consent is unnecessary will depend on such factors as the minor's age, maturity, mental status, and emancipation and the procedure involved, as well as public policy considerations.

In *Carter v. Cangello*,[17] the California Court of Appeals held that a 17-year-old girl who was living away from home, in the home of a woman who gave her free room and board in exchange for household chores, and who made her own financial decisions, legally could consent to medical procedures performed on her. The court made this decision knowing that the girl's parents provided part of her income by paying for her private schooling and certain medical care. The physician was privileged under statute to act on the minor's consent to surgery, and such privilege insulated him from liability to the parents for treating their daughter without their consent.

Many states have recognized by legislation that treatment for such conditions as pregnancy, venereal disease, and drug dependency does not require parental consent. State legislatures have reasoned that a minor is not likely to seek medical assistance when parental consent is demanded. Insisting on parental consent for the treatment of these conditions would increase the likelihood that a minor would delay or do without treatment to avoid explanation to the parents.

The Right to Choose: A Minor's Consent

Abraham Cherrix was 16 years old when he was diagnosed with Hodgkin's disease. He was treated with chemotherapy. He later learned that chemotherapy had not cured his disease. Doctors recommended a higher dosage of chemotherapy combined with radiation and culminating in stem cell therapy. The treatment program offered Abraham less than a 50% chance of survival. Abraham and his family chose to pursue alternative treatment in Mexico. Cherrix's oncologist reported the family's decision to the Department of Social Services (DSS). Cherrix's parents were accused of medical neglect by DSS. A judge granted the DSS temporary joint custody with the Cherrixes. The parents faced charges in the juvenile and domestic court for parental neglect. The family obtained a stay from the circuit court.[18] The Accomack Virginia Circuit Court judge cleared Abraham's parents of all charges of medical neglect and allowed Abraham to pursue alternative treatment under a doctor of the family's choice. The family will provide the court updates on Abraham's care every 3 months until he's cured or turns 18. The questions to be asked in this case include: Whose body is it, anyway? Did the state go too far? The judge must have thought so: "The judge agreed to allow me to see an oncologist of my choice! My alternative treatments WILL continue. He also ruled that my parents were not guilty of medical neglect, and social services no longer has any jurisdiction over my case! Free, happy, and ready to live, that's me!"[19]

Incompetent Patients

The ability to consent to treatment is a question of fact. The attending physician, who is in the best position to make the determination, should become familiar with his or her state's definition of legal incompetence. In any case in which a physician doubts a patient's capacity to consent, the consent of the legal guardian or next of kin should be obtained. If there are no relatives to consult, application should be made for a court order that would allow the procedure. It may be the duty of the court to assume responsibility of guardianship for a patient who is non compos mentis. The most frequently cited conditions indicative of incompetence are mental illness, mental retardation, senility, physical incapacity, and chronic alcohol or drug abuse.

A person who is mentally incompetent cannot legally consent to treatment. Therefore, consent of the patient's legal guardian must be obtained. When no legal guardian is available, a court that handles such matters must be petitioned to permit treatment.

Subject to applicable statutory provisions, when a physician doubts a patient's capacity to consent, even though the patient has not been judged legally incompetent, the consent of the nearest relative should be obtained. If a patient is conscious and mentally capable of giving consent for treatment, the consent of a relative without the consent of the competent patient would not protect the physician from liability.

RIGHT TO REFUSE TREATMENT

> *"[T]he individual's right to make decisions vitally affecting his private life*

> *according to his own conscience . . . is difficult to overstate . . . because it is, without exaggeration, the very bedrock on which this country was founded."*
>
> *Wons v. Public Health Trust*[20]

Adult patients who are conscious and mentally competent have the right to refuse medical care to the extent permitted by law, even when the best medical opinion deems it essential to life. If a patient rejects treatment, the hospital should take all reasonable steps to inform the patient of the risks of refusing treatment. Such a refusal must be honored whether it is grounded in religious belief or mere whim. Every person has the legal right to refuse to permit a touching of his or her body. Failure to respect this right can result in a legal action for assault and battery. Coercion through threat, duress, or intimidation must be avoided.

A patient's right to make decisions regarding his own health care is addressed in the Patient Self-Determination Act of 1990.[21] The act provides that each person has a right under state law (whether statutory or as recognized by the courts of the state) to make decisions concerning his or her medical care, including the right to accept or refuse medical or surgical treatment.

A competent patient's refusal to consent to a medical or surgical procedure must be adhered to, whether the refusal is grounded on lack of confidence in the physician, fear of the procedure, doubt as to the value of a particular procedure, or mere whim. The US Supreme Court stated that the "notion of bodily integrity has been embodied in the requirement that informed consent is generally required for medical treatment" and the "logical corollary of the doctrine of informed consent is that the patient generally possesses the right not to consent, that is, to refuse treatment."[22]

The question of liability for performing a medical or surgical procedure without consent is separate and distinct from any question of negligence or malpractice in performing a procedure. Liability can be imposed for a nonconsensual touching of a patient, even if the procedure improved the patient's health. The eminent Justice Cardozo, in *Schloendorff v. Society of New York Hospital*, stated:

> Every human being of adult years and sound mind has a right to determine what shall be done with his own body and a surgeon who performs an operation without his patient's consent commits an assault, for which he is liable in damages, except in cases of emergency where the patient is unconscious and where it is necessary to operate before consent can be obtained.[23]

The courts perform a balancing test to determine whether to override a competent adult's decision to refuse medical treatment. The courts balance state interests, such as preservation of life, protection of third parties, prevention of suicide, and the integrity of the medical profession against a patient's rights of bodily integrity and religious freedom.

The most frequently used state right to intervene in a patient's decision-making process is for the protection of third parties. In *In re Fetus Brown*,[24] the state of Illinois asserted that its interest in the well-being of a viable fetus outweighed the patient's rights to refuse medical treatment. The state argued that a balancing test should be used to weigh state interests against patient rights. The appellate court held that it could not impose a legal obligation upon a pregnant woman to consent to an invasive medical procedure for the benefit of her viable fetus.

Religious Beliefs

As part of their religious beliefs, Jehovah's Witnesses generally have refused the administration of blood, even in emergency situations. Case law over the past several decades has developed to a point where any person, regardless of religious beliefs, has the right to refuse medical treatment.

The plaintiff, Bonita Perkins, in *Perkins v. Lavin*,[25] was a Jehovah's Witness. She gave birth at the defendant–hospital on September 26, 1991, and was discharged 2 or 3 days later. After going home, she began hemorrhaging and returned to the hospital. She specifically informed the defendant's employees that she was not to be provided any blood or blood derivatives and completed and signed a form to that effect:

> I request that no blood or blood derivatives be administered to (plaintiff) during this hospitalization, notwithstanding that such treatment may be deemed necessary in the opinion of the attending physician or his assistants to preserve life or promote recovery. I release the attending physician, his assistants, the hospital and its personnel from any responsibility whatever for any untoward results due to my refusal to permit the use of blood or its derivatives.[26]

Due to the plaintiff's condition, it became necessary to perform an emergency dilation and curettage on her. She continued to bleed, and her condition deteriorated dramatically. Her blood count dropped, necessitating administration of blood products as a lifesaving measure. Her husband, who was not a Jehovah's Witness, consented to a blood transfusion, which was administered. The plaintiff recovered and filed an action against the defendant for assault and battery and intentional infliction of emotional distress. The plaintiff's claim as to assault and battery was sustained. The claim as to the intentional infliction of emotional distress was overruled.

GOOD PEOPLE: BAD DECISIONS

Sometimes good people make bad decisions. In health care, both the provider and the patient can make bad decisions. Although in the following case the hospital was exonerated from wrongdoing, an argument could be made that the hospital should have been more alert to the patient's needs. The patient, however, unwilling to wait, left the hospital without care and thus suffered harm.

The Long Wait

On August 10, 1988, Matthews had gone unassisted to the emergency department (ED) of the hospital complaining of a burning pain in her upper chest that had radiated down her right side that evening. Upon arriving at the hospital at about 11:25 p.m., Matthews was triaged by a nurse who took her vital signs, recorded her medical history, and made an assessment of her immediate medical needs. Although slightly elevated, Matthews's vital signs were within normal limits. The triage nurse classified Matthews as a "category two" patient, a nonthreatening condition. It was explained to her that she would have a long wait because the ED was busy. A social services representative (SSR) testified that he spoke to Matthews six or eight times during her wait in the ED. He indicated that she was in no apparent distress during those times that he spoke to her. Following a $4^1/_2$-hour wait, Matthews decided to leave the ED without being treated. The SSR stated that he told Matthews that a treatment room was ready for her and that she would be attended to shortly. Matthews said that she had already waited long enough and she was leaving. The SSR stated that he pleaded with her to stay but she refused, claiming that she would see her own physician in the morning. Matthews went to work the following day without having seen her physician. She died on August 12, 1988. A malpractice action was brought against the hospital arising out of the death of Matthews. The DeKalb Superior Court granted the hospital's motion for summary judgment, and an appeal was taken.

Matthews voluntarily terminated her relationship with the emergency department personnel, severing any causal relationship that might have existed between the hospital's act of classifying Matthews as a category two patient and her death. Accordingly, the hospital could not be liable for the death of the patient.[27]

RELEASE FORM

A patient's refusal to consent to treatment, for any reason, religious or otherwise, should be noted in the medical record, and a release form should be executed. The completed release provides documented evidence of a patient's refusal to consent to a recommended treatment. A release will help protect the organization and physicians from liability should a suit arise as a result of a failure to treat. The best possible care must be rendered to the patient at all times within the limits imposed by the patient's refusal.

Should a patient refuse to sign the release, documentation of the refusal should be placed on the form, and the form should be included as part of the patient's permanent medical record. Advice of legal counsel should be sought in those cases where refusal of treatment poses a serious threat to a patient's health. With the advice of legal counsel, the organization should formulate a policy regarding treatment when consent has been refused. An administrative procedure should be developed to facilitate application for a court order when one is necessary and there is sufficient time to obtain one.

INFORMED CONSENT: AVAILABLE DEFENSES

Several defenses are available to provider–defendants who have been sued on the basis of failure to provide their patients with sufficient information to make an informed decision. Some of the defenses include:

- the risk not disclosed is too commonly known to warrant disclosure
- the patient assured the medical practitioner that he or she would undergo the treatment or procedure regardless of the risk involved, or the patient assured the medical practitioner that he or she did not want to be informed of the matters to which he or she would be entitled to be informed
- consent by or on behalf of a patient was not reasonably possible
- the medical practitioner, after considering all of the attendant facts and circumstances, used reasonable discretion as to the manner and extent to which such alternatives or risks were disclosed to the patient because the practitioner reasonably believed that the manner and extent of such disclosure could reasonably be expected to adversely and substantially affect the patient's condition

A patient's condition during surgery may be recognized as different from that which had been expected and explained, requiring a different procedure than the one to which the patient initially consented. The surgeon may proceed to treat the new condition; however, the patient must have been aware of the possibility of extending the procedure.

The patient in *Winfrey v. Citizens & Southern National Bank*[28] brought a suit against the deceased surgeon's estate, alleging that during exploratory surgery, the surgeon performed a complete hysterectomy without the patient's consent. The superior court granted summary judgment for the surgeon's estate, and the patient appealed. The court of appeals held that even though the patient may not have read the consent document, when no legally sufficient excuse appeared, she was bound by the terms of the consent document that she voluntarily executed. The plain wording of the binding consent authorized the surgeon to perform additional or different operations or procedures that he might consider necessary or advisable in the course of the operation. Relevant sections of the consent signed by the patient included the following:

> 1. I authorize the performance on (patient's name) of the following operation/laparoscopy, possible laparotomy . . . .

> 2. I consent to the performance of operations and procedures in addition to or different from those now contemplated, which the above named doctor or his associates or assistants may consider necessary or advisable in the course of the operation . . . .
>
> • • •
>
> 7. I acknowledge that the nature and purpose of the operation, possible alternative methods of treatment, the risks involved, and the possibility of complications have been fully explained to me.[29]

DIALOGUE BETWEEN PHYSICIAN AND PATIENT

Informed consent is not merely a tool to avoid lawsuits; rather it is designed to allow patients to make an informed decision. The emphasis of "informed" must not be to avoid a lawsuit by meeting some legal requirement, with little regard to the patient's level of understanding of informed consent. The use of consent forms in this manner has contributed to the view that what was intended as a process of dialogue and discussion has developed into an event in which papers are signed and minimal legal requirements are satisfied. The consent form is often used as legal protection for the physician for unforeseen mishaps that might occur during surgery.

The ethical rationale underlying the doctrine of informed consent is firmly rooted in the notions of liberty and individual autonomy. Informed consent protects the basic right of the patient to make the ultimate informed decision regarding the course of treatment to which he or she knowledgeably consents. The focus of informed consent must involve the patient receiving informed consent as a result of active personal interaction with the physician. Consent forms should be used as a supplement to the oral disclosure of risks, benefits, and alternatives to the proposed procedure that a physician normally gives. Ideally, the consent should be the result of an active process of dialogue between the patient and physician.

Notes

1. 141 U.S. 250, 21 (1891).
2. In re Duran, 769 A.2d 497 (Pa. 2001).
3. 497 U.S. 261 (1990).
4. 635 A.2d 1047 (Pa. Super. Ct. 1993).
5. Mathias v. St. Catherne's Hosp., Inc., 569 N.W.2d 330 (Wis. App. 1997).
6. 733 A.2d 456 (1999).
7. 620 So. 2d 372 (La. Ct. App. 1993).
8. Id. at 380.
9. 842 S.W.2d 860 (Ky. 1992).
10. 418 A.2d 1123 (Me. 1980).
11. 534 N.E.2d 472 (Ill. App. Ct. 1989).
12. No. 04-CA-939 (La. Ct. App. 5 Cir. 1/11/05).
13. 136 N.W. 1106 (Mich. 1912).
14. 390 N.Y.S.2d 523 (N.Y. Sup. Ct. 1976).
15. 536 N.Y.S.2d 492 (N.Y. App. Div. 1989).
16. 534 A.2d 452 (Pa. 1987).
17. 164 Cal. Rptr. 361 (Cal. Ct. App. 1980).
18. My Journey, Abraham Cherrix's Page, www.abrahamsjourney.com/theHOMEpage.html.
19. Id.
20. 500 So. 2d 679, 687 (Fla. Dist. Ct. App. 1987), aff'd 541 So. 2d 96 (Fla. 1989).
21. Public Law 101-508, November 5, 1990, sections 4206 and 4751 of the Omnibus Budget Reconciliation Act.
22. Cruzan v. Director, Missouri Dep't of Health, 497 U.S. 261, 269 (1990).
23. 105 N.E. 92, 93 (N.Y. 1914).
24. 689 N.E.2d 397 (Ill. App. Ct. 1997).
25. 648 N.E.2d 839 (Ohio App. 9 Dist. 1994).
26. Id. at 840.
27. Matthews v. DeKalb County Hosp. Auth., 440 S.E.2d 743 (Ga. Ct. App. 1994).
28. 254 S.E.2d 725 (Ga. Ct. App. 1979).
29. Id. at 727.

13

LEGAL REPORTING REQUIREMENTS

This chapter provides an overview of a variety of reporting requirements mandated by both federal and state regulatory agencies. Most states have legislated a variety of mandatory reporting requirements (e.g., child abuse, diseases that pose a threat to public health and safety).

CHILD ABUSE

The physically abused or neglected child presents a medical, social, and legal problem. What constitutes an abused child is difficult to determine because it is often impossible to ascertain whether a child was injured intentionally or accidentally.

Child Abuse and Neglect

Child abuse is intentional serious mental, emotional, sexual, and/or physical injury inflicted by a family member or other person who is responsible for the child's care. Some states extend the definition to include a child who suffers from starvation. Other states include moral neglect in the definition of abuse. Others mention immoral associations; endangering a child's morals; and the location of a child in a disreputable place or in association with vagrant, vicious, or immoral persons. Sexual abuse also is enumerated as an element of neglect in the statutes of some states.

The *Child Abuse Prevention and Treatment Act* defines the term "child abuse and neglect" as any recent act or failure to act on the part of a parent or caretaker, which results in death, serious physical or emotional harm, sexual abuse or exploitation, or an act or failure to act that presents an imminent risk of serious harm.[1]

Reporting Child Abuse

Presently, all states have enacted laws to protect abused children. Most states protect the persons required to report cases of child abuse. In some states, certain identified individuals who are not required to report instances of child abuse, but who do so, are protected. Persons in the health care setting who are required to report, or cause a report to be made, when they have reasonable cause to suspect that a child has been abused include administrators, physicians, interns, registered nurses, chiropractors, social service workers, psychologists, dentists, osteopaths, optometrists, podiatrists, mental health professionals, and volunteers in residential facilities.

Detecting Abuse

An individual who reports child abuse should be aware of the physical and behavioral indicators of abuse and maltreatment that appear to be part of a pattern (e.g., bruises, burns, and broken bones). In reviewing the indicators of abuse and maltreatment, the reporter does not have to be absolutely certain that abuse or maltreatment exists before reporting. Rather, abuse and maltreatment should be reported whenever they are suspected, based on the existence of the signs of abuse and maltreatment and in light of the reporter's training and experience. Behavioral indicators include, but are not limited to, substantially diminished psychological or intellectual functioning, failure to thrive, no control of aggression, self-destructive impulses, decreased ability to think and reason, acting out and misbehavior, or habitual truancy. Such impairment must be clearly attributable to the unwillingness or inability of the person responsible for the child's care to exercise a minimum degree of care toward the child.

Good-Faith Reporting

Any report of suspected child abuse must be made with a *good-faith* belief that the facts reported are true. The definition of good faith as used in a child abuse statute may vary from state to state. However, when a health care practitioner's medical evaluation indicates reasonable cause to believe a child's injuries were not accidental and when the health care practitioner is not acting from his or her desire to harass, injure, or embarrass the child's parents, making the report will not result in liability. Statutes generally require that when a person covered by a statute is attending a child and suspects abuse, the staff member must report such concerns. Typical statutes provide that an oral report be made immediately, followed by a written report. Most states require the report to contain the following information: the child's name and address; the person(s) responsible for the child's care; the child's age; the nature and extent of the child's injuries (including any evidence of previous injuries); and any other information that might be helpful in establishing the cause of the injuries, such as photographs of the injured child and the identity of the alleged abuser.

Psychologist Immune from Liability

The psychologist in E.S. by *D.S. v. Seitz*[2] was immune from liability in a suit charging her with negligence in formulating and reporting her professional opinion to a social worker that a father had sexually abused his 3-year-old daughter. The psychologist made the report in compliance with the Wisconsin statute after having examined the child in the course of her professional duties as a mental health professional.

The patient in *Marks v. Tenbrunsel*[3] had been assured that anything he disclosed during his treatment sessions would remain confidential. During the treatment sessions, the patient disclosed that he had fondled two children under the age of 12. As a result of that disclosure, two psychologists made a good-faith report to Child Protective Services. The report caused the patient to be prosecuted for his admitted sexual misconduct. Because the patient admitted to the abuse of two children, the psychologists had reasonable cause to believe that the children currently were being abused. The psychologists were found immune from both civil and criminal liability as a result of their good-faith report.

Failure to Report Child Abuse

The criminal and civil risks for health care professionals do not lie in good faith reporting of suspected incidents of child abuse, but in failing to report such incidents. Most states have legislated a variety of civil and criminal penalties for failure to report suspected child abuse incidents.

Psychologist: Failure to Report Past Abuse

The Minnesota Board of Psychology was found to have acted properly when it placed the license of a psychologist on conditional status.[4] The psychologist argued that he was not required to report past abuse that was not ongoing, that a report made 5 weeks after the incident was not untimely, and that the reporting laws were unconstitutional because they violated the privacy rights of clients and the privilege against self-incrimination. The psychologist had failed to report incidents of sexual child abuse. The court held that there was no merit to the psychologist's contentions that the child abuse reporting laws were unclear and that they did not apply to one patient who was a grandfather responsible for the child's care at the time of the incident in question.

Nurse: Failure to Document and Report

In *State v. Brown*,[5] rescue personnel who were summoned to the scene of an emergency found a 2-year-old foster child unconscious, not breathing, and "posturing," which is an abnormal rigidity of the body and a sign of brain damage. While performing emergency medical treatment, rescue personnel discovered a series of small, round, dime- to quarter-sized bruises running parallel along the child's spine. They also noticed a red bruise under his eye. This information was relayed to the flight crew, who airlifted the child to the hospital. The flight crew then reported the information to a nurse employed at the hospital. The child recovered after treatment and was released from the hospital on August 14, 2002. Four days later, on August 18, the child was returned to the hospital where he died of abusive head trauma.

The *nurse did not document* the bruises or call the state's child abuse hotline because the boy's foster mother said the bruises were the result of the boy leaning back in a booster seat. In February 2003, the prosecutor alleged that the nurse had reasonable cause to suspect that the child had been abused or neglected. She was charged with *failure to report child abuse* to the division of family services and to a physician. The nurse sought to dismiss the charges, alleging that Missouri statutes were unconstitutionally vague. The appellate court determined that the statutes were not vague. The test for determining whether a law is void for vagueness is whether its language conveys to a person of ordinary intelligence a sufficiently definite warning as to the proscribed conduct when measured by common understanding and practices. The statute criminalizing a health professional's failure to report child abuse upon "reasonable cause to suspect" abuse was not unconstitutionally vague.

Physician Entitled to Immunity

A physician who was not the initial reporter of suspected child abuse, but who performed a medical examination of a child at the request of the department of children and families to determine whether reasonable cause existed to suspect child abuse, was entitled to the immunity from liability provided by statutory law. It was clear that the physician, a mandated reporter under the law, examined the child in the ordinary course of his employment in the emergency department. He complied with applicable statutes when he relayed his findings that there was a reasonable suspicion of child abuse to the department. Inasmuch as the plaintiffs did not allege that the physician acted in bad faith during the examination and reporting process, his actions constituted a report of suspected child abuse protected by statutory law.[6]

ELDER ABUSE AND NEGLECT

Elder abuse is any form of mistreatment that results in harm or loss to an older person. It can involve physical abuse (that results in bodily injury, pain, or impairment and includes assault, battery, and inappropriate restraint); sexual abuse (nonconsensual sexual contact of any kind with an older person); domestic violence (an escalating pattern of violence by an intimate partner where the violence is used to exercise power and control); psychological abuse (the willful infliction of mental or emotional anguish by threat, humiliation, or other verbal or nonverbal conduct); or financial abuse (the illegal or improper use of an older person's funds, property, or resources).[7] Neglect is the failure to provide the care necessary to avoid physical harm (e.g., the failure of staff to turn a patient periodically to prevent pressure sores) or mental anguish.

Most states have enacted statutes mandating the reporting of elder abuse. In general, elder abuse is less likely to be reported than child abuse. Physical and emotional neglect, as well as verbal and financial abuse, is perceived as the most prevalent form of elder abuse. Seniors often fail to report incidents of abuse because they fear retaliation and not being believed or threats of placement in a nursing home. In addition, proving such charges is often difficult. Signs of abuse or neglect include: unexplained or unexpected death; development of pressure sores; heavy medication and sedation used in place of adequate nursing staff; occurrence of broken bones; sudden and unexpected emotional outbursts, agitation, or withdrawal; bruises, welts, discoloration, burns; absence of hair and/or hemorrhaging below the scalp; dehydration and/or malnourishment without illness-related cause; hesitation to talk openly; implausible stories; unusual or inappropriate activity in bank accounts; signatures on checks and other written materials that do not resemble the patient's signature; power of attorney given or recent changes or creation of a will when the person is incapable of making such decisions; missing personal belongings such as silverware or jewelry; an untreated medical condition; and the patient is unable to speak for himself or herself, or see others, without the presence of the caregiver (suspected abuser).

Documentation

Caregivers who suspect abuse are expected to report their findings. Symptoms and conditions of suspected abuse should be defined clearly and objectively.

- Witnesses: Reporters of abuse must describe statements made by others as accurately as possible. Information should include information as to how witnesses can be contacted.
- Photographs: It may be necessary to photograph wounds or injuries. A hospital emergency room or the police department can be asked to photograph in emergency situations.

COMMUNICABLE DISEASES

Most states have enacted laws that require the reporting of actual or suspected cases of communicable diseases. The need for statutes requiring the reporting of communicable diseases is clear. If a state is to protect its citizens' health through its power to quarantine, it must ensure the prompt reporting of infection or disease.

BIRTHS AND DEATHS

All births and deaths are reportable by statute. Births occurring outside of a health care facility should be reported by the legally qualified physician in attendance at a delivery or, in the event of the absence of a physician, by the registered nurse or other attendant. The physician who pronounces death must sign the death certificate. Statutes requiring the reporting of births and deaths are necessary to maintain accurate census records.

SUSPICIOUS DEATHS

Greater than a state's interest in the recording of all births and deaths is the state's desire to review suspicious deaths that may be the result of some form of criminal activity. Unnatural deaths must be referred to the medical examiner for review. Such cases include violent deaths, deaths caused by unlawful acts or criminal neglect, and deaths that may be considered suspicious or unusual. The medical examiner may make an investigation of such cases and issue an autopsy report. The purpose of a medical examiner's investigation is to determine the actual cause of death and thereby provide assistance for any further criminal investigation that may be considered necessary.

HEALTH CARE QUALITY IMPROVEMENT ACT

Congress enacted the Health Care Quality Improvement Act (HCQIA)[8] of 1986 to improve the quality of medical care by encouraging physicians to participate in peer review and by restricting incompetent physicians' ability to move from state to state without disclosure or discovery of their previous substandard performance or unprofessional conduct. The HCQIA was enacted in part to provide those persons giving information to professional review bodies and those assisting in review activities limited immunity from damages that may arise as a result of adverse decisions that affect a physician's medical staff privileges. Prior to enacting the HCQIA, Congress found that "[t]he increasing occurrence of medical malpractice and the need to improve the quality of medical care . . . [had] become nationwide problems," especially in light of "the ability of incompetent physicians to move from State to State without disclosure or discovery of the physician's previous damaging or incompetent performance."[9] HCQIA was enacted to facilitate the frank exchange of information among professionals who conduct peer review inquiries without the fear of reprisals in civil lawsuits. The statute attempts to balance the chilling effect of litigation on peer review with concerns for protecting physicians who are improperly subjected to disciplinary action.

NATIONAL PRACTITIONER DATA BANK

The National Practitioner Data Bank (NPDB)[10] was created by Congress as a national repository of information with the primary purpose of facilitating a comprehensive review of physicians' and other health care practitioners' professional credentials. Hospitals are required to report to the NPDB professional review actions that are related to a physician's competence or conduct and that adversely affect clinical privileges for more than 30 days, and a physician's voluntary surrender or restriction of clinical privileges.

Responsibility for data bank implementation resides in the Bureau of Health Professions, Health Resources and Services Administration of the DHHS. The act authorizes the data bank to be used to collect and release information on the professional competence and conduct of physicians, dentists, and other health care practitioners. The regulations are intended to encourage good-faith professional review activities.

The NPDB presents a number of challenges to health care institutions. A major one is to educate the medical staff so that the data bank will not erode medical staff participation in risk management. The purpose of the data bank is not punishment; rather, it is prevention and deterrence.

Reporting Requirements

The regulations establish reporting requirements applicable to hospitals; health care entities; boards of medical examiners; professional societies of physicians, dentists, or other health care practitioners that take adverse licensure or professional review actions (e.g., reduction, restriction, suspension, revocation, or denial of clinical privileges or membership in a health care entity of 30 days or longer); and individuals and entities (including insurance companies) who make payments as a result of medical malpractice actions or claims. A medical malpractice action (or claim) has been defined as a written complaint or claim demanding payment based on a health care practitioner's provision of or failure to provide health care services, including the filing of a cause of action based on tort law, brought in any state or federal court or other adjudicative body.

Required Queries and Medical Staff Privileges

Health care organizations must query the data bank every 2 years on the renewal of staff privileges of physicians and dentists. The data bank serves as a flagging system whose principal purpose is to facilitate a more comprehensive review of professional credentials. As a nationwide flagging system, it provides another resource to assist state licensing boards, hospitals, and other health care entities in conducting extensive independent reviews of the qualifications of health care practitioners they seek to license or hire or to whom they wish to grant clinical privileges.

Who Should Report?

For those health care providers who question whether they are covered under this law, DHHS defines the term "entity" broadly, rather than attempting to focus on the myriad health care organizations, practice arrangements, and professional societies, to ensure that the regulations include all entities within the scope of the statute. A health care entity is an entity that provides health care services and engages in professional review activity through a formal peer-review process for the purpose of furthering quality health care or a committee of that entity. Health care practitioners include all health care practitioners authorized by a state to provide health care services by whatever formal mechanism the state uses (e.g., certification, registration, and licensure).

Data Bank Queries

Data bank queries can be made by state licensing boards, hospitals, other health care entities, and professional societies that have entered or may be entering employment or affiliation relationships with a physician, dentist, or other health care practitioner who has applied for clinical privileges or appointment to a medical staff. A plaintiff's attorney is permitted to obtain information from the data bank when a malpractice action has been filed and the practitioner on whom information has been sought is named in the suit.

Confidentiality of Data Bank Information

Information reported to the data bank is considered to be strictly confidential and cannot be disclosed except as specified in the NPDB regulations. Individuals and entities that knowingly and willfully report to or query the data bank under false pretenses or fraudulently access the data bank computer directly are subject to civil penalties.

The Privacy Act of 1974 protects the contents of federal systems of records such as those contained in the NPDB from disclosure, unless the disclosure is for a routine use of the system of records as published annually in the Federal Register. The published routine uses of NPDB information do not allow for disclosure of information to the general public.

INCIDENT REPORTING

Incident reports contain statements made by employees and physicians regarding a deviation from acceptable patient care. Some state health codes provide that hospitals and nursing facilities must investigate incidents regarding patient care and require that certain incidents must be reported in a manner prescribed by regulation. Reportable incidents often include such things as those incidents that have resulted in a patient's serious injury or death, an event such as fire or loss of emergency power, certain infection outbreaks, and strikes by employees.

Incident reports should not be placed in the medical record. They should be directed to counsel for legal advice. This will help prevent discovery on the basis of client–attorney privilege. There is conflicting case law in that some courts will not permit incident reports to be discovered whereas others will allow discovery.

State Reportable Incidents

State reportable events include the reporting of communicable diseases, infections, and unusual or an unexpected cluster of patients with symptoms/diseases or exposures suggestive of a health emergency or terrorism event.

Many states have enacted legislation requiring hospitals to report incidents that result in patient injury. The new Pennsylvania Medical Care Availability and Reduction of Error Act (MCARE Act) reporting requirements, for example, are intended to help reduce and eliminate medical errors by identifying problems and implementing solutions to improve patient safety. The MCARE Act requires health care facilities to report serious events and incidents to a newly established patient safety authority. The act defines a serious event as an event, occurrence, or situation involving the clinical care of a patient in a medical facility that results in death or compromises patient safety and results in an unanticipated injury requiring the delivery of additional health care services to the patient.

Hospital procedures for reporting patient care incidents must comply with state regulations. As with The Joint Commission requirements, the Pennsylvania law prohibits retaliatory action against the health care worker for reporting patient care incidents and provides for written notification to patients.

Individuals designated to report incidents must do so if required by a state's statute. The director of nursing at a nursing facility in *Choe v. Axelrod*[11] was fined $150 for failure to report an instance of patient neglect. An anonymous telephone call had been placed with the department of health regarding two incidents of alleged patient neglect. In one incident, a patient had been left unattended in a shower by an orderly, and the patient sprayed himself with hot water, which resulted in second-degree burns on his forehead. On a second occasion, a similar incident occurred, but no one was injured. On investigation by the department of health, a determination was made that both incidents constituted patient neglect and that failure to report these incidents was a violation of New York public health law. After a hearing by an administrative law judge, the charge in the first incident was sustained and in the second incident was dismissed. The director of nurses petitioned to annul the administrative determination. She contended that the department of health failed to establish a prima facie case of patient neglect, that the incident was an unavoidable accident, and that the department of health's proof was based on hearsay evidence. The court held that evidence supported a finding that the director of nurses failed to report an incident of patient neglect as required by statute.

Although it may not always be clear as to when an incident report should be filed, appropriate procedures should be in place to address how questionable events should be handled.

SENTINEL EVENTS

The Joint Commission encourages health care organizations to self-report sentinel events. The Joint Commission defines a *sentinel event* as "an unexpected occurrence involving death or serious physical or psychological injury, or the risk thereof. Serious injury specifically includes loss of limb or function. The phrase, 'or the risk thereof,' includes any process variation for which a recurrence would carry a significant chance of a serious adverse outcome."[12] Frequently reported sentinel events include patient suicides, medication errors, death due to delays in treatment, operative/postoperative complications, and surgical procedures on the wrong site.

Although The Joint Commission encourages but does not require the reporting of sentinel events, it does expect organizations to conduct a root-cause analysis when sentinel events occur.

Root Cause Analysis

A *root cause analysis* (RCA) is:

> a process for identifying the basic or causal factors that underlie variation in performance, including the occurrence or possible occurrence of a sentinel event. A root cause analysis focuses primarily on systems and processes, not on individual performance. It progresses from special causes in clinical processes to common causes in organizational processes and systems and identifies potential improvements in processes or systems that would tend to decrease the likelihood of such events in the future or determines, after analysis, that no such opportunities exist.[13]

The basic purpose of an RCA is to improve organizational performance outcomes. Organizations are often concerned with the possibility that RCAs could be subject to discovery by a plaintiff's attorney and could then be used against them in civil trials. To address this concern and minimize the risks of additional liability exposure, The Joint Commission continues to work on ways to prevent the disclosure of the substance of RCAs.

The RCA process involves:

- thoroughly investigating an unfortunate occurrence to determine the main cause of the event
- conducting a thorough and credible analysis
- investigating both general and special causes that instigated the event
- researching and reviewing the literature
- searching for best practices on the Internet
- contacting and consulting with other organizations that have implemented best practices to limit the likelihood of such events from occurring in the future
- identifying changes that can be made to reduce or eliminate the likelihood of similar occurrences in the future
- identifying who will be responsible for implementing changes
- pilot testing the new design/best practice prior to full implementation
- determining a time line for implementing changes
- determining how changes will be communicated to those who will be working under the new design
- educating staff, who will be responsible for operating under the newly designed practice
- determining how implementation of new processes will be monitored and evaluated

Reporting sentinel events, conducting root cause analyses, and sharing that information with The Joint Commission will be helpful to all organizations in improving patient care. For helpful information on sentinel events and root cause analyses, visit The Joint Commission's Web site (http://jointcommission.org/).

CORPORATE COMPLIANCE PROGRAMS

The federal government's initiative to investigate and prosecute health care organizations for criminal wrongdoing, coupled with strong sanctions imposed after conviction, has resulted in health care organizations establishing corporate compliance programs. These programs establish internal mechanisms for preventing, detecting, and reporting criminal conduct. Sentencing incentives are in place for organizations that establish such programs. The following paragraphs describe the elements of an effective corporate compliance program.

An "effective program to prevent and detect violations of the law" means a program that has been reasonably designed, implemented, and enforced so that it generally will be effective in preventing and detecting criminal conduct. Failure to prevent or detect the instant offense, by itself, does not mean that the program was not effective. The hallmark of an effective program to prevent and detect violations of law is that the organization exercised due diligence in seeking to prevent and detect criminal conduct by its employees and other agents. Due diligence requires that an organization will, at the very least, have implemented the following:

1. The organization must have established compliance standards and procedures to be followed by its employees and other agents that are reasonably capable of reducing the prospect of criminal conduct.
2. Specific individual(s) within high-level personnel of the organization must have been assigned overall responsibility to oversee compliance with such standards and procedures.
3. The organization must have used due care not to delegate substantial discretionary authority to individuals whom the organization knew, or should have known through the exercise of due diligence, had a propensity to engage in illegal conduct.
4. The organization must have taken steps to communicate effectively its standards and procedures to all employees and other agents, for example, by requiring participation in training programs or by disseminating publications that explain in a practical manner what is required.
5. The organization must have taken reasonable steps to achieve compliance with its standards, for example, by utilizing monitoring and auditing systems reasonably designed to detect criminal conduct by its employees and other agents and by having in place and publicizing a reporting system whereby employees and other agents could report criminal conduct by others within the organization without fear of retribution.
6. The standards must have been consistently enforced through appropriate disciplinary mechanisms, including, as appropriate, discipline of individuals who are responsible for the failure to detect an offense. Adequate discipline of individuals who are responsible for an offense is a necessary component of enforcement; however, the discipline that will be appropriate will be case specific.
7. After an offense has been detected, the organization must have taken all reasonable steps to respond appropriately to the offense and to prevent similar offenses—including any necessary modifications to its program to prevent and detect violations of the law.[14]

Notes

1. U.S. Code, Title 42, Chapter 67, Subter 1, § 5106g.
2. 413 N.W.2d 670 (Wis. Ct. App. 1987).
3. No. 1031515 (Ala. 2005).
4. 415 N.W.2d 436 (Minn. Ct. App. 1987).
5. 140 S.W.3d 51 (Mo. banc).
6. Manifold v. Ragaglia, No. SC 17150 (Conn. 2004).
7. What is Elder Abuse, National Committee for the Prevention of Elder Abuse, www.preventelderabuse.org/elderabuse/elderabuse.html.
8. PUB. L. No. 99-660, tit. IV (1986).
9. 42 U.S.C. § 11101[0].
10. http://www.npdb-hipdb.hrsa.gov/.
11. 534 N.Y.S.2d 739 (N.Y. App. Div. 1988).

12. 2007 Comprehensive Manual for Hospitals: The Official Handbook, The Joint Commission on Accreditation of Healthcare Organizations, at SE-1.
13. Id. at SE-2.
14. 56 Fed. Reg. 22,762 (May 16, 1991).

14

ISSUES OF PROCREATION

This chapter reviews a variety of issues of procreation. Primary emphasis is placed on abortion. Discussed to a lesser extent are issues relating to sterilization, artificial insemination, and wrongful birth, wrongful life, and wrongful conception.

ABORTION

Abortion is the premature termination of pregnancy. It can be classified as spontaneous or induced. It may occur as an incidental result of a medical procedure or it may be an elective decision on the part of the patient. In addition to having substantial ethical, moral, and religious implications, abortion has proven to be a major political issue and will continue as such in the future. More laws will be proposed, more laws will be passed, and more lawsuits will wind their way up to the US Supreme Court.

Right to Abortion

Roe v. Wade[1] in 1973 gave strength to a woman's right to privacy in the context of matters relating to her own body, including how a pregnancy would end. However, the Supreme Court also has recognized the interest of the states in protecting potential life and has attempted to spell out the extent to which the states may regulate and even prohibit abortions.

In *Roe v. Wade*, the US Supreme Court held the Texas penal abortion law unconstitutional, stating: "[s]tate criminal abortion statutes . . . that except from criminality only a lifesaving procedure on behalf of the mother, without regard to the stage of her pregnancy and other interests involved, is violating the Due Process Clause of the Fourteenth Amendment."[2]

First Trimester

During the first trimester of pregnancy, the decision to undergo an abortion procedure is between the woman and her physician. A woman's right to an abortion is not unqualified because the decision to perform the procedure must be left to the medical judgment of her attending physician. "For the stage prior to approximately the end of the first trimester, the abortion decision and its effectuation must be left to the medical judgment of the pregnant woman's attending physician."[3]

Second Trimester

In *Roe v. Wade*, the Supreme Court stated, "for the stage subsequent to approximately the end of the first trimester, the State, in promoting its interest in the health of the mother, may, if it chooses, regulate the abortion procedure in ways that are reasonably related to maternal health."[4] Thus, during approximately the fourth to sixth months of pregnancy, the state may regulate the medical conditions under which the procedure is performed. The constitutional test of any legislation concerning abortion during this period would be its relevance to the objective of protecting maternal health.

Third Trimester

The Supreme Court reasoned that by the time the final stage of pregnancy has been reached, the state has acquired a compelling interest in the product of conception, which would override the woman's right to privacy and justify stringent regulation even to the extent of prohibiting abortions. In the *Roe* case, the Court formulated its ruling as to the last trimester in the following words: "[f]or the stage subsequent to viability, the State in promoting its interest in the potentiality of human life, may, if it chooses, regulate, and even proscribe, abortion except where it is necessary, in appropriate medical judgment for the preservation of the life or health of the mother."[5]

Thus, during the final stage of pregnancy, a state may prohibit all abortions except those deemed necessary to protect maternal life or health. The state's legislative powers over the performance of abortions increase as the pregnancy progresses toward term.

Abortion Restrictions

1992: In *Planned Parenthood v. Casey*,[6] the Supreme Court ruling, as enunciated in *Roe v. Wade*, reaffirmed: (1) the constitutional right of women to have an abortion before viability of the fetus, as first enunciated in *Roe v. Wade;* (2) the state's power to restrict abortions after fetal viability, as long as the law contains exceptions for pregnancies that endanger a woman's life or health; and (3) the principle that the state has legitimate interests from the outset of the pregnancy in protecting the health of the woman and the life of the fetus.

The Supreme Court here also ruled that it is not an undue burden to require that: (1) a woman be informed of the nature of the abortion procedure and the risks involved; (2) a woman be offered information on the fetus and on the alternatives to abortion; (3) a woman give her informed consent before the abortion procedure; (4) parental consent be given for a minor seeking an abortion, providing for a judicial bypass option if the minor does not wish or cannot obtain parental consent; and (5) there be a 24-hour waiting period before any abortion can be performed.

Abortion Counseling

1983: The Supreme Court in *City of Akron v. Akron Center for Reproductive Health*[7] voted that the different states cannot: (1) mandate what information physicians give abortion patients, or (2) require that abortions for women more than 3 months pregnant be performed in a hospital.

With respect to a requirement that the attending physician must inform the woman of specified information concerning her proposed abortion, it is unreasonable for a state to insist that only a physician is competent to provide the information and counseling relative to informed consent.

Prohibition of Counseling Not Unconstitutional

1991: The Supreme Court in *Rust v. Sullivan*[8] determined that federal regulations that prohibit abortion counseling and referral by family planning clinics that receive funds under Title X of the Public Health Service Act were found not to violate the constitutional rights of pregnant women. The Court extended the doctrine that government need not subsidize the exercise of the fundamental rights to free speech.

Abortion Committee Requirement Too Restrictive

The Supreme Court in *Doe v. Bolton*[9] struck down four preabortion procedural requirements commonly imposed by state statutes that require: (1) residency; (2) performance of the abortion in a hospital accredited by The Joint Commission; (3) approval by an appropriate committee of the medical staff; and (4) consultations.

The Court was unable to find any constitutionally justifiable rationale for a statutory requirement of advance approval by an abortion committee of the hospital's medical staff. Insofar as statutory consultation requirements are concerned, the Court reasoned that the acquiescence of two copractitioners has no rational connection with a patient's needs and, further, unduly infringes on the physician's right to practice.

Spousal Consent Unconstitutional

1975: A Florida statute required written consent of the husband before a wife could be permitted to obtain an abortion. The husband's interest in the baby was held to be insufficient to force his wife to face the mental and physical risks of pregnancy and childbirth.[10]

In *Doe v. Zimmerman*,[11] the court declared unconstitutional the provisions of the Pennsylvania Abortion Control Act, which required that the written consent of the husband of a married woman be secured before the performance of an abortion. The court found that these provisions impermissibly permitted the husband to withhold his consent either because of his interest in the potential life of the fetus or for capricious reasons. The natural father of an unborn fetus in *Doe v. Smith*[12] was found not to be entitled to an injunction to prevent the mother from submitting to an abortion. Although the father's interest in the fetus was legitimate, it did not outweigh the mother's constitutionally protected right to an abortion.

Parental Consent

1979: The Supreme Court in *Bellotti v. Baird*[13] ruled that a Massachusetts statute requiring parental consent before an abortion could be performed on an unmarried woman under age 18 was unconstitutional. Justice Stevens, joined by Justices Brennan, Marshall, and Blackmun, concluded that the Massachusetts statute was unconstitutional because under that statute as written and construed by the Massachusetts Supreme Judicial Court, no minor, no matter how mature and capable of informed decision making, could receive an abortion without the consent of either both parents or a superior court judge, thus making the minor's abortion subject in every instance to an absolute third-party veto.

Notice Requirement for Immature Minor

1981: The Supreme Court, in *H. L. v. Matheson*,[14] upheld a Utah statute that required a physician to "notify, if possible" the parents or guardian of a minor on whom an abortion was to be performed. In this case, the physician advised the patient that an abortion would be in her best medical interest but, because of the statute, refused to perform the abortion without notifying her parents. The Supreme Court ruled that although a state may not constitutionally legislate a blanket, unreviewable power of parents to veto their daughter's abortion, a statute setting out a mere requirement of parental notice when possible does not violate the constitutional rights of an immature, dependent minor.

Consent Not Required for Emancipated Minor

1987: The trial court in *In re Anonymous*[15] was found to have abused its discretion when it refused a minor's request for waiver of parental consent to obtain an abortion. The record indicated that the minor lived alone, was within one month of her 18th birthday, lived by herself most of the time, and held down a full-time job.

Parental Notification Not Required

2000: The issue in *Planned Parenthood v. Owens*[16] is whether the Colorado Parental Notification Act, Colo. Rev. Stat. §§ 12-37.5-101, et seq. (1998), which requires a physician to notify the parents of a minor prior to performing an abortion upon her, violates the minor's rights protected by the US Constitution. The act generally prohibits physicians from performing abortions on an unemancipated minor until at least 48 hours after written notice has been delivered to the minor's parent, guardian, or foster parent. The plaintiffs claim the act is unconstitutional because it fails to provide an exception to the notice requirement when necessary to protect the health of minors short of imminent death. It was uncontested that there are situations when a physician must act promptly to protect the health or life of the minor. As a consequence, and as both parties agreed, delay in the abortion inherent in the act's notification process will result in adverse health consequences for some minors. The US District Court decided that the act violated the rights of minor women protected by the 14th Amendment.

2006: In another case, the minor in *In re Doe* was determined to be sufficiently mature to decide whether to terminate her pregnancy, thus precluding notification of her pregnancy to a parent or guardian, which placed her less than one year from being outside the scope of notification law. The minor was a good student, employed part-time, and had formulated a plan for her future. Although she admitted that her pregnancy was the result of an immature decision, her acknowledgement supported her belief that she had sufficient maturity whether or not to terminate pregnancy.[17]

Funding

Some states have placed an indirect restriction on abortion through the elimination of funding. Under the Hyde Amendment, the US Congress, through appropriations legislation, has limited the types of medically necessary abortions for which federal funds may be spent under the Medicaid program. Although the Hyde Amendment does not prohibit states from funding nontherapeutic abortions, this action by the federal government opened the door to state statutory provisions limiting the funding of abortions.

Not Required for Elective Abortions

1977: In *Beal v. Doe*,[18] the Pennsylvania Medicaid plan was challenged on the basis of the denial of financial assistance for nontherapeutic (elective) abortions. The Supreme Court held that Title XIX of the Social Security Act (Medicaid) does not require the funding of elective abortions as a condition of state participation in the program. The state has a strong interest in encouraging normal childbirth, and nothing in Title XIX suggests that it is unreasonable for the state to further that interest.

Funding Bans Unconstitutional in California

The California Supreme Court held that funding bans were unconstitutional; the court asked rhetorically:

> If the state cannot directly prohibit a woman's right to obtain an abortion, may the state by discriminatory fi-

> nancing indirectly nullify that constitutional right? Can the state tell an indigent person that the state will provide him with welfare benefits only upon the condition that he join a designated political party or subscribe to a particular newspaper that is favored by the government? Can the state tell a poor woman that it will pay for her needed medical care but only if she gives up her constitutional right to choose whether or not to have a child?[19]

Discrimination in Funding Prohibited in Arizona

The Arizona Supreme Court, in *Simat Corp. v. Arizona Health Care Cost Containment Sys.*,[20] found that the state's constitution does not permit the state and the Arizona Health Care Cost Containment System to refuse to fund medically necessary abortion procedures for pregnant women suffering from serious illness while, at the same time, funding such procedures for victims of rape or incest or when the abortion was necessary to save the woman's life. After the state has chosen to fund abortions for one group of indigent, pregnant women for whom abortions are medically necessary to save their lives, the state may not deny the same option to another group of women for whom the procedure is also medically necessary to save their health. An example is cancer, for which chemotherapy or radiation therapy ordinarily cannot be provided if the patient is pregnant, making an abortion necessary before proceeding with the recognized medical treatment. Other therapy regimens that must at times be suspended during pregnancy include heart disease, diabetes, kidney disease, liver disease, chronic renal failure, inflammatory bowel disease, and lupus. In many of the women suffering from these diseases, suspension of recognized therapy during pregnancy will have serious and permanent adverse effects on their health and lessen their life span. In such a situation, the state is not simply influencing a woman's choice but is actually conferring the privilege of treatment on one class and withholding it from another.

A woman's right to choose preservation and protection of her health, and therefore, in many cases, her life, is at least as compelling as the state's interest in promoting childbirth. The court's protection of the fetus and promotion of childbirth cannot be considered so compelling as to outweigh a woman's fundamental right to choose and the state's obligation to be evenhanded in the design and application of its health care policies. The majority of states that have examined similar Medicaid funding restrictions have determined that their state statutes or constitutions offer broader protection of individual rights than does the US Constitution, and they have found that medically necessary abortions should be funded if the state also funds medically necessary expenses related to childbirth. The case was remanded to the trial court for further proceedings consistent with this opinion.

States May Protect Viable Fetus

1979: The Supreme Court in *Colautti v. Franklin*[21] determined that the states may seek to protect a fetus that a physician has determined could survive outside the womb. Determination of whether a particular fetus is viable is, and must be, a matter for judgment of the responsible attending physician. State abortion regulations that impinge on this determination, if they are to be constitutional, must allow the attending physician the room that he or she needs to make the best medical judgment.

Viability Tests Required

1989: *Webster v. Reproductive Health Services*[22] began the Court's narrowing of abortion rights by upholding a Missouri statute providing that no public facilities or employees should be used to perform abortions and that physicians should conduct viability tests before performing abortions.

Partial-Birth Abortion: Ban Unconstitutional

2002: The US Supreme Court in *Stenberg v. Carhart*[23] struck down a Nebraska ban on partial-birth abortion, finding it an unconstitutional violation of *Roe v. Wade*. The court found these types of bans to be extreme descriptive attempts to outlaw abortion—even early in pregnancy—that jeopardize women's health. Following *Stenberg v. Carhart*, a Virginia statute that attempted to criminalize partial-birth abortion was also held to be unconstitutional, under the 14th Amendment where it lacked an exception to protect a woman's health.[24]

2006: The Partial Birth Abortion Ban Act, 18 U.S.C. Section 1531, in *National Abortion Fed'n v. Gonzages*,[25] was found to be unconstitutional because it lacked any exception to preserve the health of the mother, where such exception was constitutionally required. Also, the Act was unconstitutional because it imposed an undue burden on a woman's right to choose previability abortion, and it was constitutionally vague.

Employee Refusal to Participate in Abortions

1975: Individuals have a right to refuse to participate in abortions and can abstain from involvement in abortions as a matter of conscience or religious or moral conviction. In a Missouri case, *Doe v. Poelker*,[26] the city was ordered to obtain the services of physicians and personnel who had no moral objections to participating in abortions. The city also was required to pay the plaintiff's attorneys' fees because of the wanton disregard of the indigent woman's rights and the continuation of a policy to disregard and/or circumvent the US Supreme Court's rulings on abortion.

Physicians Feeling the Heat

Physicians are feeling the heat and are concerned about the ongoing abortion controversy. In *Beverly v. Choices Women's Medical Center*,[27] a physician, whose picture was published in an abortion calendar without her consent, brought a civil rights action against the for-profit medical center for publication of her picture. The calendar was disseminated to the public by the center. The center, among other things, performs abortions from which it derives approximately 50% of its income. The plaintiff was awarded $50,000 in compensatory damages and $25,000 in punitive damages. The physician testified that the publication of her picture caused her to suffer physical and mental injury.

Abortion Ban Overturned by Voters

South Dakota lawmakers had approved a far-reaching ban on abortion. The measure, which passed the state senate, would have made it a felony for doctors to perform any abortion, except to save the life of a pregnant woman. The bill was designed to challenge the Supreme Court's ruling in *Roe v. Wade*. South Dakota voters, however, overturned the state abortion ban that supporters had championed as the best chance to challenge a 33-year-old US Supreme Court decision legalizing abortion.

Continuing Controversy

While pro-choice advocates are arguing the rights of women to choose, they are also pointing out the fact that legalized abortions are safer. In 1972, for example, the year before *Roe v. Wade* was upheld, the number of deaths from abortions in the United States is estimated to have reached the thousands; by 1985, the figure was six. In addition, *pro-choice advocates* argue that women who have a right to an abortion when pregnancy threatens the life of the mother also have the right to an abortion when pregnancy is the result of incest or rape. *Right-to-life advocates* argue that life comes from God and that no one has a right to deny the right to life.

There will most likely be a continuing stream of court decisions, as well as political and legislative battles, well into the 21st century. Given the emotional, religious, and ethical concerns, as well as those of women's rights groups, it is unlikely that this matter will be resolved anytime soon.

STERILIZATION

Sterilization is the termination of the ability to produce offspring. Sterilization often is accomplished by a vasectomy for men and tubal ligation for women. A *vasectomy* is a surgical procedure in which the vas deferens is severed and tied to prevent the flow of the seminal fluid into the urinary canal. A *tubal ligation* is a surgical procedure in which the fallopian tubes are cut and tied, preventing passage of the ovum from the ovary to the uterus. Sterilizations are often sought because of: (1) economic necessity to avoid the additional expense of raising a child; (2) therapeutic purposes to prevent harm to a woman's health (e.g., to remove a diseased reproductive organ); and (3) genetic reasons to prevent the birth of a defective child.

Elective Sterilization

Voluntary or elective sterilizations on competent individuals present few legal problems, as long as proper consent has been obtained from the patient and the procedure is performed properly. Civil liability for performing a sterilization of convenience may be imposed if the procedure is performed in a negligent manner. The physician in *McLaughlin v. Cooke*[28] was found negligent for mistakenly cutting a blood vessel in the patient's scrotum while he was performing a vasectomy. Excessive bleeding at the site of the incision was found to have occurred because of the physician's negligent postsurgical care. On appeal, the jury's finding of negligence was supported by testimony that the physician's failure to intervene sooner and to remove a hematoma had been the proximate cause of tissue necrosis.

Regulation of Sterilization for Convenience

Like abortion, voluntary sterilization is the subject of many debates over its moral and ethical propriety. Some health care institutions have adopted policies restricting the performance of such operations at their facilities. The US Court of Appeals for the First Circuit ruled in *Hathaway v. Worcester City Hospital*[29] that a governmental hospital may not impose greater restrictions on sterilization procedures than on other procedures that are medically indistinguishable from sterilization with regard to the risk to the patient or the demand on staff or facilities. The court relied on the Supreme Court decisions in *Roe v. Wade*[30] and *Doe v. Bolton*,[31] which accorded considerable recognition to the patient's right to privacy in the context of obtaining medical services.

Therapeutic Sterilization

If the life or health of a woman may be jeopardized by pregnancy, the danger may be avoided by terminating her ability to conceive or her husband's ability to impregnate. Such an operation is a therapeutic sterilization—one performed to preserve life or health. The medical necessity for sterilization renders the procedure therapeutic. Sometimes a diseased reproductive organ has to be removed to preserve the life or health of the individual. The operation results in sterility, although this was not the primary reason for the procedure. Such an operation technically should not be classified as a sterilization because the sterilization is incidental to the medical purpose.

Involuntary/Eugenic Sterilization

The term eugenic sterilization refers to the involuntary sterilization of certain categories of persons described in statutes, without the need for consent by, or on behalf of, those subject to the procedures. Persons classified as mentally deficient, feeble minded, and, in some instances, epileptic, are included within the scope of the statutes. Several states also have included certain sexual deviates and persons classified as habitual criminals. Such statutes ordinarily are designed to prevent the transmission of hereditary defects to succeeding generations, but several statutes also have recognized the purpose of preventing procreation by individuals who would not be able to care for their offspring.

Although there have been many judicial decisions to the contrary, the US Supreme Court in *Buck v. Bell*[32] specifically upheld the validity of such eugenic sterilization statutes provided that certain procedural safeguards are observed.

At the minimum, eugenic sterilization statutes provide a grant of authority to public officials who supervise state institutions for the mentally ill or prisons and to certain public health officials to conduct sterilizations; a requirement of personal notice to the person subject to sterilization and, if that person is unable to comprehend what is involved, notice to the person's legal representative, guardian, or nearest relative; a hearing by the board designated in the particular statute to determine the propriety of the prospective sterilization; at the hearing, evidence may be presented, and the patient must be present or represented by counsel or the nearest relative or guardian; and an opportunity to appeal the board's ruling to a court.

The procedural safeguards of notice, hearing, and the right to appeal must be present in sterilization statutes to fulfill the minimum constitutional requirements of due process. An Arkansas statute was found to be unconstitutional in that it did not provide for notice to the incompetent patient and opportunity to be heard, or for the patient's entitlement to legal counsel.[33]

ARTIFICIAL INSEMINATION

Generally, *artificial insemination* is the injection of seminal fluid into a woman to induce pregnancy. The term also may include insemination that takes place outside of the woman's body, as with so-called test-tube babies. If the semen of the woman's husband is used to impregnate her, the technique is called homologous artificial insemination. If the semen comes from a donor other than the husband, the procedure is identified as heterologous artificial insemination.

The absence of answers to many questions concerning heterologous artificial insemination may have discouraged couples from seeking to use the procedure and physicians from performing it. Some of the questions concern the procedure itself; others concern the status of the offspring and the effect of the procedure on the marital relationship.

Consent

The Oklahoma heterologous artificial insemination statute specifies that husband and wife must consent to the procedure.[34] It is obvious that the wife's consent must be obtained; without it, the touching involved in the artificial insemination would constitute a battery. Besides the wife's consent, it is important to obtain the husband's consent to ensure against liability accruing if a court adopted the view that without the consent of the husband, heterologous artificial insemination was a wrong to the husband's interest for which he could sustain a suit for damages.

In states without specific statutory requirements, medical personnel should attempt to avoid such potential liability by establishing the practice of obtaining the written consent of the couple requesting the heterologous artificial insemination procedure.

WRONGFUL BIRTH, LIFE, AND CONCEPTION

Lawsuits have been brought on such theories as wrongful birth, wrongful life, and wrongful conception. Wrongful life suits are generally unsuccessful, primarily because of the court's unwillingness, for public policy reasons, to permit financial recovery for the "injury" of being born into the world.

However, some success has been achieved in litigation by the patient (and his or her spouse) who allegedly was sterilized and subsequently proved fertile. Damages have been awarded for the cost of the unsuccessful procedure; pain and suffering as a result of the pregnancy; the medical expense of the pregnancy; and the loss of comfort, companionship services, and consortium of the spouse. Again, as a matter of public policy, the courts have indicated that the joys and benefits of having the child outweigh the costs incurred in raising a child.

There have been many cases in recent years involving actions for wrongful birth, wrongful life, and wrongful conception. Such litigation originated with the California case in which a court found that a genetic testing laboratory can be held liable for damages from incorrectly reporting genetic tests, leading to the birth of a child with defects.[35] Injury caused by birth had not been previously actionable by law. The court of appeals held that medical laboratories engaged in genetic testing owe a duty to parents and their unborn child to use ordinary care in administering available tests for the purpose of providing information concerning potential genetic defects in the unborn. Damages in this case were awarded on the basis of the child's shortened life span.

Wrongful Birth

In a *wrongful birth action*, the plaintiffs claim that but for a breach of duty by the defendant(s) (e.g., improper sterilization), the child would not have been born. A wrongful birth claim can be brought by the parent(s) of a child born with genetic defects against a physician who or a laboratory that negligently fails to inform them, in a timely fashion, of an increased possibility that the mother will give birth to such a child, therefore precluding an informed decision as to whether to have the child.

Recovery for damages was permitted for wrongful birth in *Keel v. Banach*[36] where the Alabama Supreme Court held that a cause of action for wrongful birth is recognized in Alabama, and compensable losses are any medical and hospital expenses incurred as a result of the physician's negligence, physical pain suffered by the mother, loss of consortium, and mental and emotional anguish suffered by the parents. The basic rule of tort compensation is that the plaintiffs should be placed in the position where they would have been without the defendant's negligence. A jury could conclude that the defendants, in failing to inform the mother of the possibility of giving birth to a child with multiple congenital deformities, directly deprived her and her husband of the option to accept or reject a parental relationship with the child and thus caused them to experience mental distress.

Wrongful Life

A wrongful life claim was brought in *Kassama v. Magat*,[37] by the plaintiff who claimed that Dr. Magat failed to advise her of the results of a blood test that indicated a heightened possibility that her child might be afflicted with Down syndrome. Had she received that information, the plaintiff contends she would have chosen to terminate the pregnancy through an abortion.

The Supreme Court of Maryland decided that an impaired life was not worse than nonlife, and, for that reason, life itself was not, and could not, be considered an injury. There was no evidence that the child was not deeply loved and cared for by her parents or that she did not return that love. Allowing a recovery of extraordinary life expenses on a theory of fairness that the doctor or his or her insurance company should pay not because the doctor caused the injury but because the child was born ignores the fundamental issue that people afflicted with Down syndrome can lead productive and meaningful lives. They can be educated, employed, and form friendships.

Wrongful birth is based on the premise that being born, and having to live, with the affliction is a disadvantage and thus a cognizable injury. The issue here is whether Maryland law is prepared to recognize that kind of injury—the injury of life itself.

The child has not suffered any damage cognizable at law by being brought into existence. One of the most deeply held beliefs of society is that life, whether experienced with or without a major physical handicap, is more precious than nonlife. No one is perfect, and each person suffers from some ailments or defects, whether major or minor, which make impossible participation in all the activities life has to offer. Our lives are not thereby rendered less precious than those of others whose defects are less pervasive or less severe. Despite their handicaps, the Down syndrome child is able to love and be loved and to experience happiness and pleasure—emotions that are truly the essence of life and that are far more valuable than the suffering that may be endured.

The right to life and the principle that all are equal under the law are basic to our constitutional order. To presume to decide that a child's life is not worth living would be to forsake these ideals. To characterize the life of a disabled person as an injury would denigrate the handicapped themselves. Measuring the value of an impaired life as compared to nonexistence is a task that is beyond mortals.

Unless a judgment can be made on the basis of reason, rather than the emotion of any given case, that nonlife is preferable to impaired life—that the child-plaintiff would, in fact, have been better off had he or she never been born—there can be no injury, and, if there can be no injury, whether damages can or cannot be calculated becomes irrelevant.

The crucial question, a value judgment about life itself, is too deeply immersed in each person's own individual philosophy or theology to be subject to a reasoned and consistent community response in the form of a jury verdict.

The court, in deciding whether to render a verdict in the child's favor or what damages, if any, should be awarded, and a jury would be faced with an imponderable question: Is a severely impaired life so much worse than no life at all that the child is entitled to damages? The civil justice system places inestimable faith in the ability of jurors to reach a fair and just result under the law, but even a jury collectively imbued with the wisdom of Solomon would be unable to weigh the fact of being born with a defective condition against the fact of not being born at all; in other words, nonexistence. It is simply beyond the human experience to analyze this position. The court declined to recognize a cause of action for wrongful life brought by or on behalf of a child born with a congenital defect. It was untenable to argue that a child who already had been born should have the chance to prove it would have been better if he had never been born at all.[38]

Wrongful Conception or Pregnancy

A wrongful conception or pregnancy claim is based on damages sustained by the parents of an unexpected child based on an allegation that conception of the child is the result, for example, of a negligent sterilization procedure. Damages sought for a negligently performed sterilization might include: pain and suffering associated with pregnancy and birth; expenses of delivery; lost wages; father's loss of consortium; damages for emotional or psychological pain; suffering resulting from the presence of an additional family member in the household; the cost and pain and suffering of a subsequent sterilization; and damages suffered by a child who is born with genetic defects.

The most controversial item of damages claimed is that of raising a normal healthy child to adulthood. The mother in *Hartke v. McKelway*[39] had undergone sterilization for therapeutic reasons to avoid endangering her health from pregnancy. The woman became pregnant as a result of a failed sterilization. She delivered a healthy child without injury to herself. It was determined that "the jury could not rationally have found that the birth of this child was an injury to this plaintiff. Awarding child rearing expense would only give Hartke a windfall."[40]

However, the costs of raising a normal healthy child in *Jones v. Malinowski*[41] were recoverable. The plaintiff had three previous pregnancies. The first pregnancy resulted in a breech birth; the second child suffered brain damage; and the third child suffered from heart disease. For economic reasons, the plaintiff had undergone a bipolar tubal laparoscopy, which is a procedure that blocks both fallopian tubes by cauterization. The operating physician misidentified the left tube and cauterized the wrong structure, leaving the left tube intact. As a result of the negligent sterilization, Mrs. Malinowski became pregnant. The court of appeals held that the costs of raising a healthy child are recoverable and that the jury could offset these costs by the benefits derived by the parents from the child's aid, comfort, and society during the parents' life expectancy. The jury was instructed not to consider that the plaintiffs "might have aborted the child or placed the child out for adoption [because] . . . as a matter of personal conscience and choice parents may wish to keep an unplanned child."[42]

The cost of raising a healthy newborn child to adulthood was recoverable by the parents of the child conceived as a result of an unsuccessful sterilization by a physician employee at Lovelace Medical Center. The physician in *Lovelace Medical Center v. Mendez*[43] found and ligated only one of the patient's two fallopian tubes and then failed to inform the patient of the unsuccessful operation. The court held that:

> the Mendezes' interest in the financial security of their family was a legally protected interest which was invaded by Lovelace's negligent failure properly to perform Maria's sterilization operation (if proved at trial), and that this invasion was an injury entitling them to recover damages in the form of the reasonable expenses to raise Joseph to majority.[44]

Some states bar damage claims for emotional distress and the costs associated with the raising of healthy children but will permit recovery for damages related to negligent sterilizations. In *Butler v. Rolling Hills Hospital*,[45] the Pennsylvania Superior Court held that the patient stated a cause of action for the negligent performance of a laparoscopic tubal ligation. The patient was not, however, entitled to compensation for the costs of raising a normal healthy child. "In light of this Commonwealth's public policy, which recognizes the paramount importance of the family to society, we conclude that the benefits of joy, companionship, and affection which a normal, healthy child can provide must be deemed as a matter of law to outweigh the costs of raising that child."[46]

As the Court of Common Pleas of Lycoming County, Pennsylvania, in *Shaheen v. Knight*, stated:

> Many people would be willing to support this child were they given the right of custody and adoption, but according to plaintiff's statement, plaintiff does not want such. He wants to have the child and wants the doctor to support it. In our opinion, to allow such damages would be against public policy.[47]

Prevention of Wrongful Birth, Life, and Conception Lawsuits

The occurrence of an unplanned pregnancy is not necessarily the result of negligence on the part of a physician. Although slight, there is known to be a given failure rate of sterilizations. Physicians can prevent lawsuits by informing each patient both orally and through written consent as to the likelihood of an unsuccessful sterilization, as well as the inherent risks in the procedure.

Notes

1. 410 U.S. 113 (1973).
2. Id. at 164.
3. Id.
4. Id.
5. Id.
6. Planned Parenthood v. Casey, 112 S. Ct. 2792 (1992).
7. 103 S. Ct. 2481 (1983).
8. 11 S. Ct. 1759 (1991).
9. 410 U.S. 179 (1973).
10. Poe v. Gerstein, 517 F.2d 787 (5th Cir. 1975).
11. 405 F. Supp. 534 (M.D. Pa.1975).
12. 486 U.S. 1308 (1988).
13. 443 U.S. 622 (1979).
14. 101 S. Ct. 1164 (1981).
15. 515 So. 2d 1254 (Ala. Civ. App. 1987).
16. 107 F. Supp. 2d 1271 (2000).
17. 921 So.2d 753 (Fla. App. 2006).
18. 432 U.S. 438 (1977).
19. Committee to Defend Reproductive Rights v. Myers, 625 P.2d 779, 798 (Cal. 1981).
20. 56 P.3d 28 (Ariz. 2002).
21. 99 S. Ct. 675 (1979).
22. 492 U.S. 490 (1989).
23. 192 F.3d 1142 (8th Cir 1999), 120 S.Ct. 2597 (2000).
24. Richmond Med. Ctr. For Women v. Hicks, 409 F.3d 619 (C.A.4, Va. 2005).
25. 437 F.3d. 278 (C.A. 2, N.Y. 2006).
26. 515 F.2d 541 (8th Cir. 1975).
27. 565 N.Y.S.2d 833 (N.Y. App. Div. 1991).
28. 774 P.2d 1171 (Wash. 1989).
29. 475 F.2d 701 (1st Cir. 1973).
30. 410 U.S. 113 (1973).
31. 410 U.S. 179 (1973).
32. 224 U.S. 200 (1927).
33. McKinney v. McKinney, 805 S.W.2d 66 (Ark. 1991).
34. Okla. Stat. Ann. 10, §§ 551–553.
35. 165 Cal. Rptr. 477 (Cal. Ct. App. 1980).
36. 624 So. 2d 1022 (Ala. 1993).
37. 136 Md. App. 38 (2002).
38. Willis v. Wu, No. 25915 (S.C. 2004).
39. 707 F.2d 1544 (D.C. Cir. 1983).
40. Id. at 1557.
41. 473 A.2d 429 (Md. 1984).
42. Id. at 431.
43. 805 P.2d 603 (N.M. 1991).
44. Id. at 612.
45. 582 A.2d 1384 (Pa. Super. Ct. 1990).
46. Id. at 1385.
47. 11 Pa. D. & C.2d 41, 46 (Lycoming Co. Ct. Com. Pl. 1957).

15

Patient Rights and Responsibilities

Every person possesses certain rights guaranteed by the Constitution of the United States and its Amendments, including freedom of speech, religion, and association and the right not to be discriminated against on the grounds of race, creed, color, or national origin. The Supreme Court has interpreted the Constitution as also guaranteeing certain other rights not expressly mentioned, such as the right to privacy and self-determination and the right to accept or reject medical treatment. This chapter provides a brief overview of both the rights and responsibilities of all patients.

PATIENT RIGHTS

Patients of the various states have certain rights and protections guaranteed by state and federal laws and regulations. Patient rights include the right to participate in health care decisions and to understand treatment options. Patients have a right to receive a clear explanation of tests, diagnoses, treatment options, prescribed medications, and prognosis.[1]

It is recognized that a professional relationship between the physician and the patient is essential for the provision of proper medical care. The traditional physician/patient relationship takes on a new dimension when care is rendered within an organizational structure. Legal precedent has established that not only does the institution have responsibility to the patient, but that the patient also has responsibility to the institution.

Patients have the right to choose the medical care they wish to receive. As medical technology becomes more advanced, these decisions become increasingly difficult to decide. Should I have the surgery? Do I want to be maintained on a respirator? Frequently, these decisions involve not only medical questions, but moral and ethical dilemmas as well. What has the greater value, the length of life or the quality of life? What is the right choice for the patient? Although patients have a right to make their own care and treatment decisions, they often face conflicting religious and moral values. Often, it is difficult to make a choice when two roads may seem equally desirable.

Patient rights may be classified as either legal, those emanating from law, or human statements of desirable ethical principles, such as the right to health care or the right to be treated with human dignity. Both staff and patients should be aware of and understand not only their own rights and responsibilities but also the rights and responsibilities of each other.

Right to Know My Rights

Upon admission for care, patients have a right to receive a copy of an organization's patient's bill of rights and responsibilities. It is expected that observing a patient's bill of rights will contribute to more effective patient care and greater satisfaction for patients, caregivers, and health care organizations alike.

Right to Explanation of My Rights

Patients have a right to receive an explanation of their rights and responsibilities. An organization's description of patient rights and responsibilities should be viewed as a document with legal significance whether or not the state in question has adopted a similar code. The rights of patients must be respected at all times. Each patient is an individual with unique health care needs. The patient has a right to make decisions regarding his or her medical care, including the decision to discontinue treatment, to the extent permitted by law.

Organization policy should provide that upon admission, each patient will be provided with a written statement of his or her rights, responsibilities, and a privacy notice. This statement includes the rights of the patient to make decisions regarding medical care and information regarding protected health information. Patients have a right to receive an explanation of the patient's bill of rights.

Right to Admission

At the time of admission, the patient should be informed in writing of his or her rights and responsibilities. If necessary, each patient has a right to have those rights explained.

Government Facilities

Whether a person is entitled to admission to a particular governmental facility depends on the statute establishing that organization. Governmental hospitals, for example, are by definition creatures of some unit of government; their primary concern is service to the population within the jurisdiction of that unit. Military hospitals, for example, have been established to care for those persons who are active members of the military.

Although persons who are not within the statutory classes have no right of admission, hospitals and their employees owe a duty to extend reasonable care to those who present themselves for assistance and are in need of immediate attention. With respect to such persons, governmental hospitals are subject to the same rules that apply to private hospitals. For example, the patient–plaintiff in *Stoick v. Caro Community Hospital*[2] brought a medical malpractice action against a government physician in which she alleged that the physician determined that she was having a stroke and required hospitalization but that he refused to hospitalize her. The plaintiff's daughter-in-law called the defendant, Caro Family Physicians, P.C., where the patient had a 1:30 p.m. appointment. She was told to take the patient to the hospital. On arriving at the hospital, there was no physician available to see the patient, and a nurse directed her to Dr. Loo's clinic in the hospital. On examination, Loo found right-sided facial paralysis, weakness, dizziness, and an inability to talk. He told the patient that she was having a stroke and that immediate hospitalization was necessary. Loo refused to admit her because of a hospital policy that only the patient's family physician or treating physician could admit her. The plaintiff went to see her physician, Dr. Quines, who instructed her to go to the hospital immediately. He did not accompany her to the hospital. At the hospital she waited approximately 1 hour before another physician from the Caro Family Physicians arrived and admitted her. Loo claimed that he did not diagnose the patient as having a stroke and that there was no bad faith on his part.

The court of appeals reversed, holding that the plaintiff did plead sufficient facts constituting bad faith on the part of Loo. His failure to admit or otherwise treat the patient is a ministerial act for which governmental immunity does not apply and may be found by a jury to be negligence.

Right to Participate in Care Decisions

Patients have a right to participate in all aspects of their care and should be encouraged to do so. They have a right to know their treatment options and to accept or refuse care.

Right to Informed Consent

Patients have a right to receive all the information necessary to make an informed decision prior to consenting to a proposed procedure or treatment. This information should include the possible risks and benefits of the procedure or treatment. The right to receive information from the physician includes information about the illness, the suggested course of treatment, the prospects of recovery in terms that can be understood, risks of treatment, benefits of treatment, alternative care options, and proof of consent.

Right to Ask Questions

Patients have the right and should be encouraged to ask questions regarding their care ("I saw blood in my IV tubing. Is this okay? Is it infiltrating?" and "My wound dressing seems wet. Is this okay? Should the dressing be changed?").

Reducing medical errors requires that the patient actively participate in his or her care. Patients should not hesitate to ask for the following:

- Clarification of the caregiver's instructions.
- Interpretation of a caregiver's illegible handwriting.
- Instructions for medication usage (e.g., frequency, dosing, drug–drug, drug–food interactions, contraindications, side effects).
- Clarification of the physician's diet orders (e.g., "Does my iced tea contain sugar-free substitutes?").
- Explanation of the treatment plan.
- A copy of the organization's hand washing policy.
- A description of the hospital's procedures to prevent wrong site surgery (e.g., the surgical site has been appropriately marked). If the site cannot be directly marked, have the surgeon draw an arrow pointing to the surgical site.
- The opportunity to provide the organization with a copy of any advance directives that may have been executed (e.g., living will).
- The right to appoint a surrogate decision maker should you become incapacitated.
- A second opinion.

Right to Know Hospital's Adverse Events

The Florida Supreme Court in the cases *Florida Hospital Waterman, Inc., etc. v. Teresa M. Buster etc., et al.*, and *Notami Hospital of Florida, Inc., etc. v. Evelyn Bowen, et al.*,[3] ruled that hospitals under amendment 7 (approved by the voters on November 2, 2004, and codified as article X, section 25 of the Florida Constitution) must reveal their records about past acts of malpractice that have been performed at the hospital. In Florida, patients now have a right to know, ask, and get records about adverse medical incidents that have happened at the hospital.

Amendment 7 to the Florida Constitution reads in part:

> Section 25, Patients' rights to know about adverse medical incidents— . . . patients have a right to have access to any records made or received in the course of business by a health care facility or provider relating to any adverse medical incident.
>
> In providing such access the identity of patients involved shall not be disclosed, and any privacy restrictions imposed by federal law shall be maintained.

Right to Refuse Treatment

Patients have a right to refuse treatment and be told what effect such a decision could have on their health. The responsibility of caregivers requires balancing risks and benefits. This balancing can lead to situations where health care professionals view their obligations to a patient as different from the patient's own assessment. The patient may refuse a certain procedure, for example, and forcing the patient to undergo an unwanted procedure would result in a failure to respect the patient's right of self-determination.

Right to Execute Advance Directives

Patients must be informed of their right to execute advance directives. The advance directives must be honored within the limits of the law and the organization's mission, philosophy, and capabilities.

Right to Designate a Decision Maker

Patients have a right to appoint a health care decision maker to make health care decisions when the patient becomes incapacitated or is unable to make decisions on his or her behalf.

Right to Privacy and Confidentiality

Patients have a right to expect that information regarding their care and treatment will be kept confidential. Confidentiality requires that the caregiver safeguard a patient's confidences within the constraints of law. Caregivers must be careful not to discuss any aspect of a patient's case with others not involved in the case.

Right to Privacy

The phlebotomist in *Bagent v. Blessing Care Corp.*[4] revealed the results of a patient's pregnancy test to the patient's sister at a public tavern. Although there was an attempt by the hospital to have the case dismissed for the phlebotomist's breach of confidentiality, invasion of privacy, and the negligent infliction of emotional distress, the appeals court determined that there were triable issues of fact precluding dismissal of the case. It was asserted that the phlebotomist had been trained to maintain the confidentiality of patient information and that she knew that she had violated the patient's rights.

Written permission must be obtained before a patient's medical record can be made available to anyone not associated with the patient's care.

The limitations of space and financial restraints make it difficult to continuously preserve a patient's right to privacy in many hospital settings (e.g., emergency departments). Nevertheless, health care organizations have a responsibility to provide for a reasonable amount of privacy for patients.

The issues of confidentiality and privacy are both ethical and legal. Caregivers must safeguard each patient's right to privacy and the right to have information pertaining to his or her care to be kept confidential.

Patients have a right to receive "Notice of Privacy Standards," a requirement under the

Health Insurance Portability and Accountability Act.

Disclosures Permitted

The following list describes some of the ways a health care provider may disclose medical information about a patient without his or her written consent.

Patient information (e.g., diagnoses, anesthesia history, surgical and other invasive procedures, drug allergies, medication usage, lab test results, and imaging studies) may be disclosed to other providers who may be caring for the patient to provide safe health care treatment.

- Disclosure of patient information to third-party payers so that providers can obtain payment for services rendered.
- Disclosure of patient information for health care operations.
- Disclosure of patient information as may be required by a law enforcement agency.
- Disclosure of patient information as may be required to avert a serious threat to public health or safety.
- Disclosure of patient information as required by military command authorities for their medical records.
- Disclosure of patient information to worker's compensation or similar programs for processing of claims.
- Disclosure of patient information in response to a subpoena for a legal proceeding.
- Disclosure of patient information to a coroner or medical examiner for purposes of identification.

Limitations on Disclosures

Some of the individual rights a patient has regarding disclosure of access to his or her medical information are as follows:

- Right to request restrictions or limitations regarding information used or disclosed about one's treatment.
- Right to an accounting of nonstandard disclosures: The patient has a right to request a list of the disclosures made of information released regarding his or her care.
- Right to amend: If a patient believes that medical information regarding his or her care is incorrect or incomplete, he or she has a right to request that the information be corrected.
- Right to inspect and copy medical information that may be used to make decisions about one's care.
- Right to file a complaint with the provider, or the Secretary of the Department of Health and Human Services in Washington, DC, if a patient believes his or her privacy rights have been violated.
- Right to a paper copy of a notice pertaining to patient.
- Right to know of restrictions on rights.

Any restrictions on a patient's visitors, mail, telephone, or other communications must be evaluated for their therapeutic effectiveness and fully explained to and agreed upon by the patient or patient representative.

Right to Have Special Needs Addressed

Patients have a right to an interpreter whenever possible. Patients who have physical or mental disabilities, or are hearing or vision impaired, have a right to special help, such as an interpreter.

Right to Emergency Care

Patients have a right to receive emergency care in a hospital's emergency department. At the time of admission, each patient has the right to be informed in writing of his or her rights and responsibilities, including any explanations if needed.

Health care organizations must not discriminate by reason of race, creed, color, sex, religion, or national origin. Those that do discriminate violate constitutionally guaranteed rights. They also may be in violation of federal, state, and local laws. Discrimination in some states can be considered a misdemeanor and also may carry a civil penalty. Federal and state funds may be withheld from those institutions that practice discrimination.

Most federal, state, and local programs specifically require, as a condition for receiving funds under such programs, an affirmative statement on the part of the organization that it will not discriminate. For example, the Medicare and Medicaid programs specifically require affirmative assurances by health care organizations that no discrimination will be practiced.

Right to Discharge

Patients have a right to be discharged and not be detained in a health care setting merely because of an inability to pay for services rendered. An unauthorized detention of this nature could subject the offending organization to charges of false imprisonment. Although patients have a right not to be held against their will, there are circumstances where reasonable detainment can be justified (e.g., a minor's release only to a parent or authorized guardian).

Right to Transfer

Patients have a right to be transferred to an appropriate facility when the admitting facility is unable to meet a patient's particular needs. This will at times necessitate the transfer of the patient to another health care organization that has the special services the patient requires. For this reason, it is important for each organization to execute transfer agreements with other health care organizations.

Patients also have a right to choose a receiving facility, whenever possible. The Medicaid patient in *Macleod v. Miller*[5] was entitled to an injunction preventing his involuntary transfer from the nursing home. The patient had not been accorded a pretransfer hearing as was required by applicable regulations. In addition, it was determined that the trauma of transfer might result in irreparable harm to the patient. The appeals court remanded the case to the trial court with directions to enter an order prohibiting the defendants from transferring the plaintiff pending exhaustion of his administrative remedies.

Health care organizations should have a written transfer agreement in effect with other organizations to help ensure the smooth transfer of patients from one facility to another when such is determined appropriate by the attending physician(s). Generally speaking, a transfer agreement is a written document that sets forth the terms and conditions under which a patient may be transferred to a facility that more appropriately provides the kind of care required by the patient. It also establishes procedures to admit patients of one facility to another when their condition warrants a transfer.

Transfer agreements should be written in compliance with and reflect the provisions of the many federal and state laws, regulations, and standards affecting health care organizations. The parties to a transfer agreement should be particularly aware of applicable federal and state regulations.

Right to Access Records

The courts have taken the view that patients have a legally enforceable interest in the information contained in their medical records and, therefore, have a right to access their records. Some states have enacted legislation permitting patients access to their records. Patients may generally have access to review and/or obtain copies of their records, X-rays, and laboratory and diagnostic tests. Access to information includes that maintained or possessed by a health care organization and/or a health care practitioner who has treated or is treating a patient. Organizations and physicians can withhold records if it is determined that the information could reasonably be expected to cause substantial and identifiable harm to the patient (e.g., patients in psychiatric hospitals, institutions for the mentally disabled, or alcohol- and drug-treatment programs).

Hospital Peer Review Materials Discoverable: Patient's Right to Know

Florida voters, in November 2004 adopted the "Patients' Right to Know About Adverse Medical Incidents" amendment to Florida's constitution ("Amendment 7"). In a medical malpractice action in which the plaintiffs sought the production of documents relating to the investigation of the plaintiffs' decedent's death and any medical incidents of negligence, neglect, or default of any health care provider who rendered services to the decedent, the trial court properly held that the Patient's Right To Know Amendment to the state constitution was self-executing and allowed for the discovery. During the course of litigation by a patient against a health care provider, of information and documents that emanate from the self-policing processes of health care providers. However, the court's retroactive application of the Amendment was found to be improper.[6]

Right to Know Third-Party Care Relationships

Patients have a right to know the hospital's relationships with outside parties that may influence their care and treatment. These relationships may be with educational institutions, insurers, and other health care caregivers.

Right to Know the Caregivers

Patients have a right to be informed of the names, qualifications, and positions of the caregivers who will be in charge of their care in the hospital. Patients have a right to know the functions of any hospital staff involved in their care and to refuse treatment, examination, or observation by any of them. These rights include:

- Patients should know who is treating them by name, discipline, and role and responsibility in their care plan.
- Patients should know the names of all consulting physicians and hospital-designated caregivers.
- Caregivers should identify themselves to patients by name, discipline, specialty, and identification badge of the treatment team.

Right to Sensitive and Compassionate Care

Patients have a right to be free from harassment, including verbal and physical abuse. They should receive considerate and respectful care given from competent caregivers who respect the patient's personal belief systems.

Right to a Timely Response to Care Needs

Patients have a right to have their care needs responded to within a reasonable time frame. Delay in responding to patient needs can put patients' lives at risk.

Right to Pain Management

I am locked in a prison of pain,
Where doctors hold the key,
Why can't they think beyond the box,
And develop a cure for me?

Pain management is the process whereby caregivers work with the patient to develop a pain control treatment plan. The process involves educating the patient as to the importance of pain management in the healing process. With current treatments, pain can often be prevented or at least be controlled. Patients have a right to have a pain assessment and management of any pain identified. These rights include the right to:

- have pain managed to the best of existing medical knowledge

- ask questions (e.g., "How much pain can I expect?" "How severe will my pain be?" "How long will my pain last?" "Will my pain ever go away?")
- be believed when they describe their pain
- have their pain assessed using an appropriate pain scale (e.g., 0 [no pain] to 10 [worst possible pain]) to measure and assess the degree of pain

A pain rating scale is a visual tool used to help patients measure their pain. It helps the caregiver know how well treatment is working and whether changes in the treatment plan are necessary.

A patient has the right to the following with regard to pain management:

- A pain control treatment plan should be developed with the caregiver.
- Alternative and/or complementary strategies should be included in the pain management treatment plan that might help improve the efficacy of traditional treatment options (e.g., pain medications), for example, acupuncture.
- The spouse, significant other, family, and caregivers should be involved in the decision-making process.
- The patient should know what medications, anesthesia, or other treatments are planned.
- The risks, benefits, and side effects of suggested treatment(s) should be explained.
- Alternative pain treatments that are available should be discussed.
- The patient should ask for changes in treatment if pain persists.
- It is acceptable to refuse the pain treatment(s) recommended.
- Pain medication should be administered on a timely basis.

What's Wrong with This Picture?

The following is a letter that a frustrated patient with complex medical issues wrote to her consulting physician. After reviewing the contents of this letter, describe the ethical and patient rights issues that appear in the correspondence.

> When I went to your office, it was with great hopes that someone was finally going to piece together all of the bizarre symptoms I have been experiencing over the last several months and get to the cause of my pain.
>
> I was quite frankly shocked by how I was treated as a patient—especially one experiencing a health crisis.
>
> I was examined by a medical student. He wrote my history and current health problems on a small "yellow sticky pad." You were not in the room when he examined me, and then I saw you for approximately 10 minutes.
>
> You took the card of my New York doctor and said you were going to call him, and then call me regarding what you thought the next steps should be.
>
> I called you on Friday because my local doctor said that you had not called, and I was told you were on vacation until yesterday. I had asked that you call me. You never did. I called you yesterday again, but you did not answer nor did you return my call.
>
> On Monday, I received a letter from a medical student, I assume. Although I empathize with the demands on your time, I have never seen a handwritten letter, which I received, informing me of test results I provided to you prior to my appointment with you. You never mentioned the liver enzyme elevations or my February test from New York. Moreover, no mention was made regarding any plan to help me alleviate immediate problems.

> Doctor, I am not a complainer or a person with a low pain tolerance. Since moving here, I've had fainting episodes, severe chest pain and pressure, leg and arm pain and stiffness, congestion on the left side when the pain kicks in, and by 3 o'clock I have to go home and lie down because I'm so weak and tired. I cannot continue to exist like this. It is not normal. If you're too busy and don't want to take me as a patient, you will not offend me. Frankly, I need attention now to get these things resolved. Testing my cholesterol in a month will not address the problem. I've been treated for that for three years.
>
> Please call or write to me so I can get another doctor if I have to.

The physician never responded.

PATIENT RESPONSIBILITIES

Patients have responsibilities as well as rights. Patients have a responsibility to:

- Provide caregivers with information relevant to medical complaints, symptoms, past illnesses, treatments, surgical procedures, hospitalizations, and medications. Information provided must be accurate, timely, and complete. (The court of appeal in *Fall v. White*[7] affirmed the superior court's ruling that the patient had a duty to provide the physician with accurate and complete information and to follow the physician's instructions for further care or tests.)
- Report unexpected changes in condition to caregivers.
- Make it known whether one clearly understands the plan of care.
- Ask questions if they do not understand what the caregiver is describing about how to best manage their pain.
- Report their pain to their caregivers.
- Discuss pain relief treatment options with their caregivers.
- Work with their health care caregivers to develop a treatment plan for pain control.
- Adhere to the pain control plan.
- Remind those who care for them that pain management is an important part of their health care treatment.
- Inform health care caregivers about any other prescriptions or over-the-counter medicines they are taking to control their pain.
- Provide caregivers with information about pain control methods that have worked, or not worked, for them.
- Discuss concerns about taking pain medication.
- Alert caregivers of any allergies they have to any medications.
- Ask caregivers about the side effects associated with their pain management program.
- Maintain a record of the effects of medications or other pain relief measures.
- Participate with caregivers in setting a pain control goal, including their pain ratings and activities that are important to them.
- Follow the treatment plan recommended (which may include following the instructions of nurses and allied health personnel).
- Follow an institution's rules and regulations.
- Refrain from the self-administration of medications not prescribed by the physician.
- Accept responsibility for the consequences of refusing treatment or not following instructions.
- Be considerate of the rights of others, including health care personnel, in the control of noise, smoking, and limitation on number of visitors.
- Be respectful of the property of others.
- Recognize the effect of lifestyle on one's health.

- Keep appointments. (Patients have a responsibility to promptly notify caregivers whenever they are unable to keep a scheduled appointment. Failure to notify caregivers of a cancellation means longer delays for other patients who may already be finding it difficult to schedule appointments with specialists.)
- Speak up and ask questions. (Patients have a responsibility to ask questions and understand explanations. Such questions include those regarding medications, diet, and infection control-related issues.)
- Request a second opinion.
- Describe the location and severity of pain.
- With the surgeon, make sure that staff accurately marks the site of all surgical procedures to avoid confusion in the operating suite.
- Make sure that the staff is aware of your preferences for care, including who the decision maker will be in the event that you become incapacitated.
- Make sure you understand caregiver instructions.

Notes

1. Your Rights as a Hospital Patient in New York State, State of New York, Department of Health.
2. 421 N.W.2d 611 (Mich. Ct. App. 1988).
3. Supreme Court of Florida, No. SC06-912 (March 6, 2008).
4. 844 N.E.2d 649 (Ill. App. 2006).
5. 612 P.2d 1158 (Colo. Ct. App. 1980).
6. Florida Hosp. Waterman, Inc. v. Buster, 932 So.2d 344 (Fla. App. 2006).
7. 449 N.E.2d 628 (Ind. Ct. App. 1983).

16

Acquired Immune Deficiency Syndrome

The AIDS epidemic is considered to be the deadliest epidemic in human history with the first case appearing in the literature in 1981. AIDS, generally, is accepted as a syndrome—a collection of specific, life-threatening, opportunistic infections and manifestations that are the result of an underlying immune deficiency. AIDS is caused by the HIV, a highly contagious bloodborne virus, and is the most severe form of the HIV infection. It is a fatal disease that destroys the body's capacity to ward off bacteria and viruses that ordinarily would be fought off by a properly functioning immune system.

SPREAD OF AIDS

AIDS is spread by direct contact with infected blood or body fluids, such as vaginal secretions, semen, and breast milk. At the present time, there is no evidence that the virus can be transmitted through food, water, or casual body contact; HIV does not survive well outside the body. Although there is presently no cure for AIDS, early diagnosis and treatment with new medications can help HIV-infected persons remain healthy for longer periods. High-risk groups include homosexual men, intravenous drug users, and those who require transfusions of blood and blood products, such as hemophiliacs.

Blood Transfusions

Suits often arise as a result of a person with AIDS claiming that he or she contracted the disease as a result of a transfusion of contaminated blood or blood products. In blood transfusion cases, the standards most commonly identified as having been violated concern blood testing and donor screening. An injured party generally must prove that a standard of care existed, that the defendant's conduct fell below the standard, and that this conduct was the proximate cause of the plaintiff's injury.

The most common occurrences that have led to a lawsuit in the administration of blood involve: transfusion of mismatched blood; improper screening and transfusion of contaminated blood; unnecessary administration of blood; and improper handling procedures (i.e., inadequate refrigeration and storage procedures).

The risk of HIV infection and AIDS through a blood transfusion has been reduced through health history screening and blood donations testing. All blood donated in the United States has been tested for HIV antibodies since May 1985.

Historically: Transfusion Before Testing

Dismissal of a case against a hospital and the American Red Cross was ordered in *Kozup v. Georgetown University*,[1] in which it was alleged that the death of a premature infant was due to causes related to AIDS contracted through a blood transfusion given in January 1983, without the parent's informed consent. The case was dismissed on the basis that no reasonable jury would have found that the possibility of contracting AIDS from a blood transfusion in 1983 was a material risk. Dismissal also was justified on the basis that the transfusion was the only method of treating the child for a life-threatening condition.

Today: Negligence in Collecting Blood

In January 1983, a blood center knew that blood should not be drawn from homosexual or bisexual males. On April 22, 1983, Kraus, a cardiologist, discovered that Mr. B received seven units of blood. In May 1987, B had chest pain and trouble breathing. On June 5, 1987, B was hospitalized. Kraus consulted with two specialists in pulmonary medicine about the unusual pneumonia evident in X-rays of B's lungs. Because there was a possibility that the lung infection was secondary to AIDS, B was tested for HIV. Although B had not yet been formally diagnosed, physicians started him on therapy for AIDS.

B was formally diagnosed as HIV positive. His wife was then tested for HIV, and she learned that she was also HIV positive. On July 2, 1987, B expired. On April 21, 1989, the plaintiffs, Mrs. B and her son, filed suit against the blood center, alleging that her husband contracted HIV from the transfusion of a unit of blood donated at the blood center on April 19, 1983, by a donor identified at trial as Doe. The parties stipulated at trial that Doe was a sexually active homosexual male with multiple sex partners.

The plaintiffs contend that the blood center's negligence in testing and screening blood donors caused Mrs. B's contraction of HIV. At trial, the jury awarded the plaintiffs $800,000 in damages. The blood center filed an appeal arguing the evidence of causation was legally insufficient to support the jury verdict.

The Texas Court of Appeals held that evidence supported a finding that the blood center's negligence in the collection of blood was the proximate cause of B's HIV infection. The blood center, despite its knowledge about the dangers of HIV-contaminated blood, failed to reject gay men; the blood center's donor screening was inadequate; and these omissions were substantial factors in causing Mr. and Mrs. B's HIV infections. The blood center's own technical director admitted that there was "strong evidence" that the blood accepted from Doe was contaminated with HIV. Another recipient of components of Doe's blood was diagnosed as HIV positive less than 6 months within Mr. B having been diagnosed as HIV positive.[2]

AIDS-Infected Surgeon

An AIDS-infected surgeon in New Jersey was unable to recover on a discrimination claim when the hospital restricted his surgical privileges. In *Estate of Behringer v. Medical Center at Princeton*,[3] the New Jersey Superior Court held that the hospital acted properly in initially suspending a surgeon's surgical privileges, thereafter imposing a requirement of informed consent and ultimately barring the surgeon from performing surgery. The court held that in the context of informed consent, the risk of a surgical accident involving an AIDS-positive surgeon and implications thereof would be a legitimate concern to a surgical patient that would warrant disclosure of the risk.[4]

CONFIDENTIALITY

Information regarding a patient's diagnosis as being HIV positive must be kept confidential and should only be shared with other health care professionals on a need-to-know basis. Each person has a right to privacy as to his or her personal affairs. The plaintiff–surgeon, in the *Estate of Behringer v. Medical Center at Princeton*,[5] was entitled to recover damages from the hospital and its laboratory director for the unauthorized disclosure of his condition during his stay at the hospital. The hospital and the director breached their duty to maintain confidentiality of the surgeon's medical records by allowing placement of the patient's test results in his medical chart without limiting access to the chart, which they knew was available to the entire hospital community. "The medical center breached its duty of confidentiality to the plaintiff, as a patient, when it failed to take reasonable precautions regarding the plaintiff's medical records to prevent the patient's AIDS diagnosis from becoming a matter of public knowledge."[6]

The hospital in *Tarrant County Hospital District v. Hughes*[7] was found to have properly disclosed the names and addresses of blood donors in a wrongful death action alleging that a patient contracted AIDS from a blood transfusion administered in the hospital. The physician–patient privilege expressed in the Texas Rules of Evidence did not apply to preclude such disclosure because the record did not reflect that any such relationship had been established. The disclosure was not an impermissible violation of the donors' right of privacy. The societal interest in maintaining an effective blood donor program did not override the plaintiff's right to receive such information. The order prohibited disclosure of the donors' names to third parties.

Duty and the Right to Confidentiality

Health care professionals and others working with AIDS patients have a right to know when they are caring for patients with highly contagious diseases. There are times when the duty to disclose outweighs the rights of confidentiality. The US Court of Appeals for the Tenth Circuit in *Dunn v. White*[8] declared there is no Fourth Amendment impediment to a state prison's policy of testing the blood of all inmates for HIV. Under the US Supreme Court's drug-testing decisions, the proper analysis is to balance the prisoner's interest in being free from bodily intrusion inherent in a blood test against the prison's institutional rights in combating the disease. The US Court of Appeals held that in or out of prison, a person has a limited privacy interest in not having his or her blood tested. The court cited *Schmerber v. California*,[9] which rejected a Fourth Amendment challenge to the blood testing of a suspected drunken driver. Against the prisoner's minimal interest, prison authorities have a strong interest in controlling the spread of HIV.

Sexual Partners

A person has a right to know when his or her partner has tested positive for HIV. Physicians are expected to counsel an HIV-positive patient to notify his or her sexual or needle-sharing partners or to seek help in doing so from public health officials. If a patient refuses to do so, a physician may, without the patient's consent, notify a sexual partner known to be at risk of HIV infection. Some states have developed informational brochures and consent, release, and partner notification forms.

Mandatory Testing

The US District Court found that routine testing of firefighters and paramedics for the AIDS virus does not violate an individual's Fourth Amendment or constitutional privacy rights.[10]

Because the tested employees are a high-risk group for contracting and transmitting HIV to the public, the city has a compelling interest and legal duty to protect the public from contracting the virus. Firefighters and paramedics are in a higher-risk category than hospital personnel because they work in a noncontrolled setting. *Skinner v. Railway Executives Association* confirmed "society's judgment that blood tests do not constitute an unduly extensive imposition on an individual's privacy and bodily integrity."[11] However, "mandatory testing by a governmental agency for the sole purpose of obtaining a baseline to determine whether an employee contracted AIDS on the job, and thereby to determine the validity of any future worker's compensation claim, is not valid. Mandatory AIDS testing of employees can be valid only if the group of employees involved is at risk of contracting or transmitting AIDS to the public."[12]

DISCRIMINATION

Discrimination against persons who have contracted the AIDS virus often is found to be in violation of their constitutional rights. The sufferings and hardships of those who have contracted the disease extend to family as well as friends. The infringements of those infected with HIV include discrimination in access to health care, education, employment, housing, insurance benefits, and military service. Those who believe that they have been discriminated against can contact their state's human rights commission.

Access to Health Care

The need for health care for AIDS patients continues to grow, particularly for those who are homeless or have no family support system. In response to the need for nursing home care, some health departments are encouraging the development of specialized HIV/AIDS nursing homes that will combine medical services and drug treatment for AIDS patients who have become infected through drug abuse.

With 40 million people around the world infected with AIDS, the Internet provides a wealth of information as to resources for care and treatment. The greatest challenge involves the nearly 90% of AIDS patients who live in resource-poor countries. As a result of poor access to health care, former President Bill Clinton made the battle against HIV/AIDS a focal point of his foundation's activities in global health security to reach the underserved populations.[13]

Education

A school's refusal to admit students with HIV generally is considered an unnecessary restriction on an individual's liberty. However, there are circumstances where it would be unreasonable to infer that Congress intended to force institutions to accept or readmit persons who pose a significant risk of harm to themselves or others. For example, in *Doe v. Washington University*,[14] the university disenrolled a dental student based on his positive HIV status: "the circumstance surrounding plaintiff's HIV status presented little alternative to those charged with evaluating plaintiff's ability to qualify as a dental student."[15]

Employment

AIDS-related employment issues are a two-sided coin: employment discrimination on one side and the refusal of employees to care for AIDS patients on the other. The growing consensus of case law indicates employment-related discrimination is unlawful. The California Court of Appeals, Second District, in *Raytheon v. Fair Employment & Housing Commission*,[16] determined an employee with AIDS who was admitted to and treated in a hospital was unlawfully denied his right to return to work after treatment in the hospital. The court held that AIDS is a protected physical handicap under California's Fair Employment and Housing Act and that the employer failed to prove its defense of protecting the health and safety of its other workers. The employer ignored the advice of county health officials and communicable disease authorities that there was no risk to other employees at the plant.

Employees who have contracted the AIDS virus and whose symptoms warrant should not be placed in positions that threaten the health and safety of patients and employees. The court in *School Board of Nassau County v. Airline* noted that "a person who poses a significant risk of communicating an infectious disease will not be otherwise qualified for his or her job if reasonable accommodations will not eliminate the risk."[17]

In the final analysis, many competing issues (e.g., humanitarian, legal, moral, ethical, and religious) pertain to the rights of patients and caregivers who have contracted the AIDS virus, as well as those who have not, and employers.

Insurance Benefits

In *Weaver v. Reagan*,[18] Medicaid recipients who were denied benefits for AZT (zidovudine, trade name Retrovir) treatments were found to be entitled to summary judgment in their class action suit to require Missouri's authorities to provide Medicaid coverage for the cost of AZT treatments. In this case, the US Court of Appeals for the Eighth Circuit decided that states must provide Medicaid coverage for the drug AZT to HIV-infected individuals who are eligible for Medicaid and whose physicians had certified that AZT was a medically necessary treatment.

NEGLIGENCE

As noted in this section, there have been a variety of HIV- and AIDS-related lawsuits. Such suits, as described here, have involved the administration of blood and untimely diagnosis of AIDS.

Administration of Wrong Blood

The plaintiff, Mrs. Bordelon, in *Bordelon v. St. Francis Cabrini Hospital*,[19] was admitted to the hospital to undergo a hysterectomy. Prior to surgery, she provided the hospital with her own blood in case it was needed during surgery. During surgery, Bordelon did indeed need blood but was administered donor blood other than her own. Bordelon filed a lawsuit claiming that the hospital's failure to provide her with her own blood resulted in her suffering mental distress. The hospital filed a peremptory exception claiming that there was no cause of action. The Ninth Judicial District Court dismissed the suit because the plaintiff did not allege that she suffered any physical injury.

On appeal by the plaintiff, the court of appeal held that the plaintiff did in fact state a cause of action for mental distress. It is well established in law that a claim for negligent infliction of emotional distress unaccompanied by physical injury is a viable claim of action. It is indisputable that HIV can be transmitted through blood transfusions even when the standard procedure for screening for the virus is in place. Bordelon's fear was easily associated with receiving someone else's blood and therefore a conceivable consequence of the defendant's negligent act.[20] The hospital acquired a duty to ensure that Bordelon received her own blood when it accepted that as a condition of her hospitalization. It is undisputed that the hospital had a duty to administer the plaintiff's own blood. The hospital breached that duty by administering the wrong blood.

Failure to Make a Timely Diagnosis

The plaintiff, Jane Doe, had been exposed to HIV as the result of sexual contact. The plaintiff consulted her defendant physicians, but they failed to diagnose her condition as being positive for either HIV or AIDS. The disease weakened her immune system, and she developed pneumonia and was admitted to a hospital. The patient was eventually diagnosed with AIDS. The patient's infectious disease expert, Dr. Hill, claimed that proper diagnosis prior to her acute episode would have provided greater opportunity for improved long-term treatment. The defendants admitted that they negligently failed to timely diagnose the patient's condition.

The Louisiana Court of Appeal held that the evidence supported the jury's finding that the defendant failed to timely diagnose the plaintiff's condition. The medical defendants agreed that they negligently failed to timely diagnose the patient's condition. The plaintiff's expert witness testified that within the "reasonable medical probability" standard and the "more-likely-than-not" standard, if the plaintiff had been properly diagnosed she would have worked, as well as lived, for another year.[21]

Patient Wrongly Notified She Had AIDS

A service member brought an action under the Federal Tort Claims Act in *Johnson v. United States*,[22] alleging that on or about October 8, 1986, Army physicians and medical personnel negligently and wrongly advised her that she had AIDS after she had donated blood to a public blood drive sponsored by the Walter Reed Hospital, which resulted in her having an unnecessary and unwanted abortion. In November 1986, prior to being notified of this error, the plaintiff discovered that she was pregnant. On November 21, 1986, physicians at Walter Reed Hospital advised the plaintiff that her child would most certainly be born with AIDS and would not live beyond 5 years. The physicians indicated that under these circumstances it would be better for the plaintiff to have an abortion than to carry the child to term. As a result of this counseling, and for no other reason, the plaintiff had an abortion on December 4, 1986. It was not until February 3, 1987, nearly 4 months later, that a physician at Walter Reed Hospital told the plaintiff that there had been an error in the paperwork, and she did not have AIDS.

The United States moved to have the case dismissed on the grounds that the action was barred by the Feres doctrine. Under this doctrine, the United States is not liable under the Federal Tort Claims Act for injuries that arise out of or are in the course of activity incident to service. The district court held that the donation of blood was not incident to service, and, therefore, the Feres doctrine did not bar the action.

Insurance Company Fails to Disclose HIV Status

Unbeknown to a husband and wife, Mr. and Mrs. P, they were infected with HIV at the time they applied for life insurance from the Farm Bureau Life Insurance Company in 1999. At the time of the application, Farm Bureau collected the initial premium and arranged for blood tests from the husband and wife in furtherance of the application. Blood samples were forwarded for analysis to an independent laboratory, LabOne, which in turn reported the HIV status to the insurance company. On receipt of the information, Farm Bureau sent a notice of rejection to Mr. and Mrs. P and advised them that it would disclose the reason for their rejection to their physician if they so wished. No action was taken by Mr. and Mrs. P. Two years later, R.P. was diagnosed with AIDS, and on inquiry she and her husband learned that Farm Bureau records showed the HIV infection at the time of the life insurance rejection. Mr. and Mrs. P sued, alleging that the defendants were negligent in failing to tell them they were HIV positive. A federal court, balancing all the interests involved as Wyoming law requires, concluded that if an insurance company, through independent investigation by it or a third party for purposes of determining policy eligibility, discovers that an applicant is infected with HIV, the company has a duty to disclose to the applicant information sufficient to cause a reasonable applicant to inquire further.[23]

REPORTING REQUIREMENTS

AIDS is a reportable communicable disease in every state. Physicians and hospitals must report every case of AIDS—with the patient's name—to government public health authorities. Cases reported to local health authorities are also reported to the CDC, with the patients' names encoded by a system known as Soundex. CDC records come under the general confidentiality protections of the Federal Privacy Act of 1974. However, the statute permits disclosures to other federal agencies under certain circumstances.

AIDS EMERGENCY ACT

AIDS has been reported in all 50 states. Because the incidence of HIV affects different localities of the United States disproportionately, the Senate and House of Representatives enacted the Ryan White Comprehensive AIDS Resources Emergency Act of 1990.[24] The purpose of the act is to:

> provide emergency assistance to localities that are disproportionately affected by the human immunodeficiency virus epidemic and to make financial assistance available to States and other public or private nonprofit entities to provide for the development, organization, coordination and operation of more effective and cost efficient systems for the delivery of essential services to individuals and families with the HIV disease.[25]

Under the HIV Care Grants section of the act, a state may use grant funds:[26]

1. to establish and operate HIV-care consortia within areas most affected by HIV disease that shall be designated to provide a comprehensive continuum of care to individuals and families with HIV disease
2. to provide home- and community-based care services for individuals with HIV disease
3. to provide assistance to ensure the continuity of health insurance coverage for individuals with HIV disease
4. to provide treatments that have been determined to prolong life or prevent serious deterioration of health to individuals with HIV disease

OCCUPATIONAL SAFETY AND HEALTH ACT

The Occupational Safety and Health Act (OSHA) requires that health care organizations implement strict procedures to protect employees against the virus that causes AIDS. OSHA requires strict adherence to guidelines developed by the CDC. Complaints investigated by OSHA can result in the issuance of fines for failure to comply with regulatory requirements.

AIDS EDUCATION

The ever-increasing likelihood that health care workers will come into contact with persons carrying HIV demands continuing development of and compliance with approved safety precautions. This is especially important for those who come into contact with blood and body fluids of HIV-infected persons. The CDC expanded its infection control guidelines and has urged hospitals to adopt universal precautions to protect their workers from exposure to patients' blood and other body fluids. Hospitals are following universal precautions in the handling of body fluids, which is the accepted standard for employee protection.

A wide variety of AIDS-related educational materials are available on the market. One of the most important sources of AIDS information is the CDC. The process of staff education in preparing to care for patients with AIDS is extremely important and must include a training program on prevention and transmission in the work setting. Educational requirements specified by OSHA for health care employees include epidemiology, modes of transmission, preventive practices, and universal precautions. See the Center for AIDS Prevention Studies Web site for some helpful information: www.caps.ucsf.edu/siteindex.php.

Notes

1. 663 F. Supp. 1048 (D.D.C. 1987).
2. J.K. & Susie L. Wadley Research Inst. v. Beeson, 835 S.W.2d 689 (Tex. Ct. App. 1992).
3. 592 A.2d 1251 (N.J. Super. Ct. Law Div. 1991).
4. Id. at 1255.
5. 592 A.2d 1251 (N.J. Super. Ct. Law Div. 1991).
6. Id. at 1255.
7. 734 S.W.2d 675 (Tex. Ct. App. 1987).
8. No. 88-2194 (10th Cir. Aug. 1, 1989) (unpublished).
9. 384 U.S. 757 (1966).
10. Anonymous Fireman v. Willoughby, No. C88-1182 (D.C. N. Ohio Dec. 31, 1991) (unpublished).
11. 489 U.S. 602, 625 (1989).
12. Anonymous Fireman, No. C88-1182.
13. HIV/AIDS Initiatives, Clinton Foundation. www.clintonfoundation.org/ aids-initiative2.htm.
14. 780 F. Supp. 628 (E.D. Mo. 1991).
15. Id. at 628.
16. No. B035809 (Cal. Ct. App. Aug. 7, 1989) (unpublished).
17. 107 S. Ct. 1131 (1987).
18. 886 F.2d 194 (8th Cir. 1989).
19. 640 So. 2d 476 (La. App. 3d Cir. 1994).
20. Id. at 479.
21. Doe v. McNulty, 630 So. 2d 825 (La. Ct. App. 1993).
22. 735 F. Supp. 1 (D.D.C. 1990).
23. The plaintiffs in Pehle v. Farm Bureau Life Insurance Company, Inc.
24. HIV/AIDS, Rep. Henry Waxman. www.waxman.house.gov/issues/health/issues_health_HIV_legislation_sum_82_91.htm.
25. PUB. L. NO. 101-381, 1990 U.S. CODE CONG. & AD. NEWS (104 Stat.) 576.
26. Id. at 586.

17

Health Care Ethics

I expect to pass through the world but once. Any good therefore that I can do, or any kindness I can show to any creature, let me do it now. Let me not defer it, for I shall not pass this way again.

Stephen Grellet[1]

This chapter provides the reader with an overview of health care ethics and moral principles. Ethics and morals are derivatives from the Greek and Latin terms (roots) for custom. The intent here is not to burden the reader with the philosophy and arguments surrounding ethical theories, morality, principles, virtues, and values. However, as with the study of any new subject, "words are the tools of thought." Therefore, some new vocabulary is presented to the reader to apply the abstract theories and principles of ethics.

Ethics is the branch of philosophy that deals with values relating to human conduct with respect to the rightness and wrongness of actions and the goodness and badness of motives and ends. Ethics encompasses the decision-making process of determining the ultimate values and standards by which actions are judged. It involves how individuals decide to live, how they exist in harmony with the environment.

Ethical dilemmas arise when values, rights, duties, and loyalties conflict. Consequently, not everyone is satisfied with a particular decision. An understanding of the concepts presented here will help to reduce conflict when addressing ethical dilemmas and making difficult decisions.

The scope of health care ethics encompasses numerous issues, including the right to choose or refuse treatment and the right to limit the suffering one will endure. The incredible advances in technology and the resulting capability to extend life beyond the point of what some may consider to be a reasonable quality of life have complicated the process of health care decision making. The scope of health care ethics is not limited to philosophical issues but embraces economic, medical, political, and legal dilemmas.

End-of-life issues continue to cause the most controversy and debate facing health care providers. Although it is well settled that competent terminally ill patients may refuse life-sustaining treatment, physician-assisted suicide remains a major point of contention. The competing concerns of privacy, morality, patient autonomy, legislation, and states' interests swirl around those involved in the decision-making process. The numerous ethical questions involve the entire life span, from the right to be born to the right to die.

Micro-ethics involves an individual's view of what is right and wrong based on life experiences. *Macro-ethics* involves a more global view of right and wrong. Although no person lives in a vacuum, solving ethical dilemmas involves consideration of ethical issues from both a micro and macro ethical perspective.

The term "ethics" is used in three different but related ways, signifying: (1) a general pattern or "way of life," such as religious ethics (e.g., Judeo-Christian ethics); (2) a set of rules of conduct or "moral code," which involves professional ethics and unethical behavior; and (3) philosophical ethics, which involves inquiry about ways of life and rules of conduct.

ETHICAL THEORIES

Ethics seeks to understand and to determine how human actions can be judged as right or wrong. Ethical judgments can be made based upon our own experiences or based upon the nature of or principles of reason. Those who study ethics believe that ethical decision making is based upon theory. Ethical theories attempt to introduce order into the way people think about life and action. The following paragraphs provide a review of the more commonly discussed ethical theories.

Normative Ethics

The *normative theory* of ethics is the attempt to determine what moral standards should be followed so that human behavior and conduct may be morally right. Normative ethics is primarily concerned with establishing standards or norms for conduct and is commonly associated with general theories about how one ought to live. One of the central questions of modern normative ethics is whether human actions are to be judged right or wrong solely according to their consequences.

General normative ethics is the critical study of major moral precepts of such matters as what things are right, what things are good, and what things are genuine. General normative ethics is the determination of correct moral principles for all autonomous rational beings.

Applied ethics is the application of normative theories to practical moral problems. It attempts to explain and justify specific moral problems such as abortion, euthanasia, and assisted suicide.

Consequential or Teleological Ethics

The *consequentialism* or *teleological* theory of ethics emphasizes that the morally right action is whatever action leads to the maximum balance of good over evil. From a contemporary standpoint, theories that judge actions by their consequences have been referred to as consequential. Consequential ethical theories revolve around the premise that the rightness or wrongness of an action depends upon the consequences or effects of an action. The theory of consequentialism is based on the view that the value of an action derives solely from the value of its consequences. The goal of a consequentialist is to achieve the greatest good for the greatest number of people.

Nonconsequential Ethics

The *nonconsequential theory* of ethics denies that the consequences of an action or rule are the only criteria for determining the morality of an action or rule. Under this theory, and as applied to health care decision making, each situation may have a different fact pattern, thus resulting in moral decisions being made on a case-by-case basis. The values held ever so strongly in one situation may conflict with the same values given a different set of facts. For example, if your plane crashed high in the Andes mountains and the only source of food for survival would be the flesh of those who did not survive, you may, if you wish to survive, have to give up your belief that it is morally wrong to eat the flesh of another human being. Given a different set of circumstances, given an abundance of food, you would most likely find it reprehensible to eat human flesh. Thus, there are no effective hard and fast rules or guidelines to govern ethical behavior.

Deontological Ethics

The *deontological theory* of ethics focuses on one's duties to others. It includes telling the truth and keeping your promises. Deontology involves ethical analysis according to a moral code or rules, religious or secular, as presented in the following sections.

Religious Ethics

The Great Physician

Dear Lord, You are the Great Physician, I turn to you in my sickness asking for your help.

I place myself under your loving care, praying that I may know your healing grace and wholeness.

Help me to find love in this strange world and to feel your presence by my bed both day and night.

Give my doctors and nurses wisdom that they may understand my illness.

Steady and guide them with your strong hand.

Reach out your hand to me and touch my life with your peace. Amen.

University of Pennsylvania
Health System

Religious codes of ethics are based on a particular religion. Biblical ethics, for example, is God centered. Judaism is based on Old Testament scriptures. Christianity is based on both Old and New Testament scriptures. The notion of right and wrong is not so much an object of philosophical inquiry as an acceptance of divine revelation. Moses, for example, received a list of 10 laws directly from God. These laws are known as the Ten Commandments. Some of the Commandments are related to the basic principles of justice that have been adhered to by society since they were first proclaimed and published. For some societies, the Ten Commandments were a turning point where essential commands such as "thou shalt not kill" or "thou shalt not commit adultery" were accepted as law.

Secular Ethics

Unlike religious ethics, secular ethics are based on codes developed by societies that have relied on customs to formulate their codes. The Code of Hammurabi, for example, written on a black Babylonian column now located in the Louvre in Paris, depicts a mythical sun god presenting a code of laws to Hammurabi, a great military leader, administrator, and law giver. His code of laws was considered to represent the ideal.

PRINCIPLES OF HEALTH CARE ETHICS

Ethical principles are universal rules of conduct that identify what kinds of actions, intentions, and motives are valued. Ethical principles core to the ethical practice of medicine are discussed next. These principles assist caregivers in making choices based on moral principles that have been identified as standards considered worthwhile in addressing health care–related ethical dilemmas. Ethical principles provide a generalized framework within which particular ethical dilemmas can be analyzed. Caregivers, in the study of ethics, will find that difficult decisions often involve choices between conflicting ethical principles.

Beneficence

Beneficence describes the principle of doing good, demonstrating kindness, showing compassion, and helping others. In the health care setting, caregivers demonstrate beneficence by providing benefits and balancing benefits against risks. Beneficence requires one to do good. Doing good requires knowledge of the beliefs, culture, values, and preferences of the patient—what one person may believe to be good for a patient may in reality be harmful. For example, a caregiver may decide that a patient should be told frankly, "There is nothing else that I can do for you." This could be injurious to the patient if the patient really wants encouragement and information about care options from the caregiver. Compassion here requires the caregiver to tell the patient, "I am not aware of new treatments for your illness; however, I have some ideas about how I can help treat your symptoms and make you more comfortable. In addition, I will keep you informed as to any significant research that may be helpful in treating your disease processes."

Paternalism is a form of beneficence. People, often believing that they know what is best for another, often make decisions that they believe are in that person's best interest. It may involve, for example, withholding information from someone, believing that the person would be better off that way. Paternalism can occur due to one's age, cognitive ability, and level of dependency.

Medical paternalism involves making choices for patients who are capable of making their own choices. Physicians are often in situations where they can influence a patient's health care decision simply by selectively telling the patient what he or she prefers based on personal beliefs. This directly violates patient autonomy. The problem of paternalism involves a conflict between principles of autonomy and beneficence, each of which is conceived by different parties as the overriding principle in cases of conflict.

Nonmaleficence

Nonmaleficence is an ethical principle that requires caregivers to avoid causing patients harm. Nonmaleficence is not concerned with improving others' well-being but rather with avoiding the infliction of harm. Medical ethics require health care providers to "first, do no harm." In *In re Conroy*, 464 A.2d 303, 314 (N.J. Super. Ct. App. Div. 1983), a New Jersey court found that "the physician's primary obligation is . . . First do no harm." Telling the truth, for example, can sometimes cause harm. If there is no cure for a patient's disease, you may have a dilemma. Do I tell the patient and possibly cause serious psychological harm, or do I give the patient what I consider to be false hopes? Is there a middle ground? If so, what is it? To avoid causing harm, alternatives may need to be considered in solving the ethical dilemma.

The caregiver, realizing that he or she cannot help a particular patient, attempts to avoid harming the patient. This is done as a caution against taking a serious risk with the patient or doing something that has no immediate or long-term benefits.

The principle of nonmaleficence is broken when a physician is placed in the position of ending life by removing respirators, giving lethal injections, or by writing prescriptions for lethal doses of medication. Helping patients die violates the physician's duty to save lives. There needs to be a distinction between killing patients and letting them die.

Justice

Justice is the obligation to be fair in the distribution of benefits and risks. Justice demands that persons in similar circumstances be treated similarly. A person is treated justly when he or she receives what is due, is deserved, or can legitimately be claimed. Justice involves how people are treated when their interests compete with one another.

Distributive justice is a principle requiring that all persons be treated equally and fairly.

No one person, for example, should get a disproportional share of society's resources or benefits. There are many ethical issues involved in the rationing of health care. This is often due to limited or scarce resources, limited access due to geographic remoteness, or a patient's inability to pay for services combined with many physicians who are unwilling to accept patients who are perceived as "no pays" with high risks for legal suits.

Autonomy

The *principle of autonomy* involves recognizing the right of a person to make one's own decisions. Auto comes from a Greek word meaning "self" or "individual." In this context, *autonomy* means recognizing an individual's right to make his or her own decisions about what is best for himself or herself. Autonomy is not an absolute principle, meaning that the autonomous actions of one person must not infringe upon the rights of another.

Each person has a right to make his or her own decisions about health care. A patient has the right to refuse to receive health care even if it is beneficial to saving his or her life. Patients can refuse treatment, refuse to take medications, refuse blood or blood by-products, and refuse invasive procedures regardless of the benefits that may be derived from them. They have a right to have their decisions followed by family members who may disagree simply because they are unable to let go. Although patients have a right to make their own decisions, they also have a concomitant right to know the risks, benefits, and alternatives to recommended procedures.

Autonomous decision making can be affected by one's disabilities, mental status, maturity, or incapacity to make decisions. Although the principle of autonomy may be inapplicable in certain cases, one's autonomous wishes may be carried out through an advance directive and/or an appointed health care agent in the event of one's inability to make decisions.

Life or Death: The Right to Choose

Vega, a Jehovah's Witness, executed a release requesting that no blood or its derivatives be administered to her during her hospitalization. Vega's husband also signed the release. She delivered a healthy baby. Following the delivery, Vega bled heavily. Her obstetrician, Dr. Sood, recommended a dilation and curettage (D&C) to stop the bleeding. Although Vega agreed to permit Sood to perform the D&C, she refused to allow a blood transfusion.

Vega's condition continued to worsen. Because physicians involved in Vega's care believed that it was essential that she receive blood to survive, the hospital petitioned the court to issue an injunction that would permit the hospital to administer blood transfusions. The court, relying on the state's interests in preserving life and protecting innocent third parties, and noting that Vega's life could be saved by a blood transfusion, granted the hospital's request for an injunction permitting it to administer blood transfusions. Vega recovered and was discharged from the hospital.

The Connecticut Superior Court determined that the hospital had no common-law right or obligation to thrust unwanted medical care on a patient who, having been sufficiently informed of the consequences, competently and clearly declined that care. The hospital's interests were sufficiently protected by Vega's informed choice, and neither it nor the trial court was entitled to override that choice. Vega's common-law right of bodily self-determination was entitled to respect and protection.[2]

MORALITY

Morality is a code of conduct. It is a guide to behavior that all rational persons would put forward for governing their behavior. Morality describes a class of rules held by society to govern the conduct of its individual members. A moral dilemma occurs when moral ideas of right and wrong conflict.

Moral judgments are those judgments concerned with what an individual or group believes to be the right or proper behavior in a given situation. It involves assessing another person's moral character based on how he or she conforms to the moral convictions established by the individual and/or group. What is considered to be right varies from nation to nation, culture to culture, religion to religion, as well as from one person to the next. In other words, there is no universal morality.

When it is important that disagreements be settled, *morality is often legislated*. Law is distinguished from morality by having explicit rules and penalties and officials who interpret the laws and apply the penalties. There is often considerable overlap in the conduct governed by morality and that governed by law. Laws are created to set boundaries for societal behavior. They are enforced to ensure that the expected behavior happens.

VIRTUES AND VALUES

The term "virtue" is normally defined as some sort of moral excellence or beneficial quality. In traditional ethics, virtues are those characteristics that differentiate good people from bad people. Virtues, such as honesty and justice, are abstract moral principles. Properly understood, virtues serve as indispensable guides to our actions. However, they aren't ends in themselves; virtues are merely abstract means to concrete ends. The ends are values: the things in life that we aim to gain or keep. Most individuals have a tendency to focus on values and not virtues. Simply stated, most individuals find it difficult to make the connection between abstract principles (virtues) and what has value. The relationship between means and ends, principles (virtues) and practice (values) is often difficult to grasp.

A *moral value* is the relative worth placed on some virtuous behavior. What has value to one person may not have value to another. A value is a standard of conduct. Values are used for judging the goodness or badness of some action. Ethical values imply standards of worth. They are the standards by which we measure the goodness in our lives. Intrinsic value is something that has value in and of itself. Instrumental value is something that helps to give value to something else (e.g., money is valuable for what it can buy).

All people make value judgments and make choices among alternatives. The values one so dearly proclaims may change as needs change. Values are the motivating power of a person's actions and are necessary to survival, both psychologically and physically.

The reader should not get caught up in the philosophical morass of how virtues and values differ, but be aware that virtues and values have been used interchangeably. For example, whether we call compassion a virtue or a value or both, the importance for our purposes in this text is to understand what compassion is and how it is applied in the health care setting.

Pillars of Moral Strength

What are the pillars that build one's moral strength? What sets each person apart? In the final analysis, it is one's virtues and values that build moral character. Look beyond the words and ask, "Do I know their meanings?" "Do I apply their concepts?" "Do I know their value?" "Are they part of me?"

This book, this chapter, is not about memorizing words, it is about applying what we learn for the good of all whose lives we touch. We begin our discussion here with an overview of those virtues commonly accepted as having value when addressing difficult health care dilemmas.

Commitment

Commitment is the act of binding oneself (intellectually or emotionally) to a course of action. It is an agreement or pledge to do something. It can be ongoing or a pledge to do something in the future.

Compassion and Conscientiousness

Compassion is the deep awareness of and sympathy for another's suffering. The ability to show compassion is a true mark of moral character. There are those who argue that

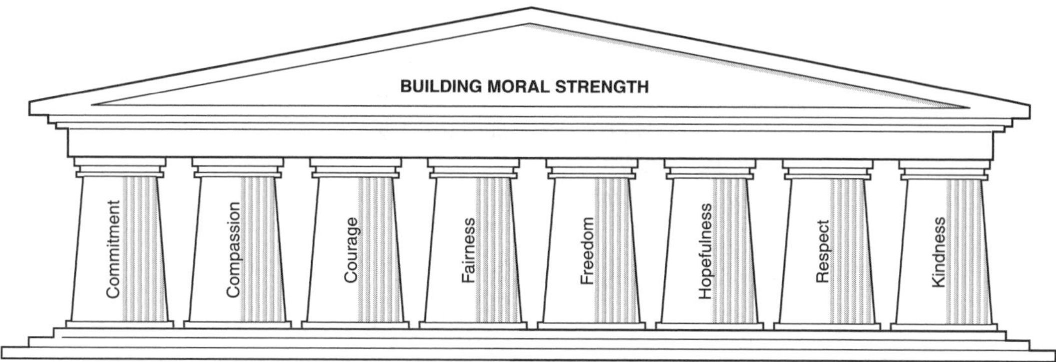

Figure 17-1 Pillars: Building Moral Strength

compassion will blur one's judgment. *Detachment*, or lack of concern for the patient's needs, however, is what often translates into mistakes that often result in patient injuries. As with all things in life, there needs to be a comfortable balance between compassion and detachment.

A *conscientious* person is one who has moral integrity and a strict regard for doing what is considered to be the right thing to do. An individual acts conscientiously if he or she is motivated to do what is right, believing it is the right thing to do. *Conscience* is a form of self-reflection on and judgment about whether one's actions are right or wrong, good or bad. It is an internal sanction that comes into play through critical reflection. This sanction often appears as a bad conscience in the form of painful feelings of remorse, guilt, or shame as the individual recognizes that his or her acts were wrong. Although a person may conscientiously object and/or refuse to participate in some action (e.g., abortion), that person must not obstruct others from performing the same act if he or she has no moral objection to it.

Courage

> *Courage is the greatest of all virtues, because if you haven't courage, you may not have an opportunity to use any of the others.*
>
> Samuel Johnson

Courage is the mental or moral strength to persevere and withstand danger.

> *Courage is the ladder on which all the other virtues mount.*
>
> Clare Booth Luce

Fairness, Fidelity, and Integrity

In ethics, fairness means being objective, unbiased, dispassionate, impartial, and consistent with the principles of ethics. *Fairness* is the ability to make judgments free from discrimination, dishonesty, or one's own bias. The virtue of *discernment* is the ability to make a good decision without personal biases, fears, and undue influences from others.

Fidelity is the virtue of faithfulness, being true to our commitments and obligations to others. A component of fidelity, veracity, implies that we will be truthful and honest in all our endeavors. It involves being faithful and loyal to obligations, duties, or observances.

Integrity involves a steadfast adherence to a strict moral or ethical code and a commitment to not compromise this code.

Freedom

Freedom is the quality of being free to make choices for oneself within the boundaries of *law*. Freedoms enjoyed by citizens of the United States include the freedom of speech, freedom of religion, and freedom from physical aggression.

Hopefulness

> *Hope is the last thing that dies in man; and though it be exceedingly deceitful, yet it is of this good use to us, that while we are traveling through life, it conducts us in an easier and more pleasant way to our journey's end.*
>
> Frans de la Rochefoucauld

Hopefulness in the patient care setting involves looking forward to something with the confidence of success. Caregivers have a responsibility to balance truthfulness while promoting hope.

Respect

> *Respect for ourselves guides our morals; respect for others guides our manners.*
>
> Laurence Sterne

Respect is an attitude of admiration or esteem. Kant was the first major Western philosopher to put respect for persons, including oneself as a person, at the center of moral theory. He believed that persons are ends in themselves with an absolute dignity, which must always be respected. In contemporary thinking, respect has become a core ideal extending moral respect to things other than persons, including all things in nature.

Kindness

> *When you carry out acts of kindness, you get a wonderful feeling inside. It is as though something inside your body responds and says, yes, this is how I ought to feel.*
>
> Harold Kushner

Kindness involves the quality of being considerate and sympathetic to another's needs.

SITUATIONAL ETHICS

A person's moral values and moral character can be compromised when faced with difficult choices. Why do good people behave differently in similar situations? Why do good people sometimes do bad things? The answer is fairly simple: One's *moral character can sometimes change* as circumstances change; thus the term "situational ethics."

Situational ethics refers to a particular view of ethics in which absolute standards are considered to be less important than the requirements of a particular situation. The standards used may, therefore, vary from one situation to another and may even contradict one another. For example, a decision not to use extraordinary means to sustain the life of an unknown 84-year-old may result in a different decision if the 84-year-old is one's mother. To better understand this concept, consider the desire to live and the extreme measures one will take to do so. Remember that ethical decision making is the process of determining the right thing to do in the event of a moral dilemma.

ORGANIZATIONAL ETHICS

The purpose of organizational ethics in the health care setting is to promote responsible behavior in the decision-making process. Recent interest in organizational ethics is, in part, the result of government regulations (e.g., Sarbanes-Oxley Act, EMTALA) and accrediting agencies (e.g., The Joint Commission), which have articulated concerns that certain unethical practices continue to plague the industry. These practices include billing scams, inappropriate advertising and marketing, and patient care issues (e.g., inappropriate patient transfers based on ability to pay, and transferring patients before they have been clinically stabilized). Commitment to organizational ethics must begin with the organization's leadership, who must develop viable accountability mechanisms for employees to follow.

According to the 2007 National Non-Profit Ethics Survey conducted by the Ethics Resource Center (www.ethics.org), when a "well implemented ethics program" is in place, levels of misconduct "drop to nearly 0 percent, and if violations do occur, 100 percent of employees report the situation to management without experiencing retaliation."

Of course, unless boards, which have been found in the study to have "high levels of misconduct," change their behavior and take advantage of their obvious influence to set and follow clear, positive ethical organizational standards, violations of the law and organizational codes of conduct will continue to rise in non-profit, for-profit, and government health care institutions.

PROFESSIONAL ETHICS

It is the direct caregivers who are frequently confronted with complex ethical dilemmas in the delivery of patient care. In response to ethical conflict, each professional's conduct should be governed by the code of ethics of one's profession, as well as by any other ethical policies, procedures, and guidelines deemed appropriate by the organization by which he or she is employed. The following cases illustrate ethical misconduct involving health professionals.

Nurse's Misconduct

The nurse's license in *Williams v. Bd. of Exam'rs for Prof. Nurses*[3] was suspended for falsifying patient records by the West Virginia Board of Examiners for Registered Professional Nurses (board) for conduct derogatory to the morals or standing of the profession of registered nursing. Pursuant to the provisions of West Virginia Code, the board has the power to deny, revoke, or suspend any license to practice registered professional nursing upon proof that he or she is guilty of conduct derogatory to the morals or standing of the profession of registered nursing. Conduct that qualifies as derogatory to the morals or standing of the nursing profession includes improperly, incompletely, or illegibly documenting the delivery of nursing care, including but not limited to treatment or medication.

On appeal, the courts determined that the evidence supported the board's 1-year suspension of the nurse's license to practice nursing for falsifying patient records.

Psychologist's Sexual Misconduct

The defendant–psychologist in *Gilmore v. Board of Psychologist Examiners*[4] had her license revoked by the board of psychologist examiners for sexual improprieties. Petitioning for judicial review, she claimed that sexual improprieties with clients did not take place during treatment sessions. She argued that therapy had terminated before the sexual relationships began. The court of appeals held that evidence supported the board's conclusion that the psychologist violated an ethical standard in caring for her patients. When a psychologist's personal interests intrude into the practitioner–client relationship, the practitioner is obliged to recreate objectivity through a third party. The board's findings and conclusions indicated that the petitioner failed to maintain that objectivity.

Attorney's and Minister's Misconduct

A minister was paid by an attorney to attend a hospital chaplain's course in furtherance of a plan by which the minister could gain access to the emergency areas of a hospital to solicit patients and their families for the purpose of aiding the attorney in gaining legal cases based on negligence and malpractice. The improper solicitations were a part of organized schemes that lasted for years with multiple offenses, including two different schemes that led to at least 22 improper solicitations. Disbarment was decided to be appropriate with respect to the attorney who hired the minister as a paralegal.[5]

ETHICS COMMITTEE

The function of an ethics committee is to analyze ethical dilemmas and to advise and educate health care providers, patients, and families. Its goal is to assist the patient and family, as appropriate, in arriving at a consensus with the options that best meet the patient's goal for care. The ethics committee enhances but does not replace the important patient/family–physician relationship, yet it affords support for decisions made within the relationship.

Ethics committees had their origins in the 1976 landmark Quinlan case,[6] where parents were granted permission by the New Jersey Supreme Court to remove their daughter, Karen, from a ventilator after she had been in a coma for a year. She died 10 years later at the age of 31, having been in a persistent vegetative state.

The Quinlan court looked to the prognosis committee to verify Karen's medical condition. It then factored in the committee's opinion with all other evidence to reach the decision to allow withdrawing her life-support equipment.

The functions of ethics committees are multifaceted and include development of policy and procedure guidelines to assist in resolving ethical dilemmas; staff and community education; conflict resolution; case reviews, support, and consultation; and political advocacy.

Always mindful of its basic orientation toward the patient's best interests, the ethics committee provides options and suggestions for resolution of ethical conflict in actual cases. Consultation with an ethics committee is not mandatory, but it is conducted at the request of a physician, patient, family member, or other health care professional.

The ethics committee strives to provide viable alternatives that will lead to the optimal resolution of ethical dilemmas involving the continuing care of the patient. It is important to remember that an ethics committee functions in an advisory capacity and should not be considered a substitute proxy for the patient.

Requests for an ethics committee consultation often involve: clarification of issues regarding decision-making capacity, informed consent, and advanced directives; do-not-resuscitate orders; withdrawal of treatment; and assistance in conflict resolution.

AUTONOMY AND REMOVAL OF LIFE SUPPORT

> *No right is held more sacred, or is more carefully guarded, by the common law, than the right of every individual to the possession and control of his own person, free from all restraint or interference of others, unless by clear and unquestioned authority of law.*[7]

The human struggle to survive and dreams of immortality have been instrumental in pushing humankind to develop means to prevent and cure illness. Advances in medicine and related technologies that have resulted from human creativity and ingenuity have given society the power to prolong life. However, the process of dying also can be prolonged. Those victims of long-term pain and suffering, as well as patients in vegetative states and irreversible comas, are the most directly affected. Rather than watching hopelessly as a disease destroys a person or as a body part malfunctions, causing death to a patient, physicians now can implant artificial body organs. Exotic machines and antibiotics are weapons in a physician's arsenal to help extend a patient's life. Such situations have generated vigorous debate.

To analyze the important questions regarding whether life-support treatment can be withheld or withdrawn from an incompetent patient, it is necessary to consider first what rights a competent patient possesses. Both statutory law and case law have presented a diversity of policies and points of view. Some courts point to common law and the early case of *Schloendorff v. Society of New York Hospital*[8] wherein the eminent Justice Cardozo stated:

> Every human being of adult years and sound mind has a right to determine what shall be done with his own body and a surgeon who performs an operation without his patient's consent commits an assault, for which he is liable in damages, except in cases of emergency where the patient is unconscious and where it is necessary to operate before consent can be obtained.[9]

This right of self-determination was emphasized in *In re Storar*[10] when the court announced that every human being of adult years and sound mind has the right to determine what shall be done with his or her own body. The Storar case was a departure from the New Jersey Supreme Court's rationale in the case of *In re Quinlan*.

The Quinlan case was the first to significantly address the issue of whether euthanasia should be permitted when a patient is terminally ill. The Quinlan court, relying on *Roe v. Wade*,[11] announced that the constitutional right to privacy protects a patient's right to self-determination. The court noted that the right to privacy "is broad enough to encompass a patient's decision to decline medical treatment under certain circumstances, in much the same way as it is broad enough to encompass a woman's decision to terminate pregnancy under certain conditions."[12]

The Quinlan court, in reaching its decision, applied a test balancing the state's interest in preserving and maintaining the sanctity of human life against Karen's privacy interest. It decided that, especially in light of the prognosis (physicians determined that Karen Quinlan was in an irreversible coma), the state's interest did not justify interference with her right to refuse treatment. Thus, Karen Quinlan's father was appointed her legal guardian, and the respirator was shut off.

Despite intense criticism by legal and religious scholars, the Quinlan decision paved the way for courts to consider extending the right to decline treatment to incompetents as well.

In the same year as the Quinlan decision, the case of *Superintendent of Belchertown State School v. Saikewicz*[13] was decided. There, the court, using the balancing test enunciated in Quinlan, approved the recommendation of a court-appointed guardian that it would be in Saikewicz's best interests to end chemotherapy treatment. Saikewicz was a mentally retarded, 67-year-old patient suffering from leukemia. The court found from the evidence that the prognosis was grim, and even though a "normal person" would probably have chosen chemotherapy, it allowed Saikewicz to die without treatment to spare him the suffering.

The Saikewicz court asserted that even though a judge might find the opinions of physicians, medical experts, or hospital ethics committees helpful in reaching a decision, there should be no requirement to seek out their advice. The court decided that questions of life and death with regard to an incompetent should be the responsibility of the courts, which would conduct detached but passionate investigations. The court took a "dim view of any attempt to shift the ultimate decision-making responsibility away from duly established courts of proper jurisdiction to any committee, panel, or group, ad hoc or permanent."[14]

Six months after Saikewicz, the Massachusetts Appeals Court narrowed the need for court intervention in *In re Dinnerstein*[15] by finding that no-code orders are valid to prevent the use of artificial resuscitative measures on incompetent, terminally ill patients. The court was faced with the case of a 67-year-old woman who was suffering from Alzheimer's disease. It was determined that she was permanently comatose at the time of trial. Further, the court decided that Saikewicz-type judicial proceedings should take place only when medical treatment could offer a reasonable expectation of affecting a permanent or temporary cure of or relief from the illness.

The Massachusetts Supreme Judicial Court attempted to clarify its Saikewicz opinion with regard to court orders in *In re Spring*.[16] It held that such different factors as the patient's mental impairment and his or her medical prognosis with or without treatment must be considered before judicial approval is necessary to withdraw or withhold treatment from an incompetent patient. The problem in all three cases is that there is still no clear guidance as to exactly when the court's approval of the removal of life-support systems would be necessary. Saikewicz seemed to demand judicial approval in every case. Spring, however, in partially retreating from that view, stated that it did not have to articulate what combination of the factors it discussed, thus making prior court approval necessary.

The inconsistencies presented by the Massachusetts cases led many courts to follow the parameters set by Quinlan, requiring judicial intervention. In cases where physicians have certified the irreversible nature of a patient's loss of consciousness, a neurological team could certify the patient's hopeless neurological condition. Then a guardian would be free to take the legal steps necessary to remove life-support systems. The main reason for the appointment of a guardian is to ensure that incompetents, like all other patients, maintain their right to refuse treatment. Most holdings indicate that because a patient has the constitutional right of self-determination, those acting on the patient's behalf can exercise that right when rendering their best judgment concerning how the patient would assert the right. The guardian's decision is sound if based on the known desires of a patient who was competent immediately before becoming comatose.

Courts adhering to the Quinlan rationale have recognized that fact, and in 1984 the highest state court of Florida took the lead and accepted the living will as persuasive evidence of an incompetent's wishes. In *John F. Kennedy Memorial Hospital v. Bludworth*,[17] the Florida Supreme Court allowed an incompetent patient's wife to act as his guardian, and, in accordance with the terms of a living will he executed in 1975, she was told to substitute her judgment for that of her husband. She asked to have a respirator removed. The court declined the necessity of prior court approval, finding that the constitutional right to refuse treatment had been decided in *Satz v. Perlmutter*.[18] The court required the attending physician to certify that the patient was in a permanent vegetative state, with no reasonable chance for recovery, before a family member or guardian could request termination of extraordinary means of medical treatment.

In keeping with *Saikewicz*, the decision maker would attempt to ascertain the incompetent patient's actual interests and preferences. Court involvement would be mandated only to appoint a guardian when: family members disagree as to the incompetent's wishes; physicians disagree on the prognosis; the patient's wishes cannot be known because he or she always has been incompetent; evidence exists of wrongful motives or malpractice; and/or no family member can serve as a guardian.

The decision in *John F. Kennedy Memorial Hospital v. Bludworth* increased the desire of the public, courts, and religious groups to know when a patient is considered to be legally dead and what type of treatment can be withheld or withdrawn. Most cases dealing with euthanasia speak of the necessity that a physician diagnose a patient as being either in a persistent vegetative state or terminally ill.

The courts have recognized that the irreversible cessation of brain function constitutes death. The American Medical Association in 1974 accepted that death occurs when there is "irreversible cessation of all brain functions including the brain stem."[19] Most states recognize brain death by statute or judicial decision.

In *In re Westchester County Medical Center ex rel. O'Connor*[20] the court determined that artificial nutrition could be withheld from O'Connor, a stroke victim who was unable to converse or feed herself. The court held that "nothing less than unequivocal proof of a patient's wishes will suffice when the decision to terminate life support is at issue."[21] The factors outlined by the court in determining the existence of clear and convincing evidence of a patient's intention to reject the prolongation of life by artificial means were the persistence of statements regarding an individual's beliefs; desirability of the commitment to those beliefs; seriousness with which such statements were made; and inferences that may be drawn from the surrounding circumstances.

The Missouri Supreme Court applied the *Westchester* ruling and held that the family of Nancy Cruzan, who was in a persistent vegetative state since 1983, could not order physicians to remove artificial nutrition.[22] In 1983, Nancy sustained injuries in a car accident, in which her car overturned, after which she was found face down in a ditch without respiratory or cardiac function. In December of 1990, Nancy was determined to be in an irreversible vegetative state. Because of the prognosis, Nancy's parents asked the hospital staff to cease all artificial nutrition and hydration procedures. The staff refused to comply with their wishes without court approval. The state trial court granted authorization for termination, finding that Nancy had a fundamental right—grounded in both the state and federal constitutions—to refuse or direct the withdrawal of death-prolonging procedures. Testimony at trial from a former roommate of Nancy indicated to the court that she had stated that if she were ever sick or injured, she would not want to live unless she could live halfway normally. The court interpreted that conversation, which had taken place when Nancy was 25 years old, as meaning that she would not want to be forced to take nutrition and hydration while in a persistent vegetative state.

The case was appealed to the Missouri Supreme Court, which reversed the lower court decision. The court held that Nancy's parents were not entitled to order the termination of her treatment. The court found that Nancy's statements to her roommate did not rise to the level of clear and convincing evidence of her desire to end nutrition and hydration.

In June 1990, the US Supreme Court heard oral arguments and held that:

- The US Constitution does not forbid Missouri from requiring that there be clear and convincing evidence of an incompetent's wishes as to the withdrawal of life-sustaining treatment.
- The Missouri Supreme Court did not commit constitutional error in concluding that evidence adduced at trial did not amount to clear and convincing evidence of Cruzan's desire to cease hydration and nutrition.
- Due process did not require the state to accept the substituted judgment of close family members, absent substantial proof that their views reflected those of the patient.[23]

Although recognizing that Missouri had enacted a restrictive law, the Supreme Court held that right-to-die issues should be decided pursuant to state law, subject to a due-process liberty interest, and in keeping with state constitutional law. After the Supreme Court rendered its decision, the Cruzans returned to Missouri probate court, where on November 14, 1990, Judge Charles Teel authorized physicians to remove the feeding tubes from Nancy. The judge determined that testimony presented to him early in November demonstrated clear and convincing evidence that Nancy would not have wanted to live in a persistent vegetative state. Several of her coworkers testified that she told them before her accident that she would not want to live like a vegetable. On December 26, 1990, 2 weeks after her feeding tubes were removed, Nancy died.

LEGISLATIVE RESPONSE

After the *Cruzan* decision, states began to rethink existing legislation and draft new legislation in the areas of living wills, durable powers of attorney, health care proxies, and surrogate decision making. Pennsylvania and Florida were two of the first states to react to the Cruzan decision. The Pennsylvania statute is applied to terminally ill or permanently unconscious patients. The statute, the *Advance Directive for Health Care Act*,[24] deals mainly with individuals who have prepared living wills. It includes in its definition of life-sustaining treatment the administration of hydration and nutrition by any means if it is stated in the individual's living will. The statute mandates that a copy of the living will be given to the physician to be effective. Further, the patient must be incompetent or permanently unconscious. If there is no evidence of the presence of a living will, the Pennsylvania probate codes allow an attorney-in-fact who was designated in a properly executed durable power of attorney document to give permission for "medical and surgical procedures to be utilized on an incompetent patient."[25]

Patient Self-Determination Act

The *Patient Self-Determination Act* of 1990 (PSDA) requires health care organizations to explain to patients their legal right to direct their own medical and nursing care as it corresponds to existing state law. A person's right to refuse medical treatment is not lost when the person's mental or physical status changes. When a person is no longer competent to exercise his or her right of self-determination, the right still exists, but the decision must be legally delegated to a surrogate decision maker. The PSDA provides that patients have a right to formulate advance directives (e.g., living wills) and to make decisions regarding their health care. Self-determination includes the right to accept or refuse medical treatment. Health care providers (including hospitals, nursing homes, home health agencies, health maintenance organizations, and hospices) that receive federal funds under Medicare are required to comply with the regulations. Providers are not entitled to reimbursement under the Medicare program if they fail to meet PSDA requirements.

PRESERVATION OF LIFE

Medical ethics do not require that a patient's life be preserved at all costs and in all circumstances. The ethical integrity of the profession is not threatened by allowing competent patients to decide for themselves whether a particular medical treatment is in their best interests. If the doctrines of informed consent and right of privacy have as their foundations the right to bodily integrity and control of one's own fate, then those rights are superior to the institutional considerations of hospitals and their medical staffs. A state's interest in maintaining the ethical integrity of a profession does not outweigh, for example, a patient's right to refuse blood transfusions.

EUTHANASIA

Originating from the Greek word euthanatos, euthanasia, meaning "good death" or "easy death," was accepted in situations in which people had what were considered to be incurable diseases. Euthanasia is defined broadly as "the mercy killing of the hopelessly ill, injured, or incapacitated." Any discussion of euthanasia obliges a person to confront humanity's greatest fear—death. The courts and legislatures have faced it and have made advances in setting forth guidelines to assist decision makers in this arena. The legal system must ensure that the constitutional rights of the patient are maintained, while at the same time protect society's interests in preserving life, preventing suicide, and maintaining the integrity of the medical profession. In the final analysis, the boundaries of patient rights remain uncertain.

Active euthanasia is commonly understood to be the intentional commission of an act, such as giving a patient a lethal drug that results in death. The act, if committed by the patient, is thought of as suicide. Moreover, because the patient cannot take his or her own life, any person who assists in the causing of the death could be subject to criminal sanction for aiding and abetting suicide.

Passive euthanasia occurs when life-saving treatment (such as a respirator) is withdrawn or withheld, allowing the patient diagnosed as terminal to die a natural death. Passive euthanasia is generally accepted pursuant to legislative acts and judicial decisions. These decisions, however, generally are based on the facts of a particular case. Regardless of the definitional differences, though, in both active and passive euthanasia, the end result is the same.

Physician-Assisted Suicide

States have been confronted with the question of whether it is ever right for a physician to provide a patient with aid in dying. Dr. Jack Kevorkian, of Michigan, for example, announced in October 1989 that he had developed a device that would end one's life quickly, painlessly, and humanely. As a result, he assisted patients in committing suicide. He was charged with first-degree murder, but the charge was later dismissed because Michigan had no law against assisted suicide.

The Michigan House approved legislation placing a temporary ban on assisted suicide. The new law, which became effective on April 1, 1993, made assisting suicide a felony punishable by up to 4 years in prison and a $2000 fine. Under the new law, assisted suicide was banned for 15 months. During this time period, a special commission studied assisted suicide and submitted its recommendations to the Michigan legislature for review and action.

Kevorkian faced prosecution for murder and for assisting in suicide. As a result, he appealed a Michigan Supreme Court ruling that found there is no right to assisted suicide.[26] The US Supreme Court rejected Kevorkian's argument that assisted suicide is a constitutional right. The high court's decision allowed the state of Michigan to move forward and prosecute Kevorkian on the pending charges. In 1999, Kevorkian was convicted of second-degree murder and for performing and assisting in patient suicide.

Oregon's Death with Dignity Act of 1994

Ironically, while Kevorkian served time in a Michigan prison, physician-assisted suicide became a legal medical option for the terminally ill residents of Oregon on October 27, 1997. The Oregon Death with Dignity Act[27] allows physicians to prescribe but not administer lethal drugs to the requester who must be terminally ill with fewer than 6 months to live. The patient must convince doctors that the decision is voluntary, sincere, and not based on being depressed. The waiting period is 15 days. The medication can only be given orally. Two physicians must examine the patient to confirm the diagnosis and prognosis. The patient must have made a witnessed request both orally and in writing. All prescriptions must be reported to the state health department.

Then, in June 1997, the US Supreme Court, in two unanimous and separate decisions, ruled that the laws in Washington and New York prohibiting assisted suicide are constitutional—yet the US Supreme Court also ruled that states can allow doctors to assist in the suicide of their terminally ill patients.

Criminalizing Assisted Suicide

The US Supreme Court determined that New York's prohibition on assisted suicide does not violate the equal protection clause of the 14th Amendment. The assisted suicide ban and the law permitting patients to refuse medical treatment do not conflict. There is a distinction between letting a patient die and making one die. In its decision, the Supreme Court determined that New York had valid reasons for distinguishing between refusing treatment and assisting suicide. Those reasons included prohibiting intentional killing and preserving life; preventing suicide; maintaining the physician's role as his or her patient's healer; and protecting vulnerable people from indifference, prejudice, and psychological and financial pressure to end their lives.[28]

In *Washington v. Glucksberg*,[29] the Supreme Court held that assisted suicide is not a liberty protected by the Constitution's due-process clause. Although a majority of states now ban assisted suicide, these rulings do not affect the right of patients to refuse treatment. It is clear that this emotionally charged issue is not settled. Legislative, judicial, and public debates continue.

ADVANCE DIRECTIVES

Advance directives allow the patient to state in advance the kinds of medical care that he or she considers acceptable or not acceptable. The patient can appoint an agent to make those decisions on his or her behalf. Patients should be asked at the time of admission to a health care facility if they have an advance directive. If a patient does not have an advance directive, the organization should provide the patient with information as to what an advance directive is and the opportunity to execute an advance directive. Every patient should clearly understand that an advance directive is a guideline for caregivers as to his or her wishes for what medical care he or she would and would not want to receive in the event he or she becomes incapacitated and unable to make decisions. This interaction should be documented in the patient's medical record. If the patient has an advance directive, a copy should be requested for insertion into the patient's record. If the patient does not have a copy of the advance directive with him or her, documentation in the medical record should include the location of the advance directive, the name and telephone number of the designated health care agent, and any information that might be helpful in the immediate care situation (e.g., patient's desire for food and hydration). The purpose of such documentation should not be considered as a need to recreate a new directive but should be considered as a desire to adhere to a patient's wishes in the event some untoward event occurs while waiting for a copy of the directive.

Guardianship

Guardianship is a legal mechanism by which the court declares a person incompetent and appoints a guardian. The court transfers the responsibility for managing financial affairs, living arrangements, and medical care decisions to the guardian.

The right to refuse medical treatment on behalf of an incompetent person is not limited to legally appointed guardians but may be exercised by health care proxies or surrogates such as close family members or friends. When a patient has not expressed instructions concerning his or her future health care in the event of later incapacity but has merely delegated full responsibility to a proxy, designation of a proxy must have been made in writing.

When a person has been declared incompetent as a result of being in a persistent vegetative state and has left no advance directive, life-sustaining decisions become more complex. Since 1990, Terri Schiavo from Clearwater, Florida, had been in a persistent vegetative state after a heart attack cut off the supply of oxygen to her brain. Her husband, Michael, became her legal guardian and fought to have her feeding tube removed, which was against her parents' wishes. Michael argued that Terri had articulated her desire not to be kept alive by artificial means.

In an unprecedented move, on October 21, 2003, Governor Jeb Bush signed an order based on a hastily passed law called Terri's Law, mandating the reinsertion of Ms. Schiavo's feeding tube, which had been removed 6 days earlier. Mr. Schiavo filed an appeal based upon a violation of his wife's right to privacy under the Florida Constitution, asserting that the law intruded upon the separation of powers. This case is the first time a governor and legislative branch of government have usurped not only the authority of the judiciary, but the rights of legal guardians to make decisions.

The law was narrowly tailored to fit Terri Schiavo's circumstances in which a patient has not left a living will, is in a persistent vegetative state, has had feeding tubes removed, and a family member challenges the removal. Florida law Chapter 2003-418 was passed by the Florida legislature. It directly affected Terri Schiavo. The act provided that the governor shall have authority to issue a one-time stay to prevent the withholding of nutrition and hydration from the patient. The act was determined to be unconstitutional as applied in the Schiavo case. The Supreme Court of Florida in Schiavo concluded:

> As the Second District noted in one of the multiple appeals in this case, we "are called upon to make a collective, objective decision concerning a question of law. Each of us, however, has our own family, our own loved ones, our own children. . . . But in the end, this case is not about the aspirations that loving parents have for their children." . . . Schiavo IV, 851 So.2d at 186. Rather, as our decision today makes clear, this case is about maintaining the integrity of a constitutional system of government with three independent and coequal branches, none of which can either encroach upon the powers of another branch or improperly delegate its own responsibilities.
>
> The trial court's decision regarding Theresa Schiavo was made in accordance with the procedures and protections set forth by the judicial branch and in accordance with the statutes passed by the Legislature in effect at that time. That decision is final and the Legislature's attempt to alter that final adjudication is unconstitutional as applied to Theresa Schiavo. Further, even if there had been no final judgment in this case, the Legislature provided the Governor constitutionally inadequate standards for the application of the legislative authority delegated in chapter 2003-418. Because chapter 2003-418 runs afoul of article II, section 3 of the Florida Constitution in both respects, we affirm the circuit court's final summary judgment.[30]

The US Supreme Court, on January 24, 2005, denied an appeal by Florida Governor Jeb Bush to overturn a decision by the Florida Supreme Court, which ruled Terri's Law unconstitutional.

Durable Power of Attorney

Power of attorney is a legal device that permits one individual, known as the "principal," to give to another person, called the "attorney-in-fact," the authority to act on the principal's behalf. The *attorney-in-fact* is authorized to handle banking and real estate affairs, incur expenses, pay bills, and handle a wide variety of legal affairs for a specified period of time. The power of attorney may continue indefinitely during the lifetime of the principal as long as that person is competent and capable of granting power of attorney. If the principal becomes comatose or mentally incompetent, the power of attorney automatically expires, just as it would if the principal dies.

Because a power of attorney is limited by the competency of the principal, some states have authorized a special legal device for the principal to express intent concerning the durability of the power of attorney, to allow it to survive disability or incompetency. The durable power of attorney is more general in scope, and the patient does not have to be in imminent danger of death as is necessary in a living will situation. Although it need not delineate desired medical treatment specifically, it must indicate the identity of the principal's attorney-in-fact and that the principal has communicated his or her health care wishes to the attorney-in-fact. Although the laws vary from state to state, all 50 states and the District of Columbia have durable power of attorney statutes. This legal device is an important alternative to guardianship, conservatorship, or trusteeship.

Health Care Proxy

A *health care proxy* is a legal document that allows a person to appoint a health care agent to make treatment decisions in the event he or she becomes incapacitated and is unable to make decisions. The agent must be made aware of the patient's wishes regarding nutrition and hydration to be allowed to make a decision concerning withholding or withdrawing them. In contrast to a living will, a health care proxy does not require a person to know about and consider in advance all situations and decisions that could arise. Rather, the appointed agent would know about and interpret the expressed wishes of the patient and then make decisions about the medical care and treatment to be administered or refused. The Cruzan decision indicates that the Supreme Court views advance directives as clear and convincing evidence of a patient's wishes regarding life-sustaining treatment.

Although most of the statutes fail to cover incompetents, cases such as Quinlan and Saikewicz created a constitutionally protected obligation to terminate the incurable incompetent's life when guardians use the doctrine of substituted judgment. Further, some states provide for proxy consent in the form of durable power-of-attorney statutes. Generally, these involve the designation of an agent to speak on the incompetent incurable's behalf. They represent a combination of the intimate wishes of the patient and the medical recommendations of the physicians.

Before exercising an incompetent patient's right to forgo medical treatment, the surrogate decision maker must satisfy the following conditions:

1. The surrogate must be satisfied that the patient executed a document (e.g., Durable Power of Attorney for Health Care and Health Care Proxy) knowingly, willingly, and without undue influence, and that the evidence of the patient's oral declaration is reliable.
2. The patient must not have reasonable probability of recovering competency so that the patient could exercise the right.
3. The surrogate must take care to ensure that any limitations or conditions expressed either orally or in written declarations have been considered carefully and satisfied.

Determining Incapacity

Before declaring an individual incapacitated, the attending physician must find with a reasonable degree of medical certainty that the patient lacks capacity. A notation should be placed in the patient's medical record describing the cause, nature, extent, and probable duration of incapacity. Before withholding or withdrawing life-sustaining treatment, a second physician must confirm the incapacity determination and make an appropriate entry on the medical record before honoring any new decisions by a health care agent.

Agent's Rights

A health care agent's rights are no greater than those of a competent patient. However, the agent's rights are limited to any specific instructions included in the proxy document. An agent's decisions take priority over any other person except the patient. The agent has the right to consent or refuse to consent to any service or treatment, routine or otherwise; to refuse life-sustaining treatment; and to access all of the patient's medical information to make informed decisions. The agent must make decisions based on the patient's moral and religious beliefs. If a patient's wishes are not known, decisions must be based on a good-faith judgment of what the patient would have wanted.

Living Will

A living will, also referred to in many states as a directive or declaration, is the instrument or legal document that describes those treatments an individual wishes or does not wish to receive should he or she become incapacitated and unable to make medical decisions. Typically, a living will allows a person, when competent, to inform caregivers in writing of his or her wishes with regard to withholding and withdrawing life-supporting treatment, including nutrition and hydration. The living will is helpful to health care professionals because it provides guidance about a patient's wishes for treatment, provides legally valid instructions about treatment, and protects the patient's rights and the provider that honors them.

The living will should be signed and dated by two witnesses who are not blood relatives or beneficiaries of property. A living will should be discussed with the patient's physician, and a signed copy should be placed in the patient's medical record. A copy also should be given to the individual designated to make decisions in the event the patient is unable to do so. A person who executes a living will when healthy and mentally competent cannot predict how he or she will feel at the time of a terminal illness. Therefore, it should be updated regularly so that it accurately reflects a patient's wishes. The written instructions become effective when a patient is either in a terminal condition, permanently unconscious, or suffering irreversible brain damage.

FUTILITY OF TREATMENT

> *. . . When we finally know we are dying,*
> *And all other sentient beings are dying with us,*
> *We start to have a burning, almost heartbreaking sense of the fragility and preciousness of each moment and each being, and from this can grow a deep, clear, limitless compassion for all beings.*
>
> Sogyal Rinpoche

Futility of treatment, as it relates to medical care, occurs when the physician recognizes that the effect of treatment will be of no benefit to the patient. Morally, a physician has a duty to inform the patient when there is little likelihood of success. The determination as to futility of medical care is a scientific decision.

After a diagnosis has been made that a person is terminally ill with no hope of recovery and is in a chronic vegetative state with no possibility of attaining cognitive function, a state generally has no compelling interest in maintaining life. The decision to forgo or terminate life-support measures is, at this point, simply a decision that the dying process will not be artificially extended. Although the state has an interest in the prolongation of life, it has no interest in the prolongation of dying, and although there is a moral and ethical decision to be made to end the process, that decision can be made only by the surrogate. The decision whether to end the dying process is a personal decision for family members or those who bear a legal responsibility for the patient.

A determination as to the futility of medical care is a decision that must be made by a physician. Even if death is not imminent but a patient's coma is irreversible beyond doubt and there are adequate safeguards to confirm the accuracy of the diagnosis with the concurrence of those responsible for the patient's care, it is not unethical to discontinue all means of life-prolonging medical treatment.

WITHDRAWAL OF TREATMENT

Withdrawal of treatment is a decision not to initiate treatment or medical interventions for the patient. When death is imminent and cannot be prevented by available treatment, it is morally permissible to withhold treatment that can yield only a precarious prolongation of life that may involve a great burden for the patient or family. Palliative care should be encouraged in end-of-life situations.

Withdrawal of treatment should be considered when: (1) the patient is in a terminal condition and there is a reasonable expectation of imminent death of the patient; (2) the patient is in a noncognitive state with no reasonable possibility of regaining cognitive function; and/or (3) restoration of cardiac function will last for a brief period.

Theologians and ethicists have long recognized a distinction between ordinary and extraordinary medical care. The theological distinction is based on the belief that life is a gift from God that should not be destroyed deliberately by humans. Therefore, extraordinary therapies that extend life by imposing grave burdens on the patient and family are not required. A patient, however, has an ethical and moral obligation to accept ordinary or life-sustaining treatment. Although the courts have accepted decisions to withhold or withdraw extraordinary care, especially the respirator, from those who are comatose or in a persistent vegetative state with no possibility of emerging, they have been unwilling until now to discontinue feeding, which they have considered to be ordinary care.

The American Medical Association, on March 17, 1986, changed its code of ethics on comas,[31] allowing physicians to withhold food, water, and medical treatment from patients in irreversible comas or persistent vegetative states with no hope of recovery—even if death is not imminent. Although physicians can consider the wishes of the patient and family or the legal representatives, they cannot cause death intentionally. The wording is permissive, so those physicians who feel uncomfortable withdrawing food and water may refrain from doing so. The AMA's decision does not comfort those who fear abuse or a mistake in euthanasia decisions nor does it have any legal value as such.

The Illinois Supreme Court, in *In re Estate of Longeway*,[32] found that the authorized guardian of a terminally ill patient in an irreversible coma or persistent vegetative state has a common-law right to refuse artificial nutrition and hydration. The court found that there must be clear and convincing evidence that the refusal is consistent with the patient's interest. The court also required the concurrence of the patient's attending physician and two other physicians. Court intervention is also necessary to guard against the possibility that greed may taint the judgment of the surrogate decision maker. Although there may be a duty to provide life-sustaining equipment in the immediate aftermath of cardiopulmonary arrest, there is no duty to continue its use when it has become futile and ineffective to do so in the opinion of qualified medical personnel.

DO-NOT-RESUSCITATE ORDERS

Do-not-resuscitate (DNR) orders, given by a physician, indicate that in the event of a cardiac or respiratory arrest, no resuscitative measures should be used to revive the patient. A DNR order is an extremely difficult decision to make for both the patient and family. It is generally made when one's quality of life has been so diminished that heroic rescue methods are no longer in the patient's best interests.

DNR orders must be in writing, signed, and dated by the physician. Appropriate consents must be obtained from the patient or his or her health care agent. Many states have acknowledged the validity of DNR orders in cases involving terminally ill patients in which the patients' families make no objections to such orders.

DNR orders must comply with statutory requirements, be of short duration, and be reviewed periodically to determine whether the patient's condition or other circumstances (e.g., change of mind by the patient or family) surrounding the no-code[33] orders have changed. Presently, it is generally accepted that if a patient is competent, a DNR order is considered to be the same as other medical decisions in which a patient may choose to reject life-sustaining treatment. In the case of an incompetent, absent any advance written directives, the best interests of the patient must be considered.

AUTOPSY

Autopsies, or postmortem examinations, are conducted to ascertain the cause of a person's death, which, in turn, may resolve several legal issues. An autopsy may reveal whether death was the result of criminal activity, whether the cause of death was one for which payment must be made in accordance with an insurance contract, whether the death is compensable under workers' compensation and occupational disease acts, or whether death was the result of a specific act or a culmination of several acts. Aside from providing answers to these specific questions, the information gained from autopsies adds to medical knowledge. As such, medical schools have an interest in autopsies for educational purposes.

In those instances when the death of a patient is the result of criminal activity or unusual or suspicious circumstances, the patient's death must be reported to the medical examiner. Deaths resulting from natural causes within 24 hours of admission to a hospital do not need to be reported as long as the patient was in the hospital at the time of death and as long as an appropriate physician signs the death certificate and records the cause of death.

Deaths that occur during a surgical procedure are generally reportable events to the medical examiner. If an autopsy for medical evaluation is desired by the hospital, consent must be obtained from the next of kin. An unauthorized autopsy may disturb persons whose religious beliefs prohibit such a procedure as well as those persons who have a general aversion to the procedure. When autopsies are performed without statutory authorization and without the consent of the decedent, the surviving spouse, or an appropriate relative, liability may be imposed.

ORGAN DONATION

Federal regulations require that hospitals have, and implement, written protocols regarding the organization's organ procurement policy. The regulations impose specific notification duties, as well as other requirements concerning informing families of potential donors. It encourages discretion and sensitivity in dealing with the families and in educating hospital staff on a variety of issues involved with donation matters to facilitate timely donation and transplantation.

Developments in medical science have enabled physicians to take tissue from persons immediately after death and use it to replace or rehabilitate diseased or damaged organs or other parts of living persons. Success rates have increased because of improved patient selection, improved clinical and operative skills, and the development of immunosuppressant drugs to aid in decreasing the incidence of tissue rejection. Progress in this field of medicine has created the problem of obtaining a sufficient supply of replacement body parts. Fear that people would buy and sell organs led to enactment of the National Organ Procurement Act in 1984, making it illegal to buy or sell organs. Throughout the country, there are tissue banks and other facilities for the storage and preservation of organs and tissue that can be used for transplantation and for other therapeutic services.

The ever-increasing success of organ transplants and the demand for organ tissue require the close scrutiny of each case, making sure that established procedures have been followed in the care and disposal of all body parts. Section 1138, Title XI, of the Omnibus Budget Reconciliation Act of 1986 requires hospitals to establish organ procurement protocols or face a loss of Medicare and Medicaid funding. Physicians, nurses, and other paramedical personnel assigned with this responsibility often are confronted with several legal issues. Liability can be limited by complying with applicable regulations. Organs and tissues to be stored and preserved for future use must be removed immediately after death. Therefore, it is imperative that an agreement or arrangement for obtaining organs and tissue from a body be completed before death, or very soon after death, to enable physicians to remove and store the tissue promptly.

The Uniform Anatomical Gift Act drafted by the Commission on Uniform State Laws has been enacted by all 50 states and has many detailed provisions that apply to a wide variety of issues raised in connection with the making, acceptance, and use of anatomic gifts. The act allows a person to make a decision to donate organs at the time of death and allows potential donors to carry an anatomical donor card. State statutes regarding donation usually permit the donor to execute the gift during his or her lifetime. Virtually all states have based their enactments on the Uniform Anatomical Gift Act, but it should be recognized that in some states there are deviations from this act or laws dealing with donation.

Individuals who are of sound mind and 18 years of age or older are permitted to dispose of their own bodies or body parts by will or other written instrument for medical or dental education, research, advancement of medical or dental science, therapy, or transplantation. Among those eligible to receive such donations are any licensed, accredited, or approved hospitals; accredited medical or dental schools; surgeons or physicians; tissue banks; or specified individuals who need the donation for therapy or transplantation. The statute provides that when only a part of the body is donated, custody of the remaining parts of the body shall be transferred to the next of kin promptly after removal of the donated part.

A donation by will becomes effective immediately on the death of the testator, without probate, and the gift is valid and effective to the extent that it has been acted on in good faith. This is true even if the will is not probated or is declared invalid for testimonial purposes.

RESEARCH AND EXPERIMENTATION

The science of medicine, by the very nature of the object that it studies, the human body, is often prevented from making progress through direct experimentation. It must resort to necessary tests in laboratories and on animals, whose reactions are similar to humans—but most of all, it advances through observation of functions of the body in health and in disease. It is natural that much of this laboratory experimentation and clinical observation should be done in the hospital.

To increase the possibility of advancement by observation, clinical records must be accurate and complete in every case, no matter how trivial, and they should be preserved in such a manner as to be available for the study of similar cases. New remedies of all kinds should be tried under conditions that favor accurate observation. Laboratories should be available under the direction of physicians, and results of examinations should be carefully compiled and studied.

Systematized research is possible only when directed by a physician with a scientific specialty, and it is rare not to find one such individual working in most hospitals.

Federal regulations control federal grants that apply to experiments involving new drugs, new medical devices, stem cell research and human cloning, or new medical procedures. Generally, a combination of federal and state guidelines and regulations ensures proper supervision and control over experimentation that involves human subjects. For example, federal regulations require hospital-based researchers to obtain the approval of an institutional review board prior to conducting clinical trials. This board functions to review proposed research studies and conduct follow-up reviews on a regular basis.

Federal and state regulations impose several other requirements on experiments involving human subjects. Institutions conducting medical research on human subjects must disclose fully the inherent risks to the patient; make a proper determination that the patient is competent to consent; identify treatment alternatives; and obtain written consent from the patient.

Written Consent

Written consent should be obtained from each patient who agrees to participate in a clinical trial. Consent should include the risks, benefits, and alternatives to the proposed treatment protocol. The consent form should be signed, witnessed, and dated. The consent form must not contain any coercive or exculpatory language through which the patient is forced to waive his or her legal rights, including the release of the investigator, sponsor, or organization from liability for negligent conduct.

Federal regulations require that the nature of experimental drugs and possible adverse consequences must be explained to the patient. Failure to obtain consent for the administration of experimental drugs can give rise to a lawsuit. The district court in *Blanton v. United States*[34] held that when a new drug of unknown effectiveness was administered to a patient at a Navy medical center, despite the availability of other drugs of known effectiveness, the hospital violated the accepted medical standards and its duty of due care, so that in the absence of the patient's consent to the experiment, the United States was liable for the resulting injury.

Institutional Review Board

Each organization conducting medical research should have a mechanism in place for approving and overseeing the use of investigational protocols. This is often accomplished through the establishment of an institutional review board (IRB). The IRB should include community representation. The IRB is responsible for reviewing, monitoring, and approving clinical protocols for investigations of drugs and medical devices involving human subjects. The IRB is responsible for ensuring that the rights of each individual are protected and that all research is conducted within appropriate state and federal guidelines (e.g., FDA guidelines).

Notes

1. French/American religious leader (1773–1855).
2. Stamford Hosp. v. Vega, 674 A.2d 821 (Conn. Super. Ct. 1996).
3. No. 31328 (W.Va. 2004).
4. 725 P.2d 400 (Or. Ct. App. 1986).
5. Florida Bar v. Barrett, No. SC03-375 (Fla. 2005).
6. In re Quinlan, 355 A.2d 647 (N.J. 1976).
7. Union Pac. Ry. Co. v. Botsford, 141 U.S. 250, 251 (1891).
8. 105 N.E. 92, 93 (N.Y. 1914).
9. Id.
10. 438 N.Y.S.2d 266, 272 (N.Y. 1981).
11. 410 U.S. 113 (1973).
12. Supra note 6.
13. 370 N.E.2d 417 (Mass. 1977).
14. Id. at 434.
15. 380 N.E.2d 134 (Mass. 1978).
16. 405 N.E.2d 115 (Mass. 1980).
17. 452 So. 2d 925 (Fla. 1984).
18. 362 So. 2d 160 (Fla. Dist. Ct. App. 1978).
19. Statement of Medical Opinion Re: "Brain Death," A.M.A. House of Delegates Res. (June 1974).
20. 534 N.E.2d 886 (N.Y. 1988).
21. Id. at 891.
22. Cruzan v. Harman, 760 S.W.2d 408 (Mo. 1988).
23. Cruzan v. Director of the Mo. Dep't of Health, 497 U.S. 261 (1990).
24. Pa. S.646, Amendment A3506, Printer's No. 689, Oct. 1, 1990.
25. 20 PA. Cons. Stat. Ann. § 5602(a)(9) (1988).
26. Hobbins v. Attorney Gen. of Mich., No. 94-1473 (Mich. 1994); Kevorkian v. Michigan, No. 94-1490 (Mich. 1994).
27. Or. Rev. Stat. Sects. 127.800-897.
28. Quill v. Vacco, 117 S. Ct. 2293 (1997).
29. 117 S. Ct. 2258 (1997).
30. Bush v. Schiavo, No. SC04-925 (Fla. App. 2004).
31. AMA Changes Code of Ethics on Comas, Newsday, Mar. 17, 1986, at 2.
32. 549 N.E.2d 292 (Ill. 1989).
33. John F. Kennedy Mem'l Hosp. v. Bludworth, 452 So. 2d 921, 925 (Fla. 1984) (citing In re Welfare of Colyer, 660 P.2d 738 (Wash. 1983), in which the court found prior court approval to be "unresponsive and cumbersome").
34. 428 F. Supp. 360 (D.D.C. 1977).

18

Professional Liability Insurance

I never was ruined but twice—once when I gained a lawsuit, and once when I lost one.

Francois Marie de Voltaire
(1694–1778)

This chapter introduces the reader to some of the basic concepts related to liability insurance. The purpose of liability insurance is to spread the risk of economic loss among members of a group who share common risks. For example, an obstetrician would share risk with other obstetricians. As risks increase, premiums increase to cover associated risks. The premiums are placed in a shared risk fund from which funds are drawn to cover the costs of lawsuits. As high awards are paid out of the fund, there is a danger that patients will have a more difficult time to find physicians willing to accept them as patients. Some physicians, because of skyrocketing malpractice premiums, find it too costly to maintain a private practice. As a result, they often limit their practice to less costly procedures.

Medical malpractice insurance, as in all insurance, is subject to the cyclical nature of the insurance market. Problems intrinsic in malpractice insurance include the uncertainty of the US legal system, the affects of inflation on ultimate claim values, emerging technology, and new treatments.

THE INSURANCE POLICY

Insurance is a contract that creates legal obligations on the part of both the insured and the insurer. It is a contract in which the insurer agrees to assume certain risks of the insured for consideration or payment of a premium. Under the terms of the contract, also known as the insurance policy, the insurer promises to pay a specific amount of money if a specified event takes place. An insurance policy contains three necessary elements:

1. identification of the risk covered
2. the specific amount payable
3. the specified occurrence

Insurance companies are required by the laws of the different states to issue only policies that contain certain mandated provisions and to maintain certain financial reserves to guarantee to policyholders that their expectations will be met when coverage is needed. The basic underlying concept of insurance is the spreading of risk. By writing coverage for a large enough pool of individuals, the company has determined actuarially that a certain number of claims will arise within that pool, and if the premium structure has been established correctly and the prediction of claims made accurately, the company ought to be able to meet those claims and return a profit to its shareholders.

Risk Categories

A risk is the possibility that a loss will occur. The main function of insurance is to provide security against this loss. Insurance does not prevent or hinder the occurrence of the loss, but it does compensate for the damages.

An insured individual may be exposed to three categories of risk: (1) property loss or damage, (2) personal injury or loss of life, and (3) incurring legal liability. Property risk is the possibility that an insured's property may be damaged or destroyed by fire, flood, tornado, hurricane, or other catastrophe. Personal risk is the possibility that the insured may be injured in an accident or may become ill; the possibility of death is a personal risk covered in the typical life insurance plan. Legal liability risk is the possibility that the insured may become legally liable to pay money damages to another and includes accident and professional liability insurance.

Types of Policies

Insurance policies include *occurrence* policies, which cover all incidents that arise during a policy year, regardless of when they are reported to the insurer; and *claims-made* policies, which cover only those claims made or reported during the policy year. *Tail* coverage policies provide for an uninterrupted extension of an insurance policy period. *Umbrella* policies cover awards over the amount provided in the basic policy coverage. The dollar amount of coverage is specified in the policy dollar.

LIABILITY OF THE PROFESSIONAL

An individual who provides professional services to another person may be legally responsible for any harm the person suffers as a result of negligence. Many professionals protect themselves from their exposure to a legal loss by acquiring a professional liability insurance policy.

All Professionals Need Insurance

All health care professionals should carry liability insurance. Even though a hospital, for example, as an employer can be held liable for the acts of its employees under the doctrine of respondeat superior, the employee can be financially liable to the employer for his or her own negligent acts. From a cost–benefit standpoint, the answer to the question "Do I really need insurance?" is yes. Insurance premiums for allied health professionals are relatively reasonable.

Malpractice insurance coverage is especially important if a caregiver is working:

- as a volunteer at a clinic or health fair not sponsored by his or her employer
- as an independent contractor providing a service in a patient's home
- for an independent agency or registry
- for an organization that is covered by an insurance policy that has an exclusionary provision by which the insurance company disclaims liability for malpractice actions brought against the insured organization

THE INSURANCE POLICY

Health care organizations, nurses, physicians, and other health care practitioners who are covered by an insurance policy must recognize the rights and duties inherent in the policy. The professional being insured should be able to identify the risks that are covered, the amount of coverage, and the conditions of the contract.

Although the policies of different insurance companies may vary, the standard policy usually provides that the insurance company will pay on behalf of the insured all sums that the insured shall become legally obligated to pay as damages because of injury arising out of malpractice error or mistake in rendering or failing to render professional services. A standard liability insurance policy has five distinct parts:

1. insurance agreement
2. defense and settlement
3. policy period
4. amount payable
5. conditions of the policy

The insurer, under the terms of the policy, has a legal obligation to pay the sum that has been agreed to or determined by a court, up to the policy limit, including legal fees. Under a professional liability policy, the professional is protected from damages arising from rendering or failing to render professional services. Thus, a professional who performs a negligent act resulting in legal liability or who fails to perform a necessary act (thereby incurring damages) is personally protected from paying an injured party. The insurer makes payment of damages to the injured party.

Defense and Settlement

In the defense and settlement portion of the insurance policy, the insured and the insurance company agree that the company will defend any lawsuit against the insured arising from performance or nonperformance of professional services. The insurance company is delegated the power to effect a settlement of any claims as it deems necessary. In a professional liability policy, the duty of the insurer under this clause is limited to the defense of lawsuits against the insured that are a consequence of professional services.

The insurance company fulfills its obligation to provide a defense by engaging the services of an attorney on behalf of the insured. The obligation of the attorney is to the insured directly because the insured is the attorney's client. Here is, to some extent, a divided loyalty because the attorney looks to the insurance company to obtain business. Nevertheless, the attorney–client relationship exists between only the attorney and the insured, and the insured has the right to expect the attorney to fulfill the requirements of such a relationship.

If an insurance company has established the right to obtain a settlement of any claim prior to trial, the company's only obligation is to act reasonably and not to the detriment of the insured.

Policy Period

The period of the policy is stated in the insurance contract. Under an occurrence policy, the contract provides protection only for claims that occur during the time frame within which the policy is stated to be in effect. Any incident that occurs before or after the policy period would not be covered under the insuring agreement. Occurrence policies provide coverage for all claims that may arise out of a policy period. The actual reporting time has no bearing on the validity of the claim, so long as it is filed before the applicable statute of limitations tolls. Although the reporting time has no bearing on the validity of the claim from the standpoint of coverage under the policy, the conditions of the policy will require notice within a specified time. Failure to provide such notice could void the insurer's obligation under the policy if it can be demonstrated that the carrier's position was compromised as a result of filing an untimely claim or report.

A claims-made policy provides coverage for only those claims instituted during the policy period. Notice of a claim is required during the policy period. Failure to give notice of a claim to the insurer in a claims-made policy until after the policy expires can result in denial by the insurance company to cover the claim.

Coverage: The Amount Payable

The amount to be paid by an insurer is determined by the amount of damages incurred by the injured party. The insurance company and the injured party may negotiate a settlement prior to or during trial. Some states have provisions mandating that consent of the court must be obtained prior to the settlement of a negligence claim on behalf of a minor.

In any event, the insurance company will pay the injured party no more than the maximum limit stated in the insurance policy. The insured professional must personally pay any damages that exceed the policy limits. For example, under a policy with a maximum coverage of $1 million for each claim and $3 million for aggregate claims (the total amount payable to all injured parties), the insured must pay any amount over $1 million on each individual claim and any amount over $3 million in a policy period.

Uninsured Claims

An insurer has no duty to defend or provide coverage for intentional torts. Contracts insuring against loss from intentional wrongs are generally void as being against public policy.

Criminal Acts: Sexual Assault

Sexual assault does not constitute rendering professional services within the coverage provisions of insurance policies. As a result, malpractice insurers are not required to indemnify the insured for liability resulting from the sexual assault. The Medical Protective Company, in *R.W. v. Schrein*,[1] a physician's professional liability insurer, sought a judgment determining that it had no duty to defend or indemnify the physician with respect to five former patients who claimed that they were sexually abused during examination and treatment. The Supreme Court of Nebraska held that there is no clearly articulated public policy that would permit or require the court to disregard the fact that the physician's acts did not fall within the coverage provided. The physician's liability to the appellants was not based on the provision or failure to provide professional services.

Conditions of an Insurance Policy

Each insurance policy contains a number of important conditions. Failure to comply with these conditions may cause forfeiture of the policy and nonpayment of claims against it. Generally, insurance policies contain the following conditions:

- notice of occurrence—When the insured becomes aware that an injury has occurred as a result of acts covered under the contract, the insured must notify the insurance company promptly. The form of notice may be either oral or written, as specified in the policy.
- notice of claim—Whenever the insured receives notice that a claim or suit is being instituted, prompt notice must be sent by the insured to the insurance company. This provides the insurance company with an opportunity to investigate the facts of a case. The policy will specify what papers are to be forwarded to the company. The mere failure to advise in a timely manner may be in and of itself a breach of the insurance contract, entitling the insurer to decline coverage. It may not matter that the insurer has in no way been prejudiced by the late notification. The mere fact that the insured failed to carry out obligations under the policy may be sufficient to permit the insurer to avoid its obligations. When the insurer

has refused to honor a claim because of late notice and the insured wishes to challenge such refusal, an action can be brought, asking a court to determine the reasonableness of the insurer's position.

- assistance of the insured—The insured must cooperate with the insurance company and render any assistance necessary to reach a settlement.
- other insurance—If the insured has pertinent insurance policies with other insurance companies, the insured must notify the insurance company so that each company may pay the appropriate amount of the claim.
- assignment—The protections contracted for by the insured may not be transferred unless the insurance company grants permission. Because the insurance company was aware of the risks the insured would encounter before the policy was issued, the company will endeavor to avoid protecting persons other than the policyholder.
- subrogation—This is the right of a person who pays another's debt to be substituted for all rights in relation to the debt. When an insurance company makes a payment for the insured under the terms of the policy, the company becomes the beneficiary of all the rights of recovery the insured has against any other persons who also may have been negligent. For example, if several nurses were found liable for negligence arising from the same occurrence and the insurance company for one nurse pays the entire claim, the company will be entitled to the rights of that nurse and may collect a proportionate share of the claim from the other nurses.
- changes—The insured cannot make changes in the policy without the written consent of the insurance company. Thus, an agent of the insurance company ordinarily cannot modify or remove any condition of the liability contract. Only the insurance company, by written authorization, may permit a condition to be altered or removed.
- cancellation—A cancellation clause spells out the conditions and procedures necessary for the insured or the insurer to cancel the liability policy. Written notice usually is required. The insured person's failure to comply with any terms of the policy can result in cancellation and possible nonpayment of a claim by the insurance company. As a legal contract, failure to meet the terms and conditions of an insurance policy can result in a breach of contract and voidance of coverage.

MEDICAL LIABILITY INSURANCE

The fundamental tenets of insurance law and their application to the typical liability insurance policy are pertinent to the provisions of medical professional liability insurance as applied to individuals and institutions. Professional liability policies vary in the broadness, the exclusions from coverage, and the interpretations a company places on the language of the contract.

There are three medical professional liability classes:

1. individuals including (but not limited to) physicians, surgeons, dentists, nurses, osteopaths, chiropractors, opticians, physiotherapists, optometrists, and different types of medical technicians (This category may include medical laboratories and blood banks.)
2. health care institutions, such as hospitals, extended-care facilities, homes for the aged, institutions for the mentally ill, and other health care facilities where bed and board are provided for patients or residents
3. outpatient facilities and clinics where there are no regular bed or board facilities (These institutions may be related to industrial or commercial enterprises; however, they are to be distinguished

from facilities operated by dentists or physicians, which usually are covered under individual professional liability contracts.)

The insuring clause usually will provide for payment on behalf of the insured if an injury arises from either of the following:

- malpractice, error, or mistake in rendering or failing to render professional services in the practice of the insured's profession during the policy period
- acts or omissions on the part of the insured during the policy period as a member of a formal accreditation or similar professional board or committee of a health care facility or a professional society

Although injury is not limited to bodily injury or property damage, it must result from malpractice, error, mistake, or failure to perform acts that should have been performed.

The most common risks covered by medical professional liability insurance are

- negligence
- assault and battery as a result of failing to obtain consent to a medical or surgical procedure
- libel and slander
- invasion of privacy for betrayal of professional confidences

Coverage may vary from company to company, but standards of policy coverage generally are followed. Rates will differ for individuals by profession and specialty and by type of health care facility (e.g., nursing facility and hospital).

SELF-INSURANCE

Exorbitant malpractice insurance premiums often have produced situations in which the premium cost of insurance has approached and, on occasion, reached the face amount of the policy. Because of the extremely high cost of maintaining such insurance, some institutions have sought alternatives to this conventional means of protecting against medical malpractice. One alternative is self-insurance. When a health care facility self-insures its malpractice risks, it no longer purchases a policy of malpractice insurance but instead periodically sets aside a certain amount of its own funds as a reserve against malpractice losses and expenses. An institution that self-insures generally retains the services of a self-insurance consulting firm and of an actuary to determine the proper level of funding that the institution should maintain.

A self-insurance program need not involve the elimination of insurance coverage in its entirety. A health care organization may find it prudent to purchase excess coverage whereby the organization self-insures the first agreed-on dollar amount of risk and the insurance carrier insures the balance. For example, in a typical program the organization may self-insure the first $1 million of professional liability risk per year. Because most claims will be disposed of within such limitation, the cost of excess insurance may be quite reasonable.

Before a corporation makes a decision to self-insure, not only must it determine the economic aspects of such a decision and the necessary funding levels to maintain an adequate reserve for future claims, but it also must determine whether there are any legal impediments to such a program. A corporation that has obtained funding from governmental sources or that has issued bonds or other obligations containing certain covenants may find itself unable to self-insure because of these prior commitments. Health care organizations should consult legal counsel to review appropriate and applicable documentation before making the self-insurance decision.

TRUSTEE COVERAGE

Trustees should be covered by liability insurance just as physicians and other health care professionals. Such coverage is generally provided for by the organization. Such coverage is helpful in attracting qualified board members. Before an insurer that writes a trustee policy (generally known as directors' and officers' liability insurance) will respond to defend or pay a claim on behalf of a trustee, it must be shown that the trustee acted in good faith and within the scope of his or her responsibilities. Ordinarily, coverage would not be afforded when a trustee is accused of acting improperly in his or her relationship with the corporation. Also, insurance coverage for officers' and directors' liability generally excludes as a covered event the failure to obtain other necessary insurance for the institution (e.g., fire insurance).

MANDATED MEDICAL STAFF INSURANCE COVERAGE

Physicians often are required by health care organizations to carry their own malpractice insurance. Physicians who fail to maintain such coverage can be suspended from a hospital's medical staff. A federal district court in *Pollack v. Methodist Hospital*[2] ruled that a hospital has the legal right to suspend a staff physician for failing to comply with its requirement that physicians carry medical malpractice insurance coverage. The decision resulted from a suit brought against a hospital by a physician whose staff privileges were suspended because he failed to comply with a newly adopted hospital requirement that all staff physicians provide proof of malpractice coverage of at least $1 million. The court rejected the physician's charges that the requirement violated his civil rights and antitrust laws.

As held in *Wilkinson v. Madera Community Hospital*,[3] a health care organization can require its medical staff to show evidence of professional liability insurance. The physician in this case was refused reappointment because he failed to maintain malpractice insurance with a recognized insurance company as required by the hospital.

INVESTIGATION AND SETTLEMENT OF CLAIMS

An injured party may request settlement of a claim prior to instituting legal action. As a first step toward settlement of a claim, the insurance carrier may have an investigator interview a claimant regarding the details of the alleged occurrence that led to the injury. After an investigation, the insurance company may agree to a settlement if liability is questionable and the risks of proceeding to trial are too great. Should settlement negotiations fail, an attorney may be employed by the injured party to negotiate a settlement. If the attorney fails to obtain a settlement, either the claim can be dropped or legal action commenced.

When a claim is settled, a general release, signed by the plaintiff, surrenders the right of action against the defendant. If the claimant is married, a general release also should be obtained from the spouse because there may be a cause of action due to loss of the injured spouse's services (e.g., companionship). A parent's release surrenders only a parental claim. Approval of a court may be necessary to release a child's claim. A release by a minor, in some instances, may be repudiated by the minor upon reaching majority.

Notes

1. 263 Neb. 708, 642 N.W.2d 505 (2002).
2. 392 F. Supp. 393 (E.D. La. 1975).
3. 192 Cal. Rptr. 593 (Cal. Ct. App. 1983).

19

Labor Relations

Federal and state regulations generally pervade all areas of employer–employee relationships. The most significant piece of federal legislation dealing with labor relations is the National Labor Relations Act. Although federal laws generally take precedence over state laws when there is a conflict between the state and the federal laws, state laws are applicable and must be considered, especially when state regulations are more rigid than federal legislation. This chapter provides an overview of those laws affecting the health care industry.

US DEPARTMENT OF LABOR

The US Department of Labor is a department within the executive branch of government. The secretary of labor advises the president on labor policies and issues. The functions of the department of labor are to foster, promote, and develop the welfare of wage earners, to improve working conditions, and to advance opportunities for profitable employment. In carrying out this mission, the department administers a variety of federal labor laws guaranteeing workers' rights to safe and healthful working conditions, a minimum hourly wage and overtime pay, freedom from employment discrimination, unemployment insurance, and workers' compensation. As the department seeks to assist all Americans who need and want to work, special efforts are made to meet the unique job market problems of older workers, youths, minority group members, women, the handicapped, and other groups. Within the department of labor are various agencies responsible for carrying out the purpose of the department (e.g., Occupational Safety and Health Administration).

UNIONS AND HEALTH CARE ORGANIZATIONS

Many labor organizations attempt to become the recognized collective bargaining representatives for employees in health care settings. Craft unions devote their primary organizing efforts to skilled employees, such as carpenters and electricians, and industrial unions and unions of governmental employees seek to represent large groups of unskilled or semiskilled employees. Professional and occupational associations, such as state nurses' associations, historically known for their social and academic efforts, have involved themselves in collective bargaining for their professions. To the extent that the professional organizations seek goals directly concerned with wages, hours, and other employment conditions and engage in bargaining on behalf of employees, they perform the functions of labor unions.

NATIONAL LABOR RELATIONS ACT

The National Labor Relations Act (NLRA)[1] was enacted by Congress in July 1935 to govern the labor–management relations of business firms engaged in interstate commerce. The act is generally known as the Wagner Act, after Senator Robert R. Wagner of New York. The act defines certain conduct of employers and employees as unfair labor practices and provides for hearings on complaints that such practices have occurred. The NLRA was modified by the Taft-Hartley amendments of 1947 and the Landrum-Griffin amendments of 1959.

National Labor Relations Board

The National Labor Relations Board (NLRB), which is entrusted with enforcing and administering the NLRA, has jurisdiction over matters involving proprietary and not-for-profit health care organizations. The NLRB is an agency, independent of the department of labor, that is responsible for preventing and remedying unfair labor practices by employers and labor organizations or their agents. The NLRB conducts secret ballot elections among employees in appropriate collective bargaining units to determine whether they desire to be represented by a labor organization and among employees under union-shop agreements to determine whether they wish to revoke their union's authority. The general counsel of the NLRB has final authority to investigate charges of unfair labor practices, issue complaints, and prosecute such complaints before the NLRB. There are regional directors, under the direction of the general counsel, who are responsible for processing representation, unfair labor practice, and jurisdictional dispute cases.

An exemption for governmental institutions was included in the 1935 enactment of the NLRA, and charitable health care institutions were exempted in 1947 by the Taft-Hartley Act amendments to the NLRA. However, a July 1974 amendment to the NLRA extended coverage to employees of nonprofit health care organizations that previously had been exempted from its provisions. In the words of the amendment, a health care facility is "any hospital, convalescent hospital, health maintenance organization, health clinic, nursing home, extended care facility, or other institution devoted to the care of the sick, infirm or aged."[2]

The amendment also enacted unique, special provisions for employees of health care organizations who oppose unionization on legitimate religious grounds. These provisions allow a member of such an organization to make periodic contributions to one of three nonreligious charitable funds selected jointly by the labor organization and the employing institution rather than paying periodic union dues and initiation fees. If the collective bargaining agreement does not specify an acceptable fund, the employee may select a tax-exempt charity.

Elections

The NLRA sets out the procedures by which employees may select a union as their collective bargaining representative to negotiate with health care organizations over employment and contract matters. A health care organization may choose to recognize and deal with the union without resorting to the formal NLRA procedure. If the formal process is adhered to, employees may vote on union representation in an election held under NLRB supervision.

The NLRA provides that the representative, having been selected by a majority of employees in a bargaining unit, is the exclusive bargaining agent for all employees in the unit. The scope of the bargaining unit is often the subject of dispute, for its boundaries may determine the outcome of the election, the employee representative's bargaining power, and the level of labor stability.

Unfair Labor Practices

The NLRA prohibits health care organizations from engaging in certain conduct classified as employer unfair labor practices. For example, discriminating against an employee for holding union membership is not permitted. The NLRA stipulates that the employer must bargain in good faith with representatives of the employees; failure to do so constitutes an unfair labor practice. The NLRB may order the employer to fulfill the duty to bargain.

The NLRA places duties on labor organizations and prohibits certain employee activities that are considered to be unfair labor practices. Coercion of employees by the union constitutes an unfair labor practice; such activities as mass picketing, assaulting nonstrikers, and following groups of nonstrikers away from the immediate area of the facility plainly constitute coercion and can be ordered stopped by the NLRB.

Unlawful Interrogation

Ms. Welton attended a union organization meeting on July 5. At a hearing before an administrative law judge (ALJ), she testified that the day after the meeting her supervisor asked whether she or anyone from the dietary department attended the meeting. Welton's supervisor denied having any conversation with Welton about the union meeting. The NLRB found that the questioning of Welton constituted unlawful interrogation.

Mr. Hopkins worked as a janitor for the nursing facility. He also attended the meeting on July 5. He testified that his supervisor approached him at work and questioned him as to whether any of the nurses or aides harassed him about the union. The board credited Hopkins's and Welton's version of the events, noting that they had nothing to gain by fabricating their testimony.

On July 18, the facility circulated a memorandum to all employees that stated: "This is to advise that the NLRB has tentatively set a hearing on Wednesday, July 25th, to decide who can vote in a union election. Our position is that supervisors, RNs, and LPNs cannot vote. We will keep you advised."

On July 19, the facility held a mandatory meeting for all nurses and supervisors. The facility's administrator, Mr. Wimer; the facility's attorney, Mr. Yocum; and the chief executive officer, Mr. Colby, told the nurses that, in the facility's opinion, nurses could not vote in the upcoming election but must remain loyal to the facility. When asked by Sands, a union supporter, what he meant by loyalty, Yocum replied that all nurses were prohibited from engaging in union activities. When asked by Sands why the facility opposed the union, Yocum responded, "Well, for one thing, they cost too . . . much money. . . . Do you think those dues come out of thin air?"

The board concluded that the facility, through Yocum, violated the National Labor Relations Act by telling nurses present at the meeting that they could not vote in the upcoming union election or participate in union activities, and that such activities could subject them to dismissal.

The US Court of Appeals for the Seventh Circuit found that the employer's interrogation of nursing facility employees about a union meeting constituted an unfair labor practice. On the record as a whole, substantial evidence supported the board's conclusions that the questioning of Welton and Hopkins amounted to unlawful interrogation.[3]

Hospital's Unfair Labor Practice

The National Labor Relations Board, in *St. John's Mercy Health Systems v. National Labor Relations Board*[4] was found to have properly upheld a union's unfair labor practice charge against a hospital that had refused to discharge registered nurses who had not paid union dues, as required by the applicable collective bargaining agreement (CBA). There was no public policy of Missouri that prevented enforcement of union-security provision of the CBA, notwithstanding statistical evidence of a regional or national nursing shortage that would make it difficult to replace nurses. In addition, the hospital was not exempt from the NLRA union-security provisions.

NORRIS-LAGUARDIA ACT

Congress enacted the Norris-LaGuardia Act[5] to limit the power of federal courts to issue injunctions in cases involving or growing out of labor disputes. The act's strict standards must be met before such injunctions can be issued. Essentially, a federal court may not apply restraints in a labor dispute until after the case is heard in open court and the finding is that unlawful acts will be committed unless restrained and that substantial and irreparable injury to the complainant's property will follow.[6]

The Norris-LaGuardia Act is aimed at reducing the number of injunctions granted to restrain strikes and picketing. An additional piece of legislation designating procedures limiting strikes in health care institutions is the 1974 amendment to the NLRA. This amendment sets out special procedures for handling labor disputes that develop from collective bargaining at the termination of an existing agreement or during negotiations for an initial contract between a health care institution and its employees. The procedures were designed to ensure that the needs of patients would be met during any work stoppage (strike) or labor dispute in such an institution.

More significantly, 10 days' notice is required in advance of any strike, picketing, or other concerted refusal to work, regardless of the source of the dispute. This allows the NLRB to determine the legality of a strike before it occurs and also gives health care institutions ample time to ensure the continuity of patient care.

In summary, the amendment's provisions are designed to ensure that every possible approach to a peaceful settlement is explored fully before a strike is called.

LABOR-MANAGEMENT REPORTING AND DISCLOSURE ACT

The Labor-Management Reporting and Disclosure Act of 1959[7] was enacted to place controls on labor unions and the relationships between unions and their members. Also, the Act requires that employers report payments and loans made to officials or other representatives of labor organizations or any promises to make such payments or loans. Expenditures made to influence or restrict the way employees exercise their rights to organize and bargain collectively are illegal unless the employer discloses them. Agreements with labor consultants, under which such persons undertake to interfere with certain employee rights, also must be disclosed.

FAIR LABOR STANDARDS ACT

The Fair Labor Standards Act (FLSA)[8] of 1938 established a national minimum wage, guaranteed time and one-half for overtime, and maximum hours of employment and prohibited most employment for minors. The FLSA is administered by the Wage & Hour Division of the US Department of Labor, which conducts audits and workplace inspections. The FLSA provides for direct federal actions by employees and offers substantial financial incentives for private litigants and their counsel.

Employees of all governmental, charitable, and proprietary health care organizations are covered by the FLSA. Employers must conform to the minimum wage and overtime pay provisions. However, bona fide executive, administrative, and professional employees are exempted from the wage and hour provisions.

The law permits employers to enter into agreements with employees, establishing a work period of 14 consecutive days as an alternative to the usual 7-day week. If the alternative period is chosen, the employer must pay the overtime rate only for hours worked in excess of 80 hours during the 14-day period. The alternative 14-day work period does not relieve a facility from paying overtime for hours worked in excess of 8 hours in any one day even if no more than 80 hours are worked during the period.

CIVIL RIGHTS ACT

Title VII of the Civil Rights Act of 1964, as amended by the Equal Employment Opportunity Act of 1972,[9] prohibits private employers and state and local governments from discrimination in employment in any business on the basis of race, color, religion, sex, or national origin. The act prohibits harassment based on one's affiliation (e.g., religion), physical and cultural traits and clothing (e.g., skin color, headscarf), perception (e.g., due to national origin: He is from Pakistan and must, therefore, be a terrorist), and association (e.g., discrimination based on association with an individual or organization). The federal antidiscrimination law provides that it is unlawful for most public and private employers to discriminate against, fail or refuse to hire, or to discharge any individual, with respect to his or her compensation, terms, conditions, or privileges of employment because of such individual's race, color, religion, sex (including pregnancy), or national origin.

Title VII also prohibits retaliation against employees who oppose such unlawful discrimination. The Equal Employment Commission (EEOC) enforces Title VII. The EEOC investigates, mediates, and sometimes files lawsuits on behalf of employees. Title VII also provides that an individual can bring a private lawsuit.

An exception to prohibited employment practices may be permitted when religion, sex, or national origin is a bona fide occupational qualification necessary to the operation of a particular business or enterprise.

OCCUPATIONAL SAFETY AND HEALTH ACT

OSHA's mission is to assure the safety and health of America's workers by setting and enforcing standards; providing training, outreach, and education; establishing partnerships; and encouraging continual improvement in workplace safety and health.[10]

Congress enacted the Occupational Safety and Health Act of 1970[11] (OSHA) to establish administrative machinery for the development and enforcement of standards for occupational health and safety. The legislation was enacted based on congressional findings that personal injuries and illnesses arising out of work situations impose a substantial burden on and are substantial hindrances to interstate commerce in terms of lost production, wage loss, medical expenses, and disability compensation payments. Congress declared that its purpose and policy were to ensure, so far as possible, every working man and woman in the nation safe and healthful working conditions and to preserve human resources by, for example, encouraging employers and employees in their efforts to reduce the number of occupational safety and health hazards at their places of employment, and stimulating employers and employees to institute new and to perfect existing programs for providing safe and healthful working conditions.[12]

Promulgation and Enforcement of OSHA Standards

OSHA develops and promulgates occupational safety and health standards for the workplace. It develops and issues regulations, conducts investigations and inspections to determine the status of compliance, and issues citations and proposes penalties for noncompliance. Inspections are conducted without advance notice.

Employers are responsible for becoming familiar with standards applicable to their businesses and for ensuring that employees have and use personal protective equipment when required for safety. Employees must comply with all rules and regulations that are applicable to their work environment. Where OSHA has not promulgated specific standards, the employer is responsible for following the act's general-duty clause. The general-duty clause states that each employer must furnish a place of employment that is free from recognized hazards that are causing or likely to cause death or serious physical harm.

Recordkeeping

Employers of 11 or more employees are required to maintain records of occupational injuries and illnesses. The purpose of maintaining records is to permit the Bureau of Labor Statistics to help define high-hazard industries and to inform employees of the status of their employer's record.

Education

Employers are responsible for keeping employees informed about OSHA and about the various safety and health matters with which they are involved. OSHA requires that employers post certain material at a prominent location in the workplace (e.g., a job safety and health protection workplace poster informing employees of their rights and responsibilities under the act).

Infectious Body Fluids

OSHA issued standards on December 2, 1991, that are to be followed by employers to protect employees from bloodborne infections. Universal precautions are mandatory, and employees who are likely to be exposed to body fluids must be provided with protective clothing (e.g., masks, gowns, and gloves). In addition, postexposure testing must be available to employees who have been exposed to body fluids.

Employee Complaints

Employees should inform their supervisors if they suspect or detect a dangerous situation in the workplace. Employers are expected to address reported hazards in the workplace. Employees or their representatives have the right to file complaints with an OSHA office and request a survey when they believe that conditions in the workplace are unsafe or unhealthy. If a violation of the act is found at the time of a survey, the employer may receive a citation stating a time frame within which the violation must be corrected.

State Regulation

The states have statutes charging employers with the duty to furnish employees with a safe working environment. The city and county in which a health care facility is located also may prescribe rules regarding the health and safety of employees. Many communities have enacted sanitary and health codes that require certain standards.

Legal Liability

From a liability point of view, an employer can be held legally liable for damages suffered by employees through exposure to dangerous conditions that are in violation of OSHA standards. Proof of an employee's exposure to noncompliant conditions is generally necessary to find an employer liable.

REHABILITATION ACT

The essential purpose of the Rehabilitation Act of 1973[13] provides protection to handicapped people from discrimination. The law basically is administered by the Department of Health and Human Services (DHHS), which derives its jurisdiction from the fact that health care organizations participate in such federal programs as Medicare, Medicaid, and Hill-Burton. The law therefore is applied to both public and private organizations because both participate in these programs.

Since July 1977, all institutions receiving federal financial assistance from DHHS have been required to file assurances of compliance forms. Each employer must designate an individual to coordinate compliance efforts. A grievance procedure should be in place to address employee complaints alleging violation of the regulation. All employment decisions must be made without regard to physical or mental handicaps that are not disqualifying (e.g., an employer is not obligated to employ a person with a highly contagious disease that can be easily transmitted to others).

Jobs should not be purposely designed to eliminate the hiring of disabled persons. Employers, however, are not required to change the essential elements of a job to create a position for a disabled person. The Iowa Supreme Court, in *Schlitzer v. U of I Hosp and Clinics*,[14] decided that an employer is not required to create a vacancy or a job for a disabled person. The court found that a nurse's 20-pound lifting restriction, due to a car accident, limited her ability to lift, thus making the demands of her job incompatible with her physical disability. The law does not require that an employer change the essential elements of a job to meet a claimant's disability. In this case, the job required that the nurse be able to work with severely disabled persons. The 20-pound limitation, in this case, was an impossible hurdle to overcome.

FAMILY AND MEDICAL LEAVE ACT

The Family and Medical Leave Act of 1993 (FMLA) was enacted to grant temporary medical leave to employees under certain circumstances. The act provides that covered employers must grant an eligible employee up to a total of 12 workweeks of unpaid leave during any 12-month period for one or more of the following reasons: the birth and care of an employee's child; placement of an adopted or foster child with the employee; for the care of an immediate family member (spouse, child, or parent) with a serious health condition; or inability to work because of a serious health condition. It is illegal to terminate health insurance coverage for an employee on FMLA leave. Following an FMLA leave, the employee's job—or an equivalent job with equivalent pay, benefits, and other terms and conditions of employment—must be restored.

STATE LABOR LAWS

The federal labor enactments serve as a pattern for many state labor laws that comprise the second labor regulation system touching health care organizations. State labor acts vary from state to state. Therefore, it is important that each institution familiarize itself not only with federal regulations but also with state regulations affecting labor relations within the institution.

Because the NLRA excludes from coverage health care organizations operated by the state or its political subdivisions, regulation of labor–management relations in these organizations is left to state law. Unless the constitution in such a state guarantees the right of employees to organize and imposes the duty of collective bargaining on the employer, health care organizations do not have to bargain collectively with their employees. However, in states that do have labor relations acts, the obligation of an organization to bargain collectively with its employees is determined by the applicable statute.

State laws vary considerably in their coverage, and often employees of state and local governmental organizations are covered by separate public employee legislation. Some of these statutes cover both state and local employees, whereas others cover only state or only local employees.

Some of the states that have labor relations acts granting employees the right to organize, join unions, and bargain collectively have specifically prohibited strikes and lockouts and have provided for compulsory arbitration whenever a collective bargaining contract cannot otherwise be executed amicably. Anti-injunction statutes would not forbid injunctions to restrain violations of these statutory provisions.

The doctrine of federal preemption, as applied to labor relations, displaces the states' jurisdiction to regulate an activity that is arguably an unfair labor practice within the meaning of the NLRA. Nonetheless, the US Supreme Court has ruled that states can still regulate labor relations activity that also falls within the jurisdiction of the NLRB when deeply rooted local feelings and responsibility are affected.

Union Security Contracts and Right-to-Work Laws

Labor organizations frequently seek to enter union-security contracts with employers. Such contracts are of two types: (1) the closed-shop contract, which provides that only members of a particular union may be hired, and (2) the union-shop contract, which makes continued employment dependent on membership in the union, although the employee need not have been a union member when applying for the job.

Various states have made such contracts unlawful. Statutes forbidding such agreements generally are called right-to-work laws on the theory that they protect everyone's right to work even if a person refuses to join a union. Several state statutes or court decisions purport to restrict union-security contracts or specify procedures to be completed before such agreements may be made.

Wage and Hour Laws

When state minimum wage standards are higher than federal standards, the state's standards are applicable.

Child Labor Acts

Many states prohibit the employment of minors younger than a specified age and restrict the employment of other minors. Child labor legislation commonly requires that working papers be secured before a child may be hired, forbids the employment of minors at night, and prohibits minors from operating certain types of dangerous machinery.

Workers' Compensation

Workers' compensation is a program by which an employee can receive certain wage benefits because of work-related injuries. An employee who is injured while performing job-related duties is generally eligible for workers' compensation. Workers' compensation programs are administered by the states.

State legislatures have recognized that it is difficult and expensive for employees to recover from their employers and therefore have enacted workers' compensation laws. Employers are required to provide workers' compensation as a benefit. Workers' compensation laws give the employee a legal way to receive compensation for injuries on the job. The acts do not require the employee to prove that the injury was the result of the employer's negligence. Workers' compensation laws are based on the employer–employee relationship and not on the theory of negligence.

Job Stress

Workers' compensation has been awarded for depression related to job stress. In *Elwood v. SAIF*,[15] a registered nurse filed a workers' compensation claim for an occupational disease based on depression. The referee and the workers' compensation board affirmed the insurer's denial of the claim, and the claimant sought judicial review. Questions that needed to be answered to determine job stress included:

- What were the "real" events and conditions of plaintiff's employment?

- Were the real stressful events and conditions the major contributing cause of plaintiff's mental disorder?

The record established that many events and conditions of her employment, including her termination, were real and capable of producing stress when viewed objectively. The claimant's treating physician advised her that she was suffering from anxiety, depression, and stress and advised her to seek a psychiatric evaluation. The court held that the claimant established that her condition was compensable.

LABOR RIGHTS

Rights and responsibilities run concurrently. Employee rights include such things as the right to:

- organize and bargain collectively
- solicit and distribute union information during nonworking hours (i.e., mealtimes and coffee breaks)
- picket
- strike

MANAGEMENT RIGHTS

As with labor, management also has certain rights and responsibilities. Specific management rights are reviewed here.

- right to receive a strike notice
- right to hire replacement workers
- right to restrict union activity to prescribed areas
- right to prohibit union activity during working hours
- right to prohibit supervisors from participating in union activity

Congress excluded supervisors from participating in union activity to assure management the loyalty of its supervisory personnel by making sure that no employer would have to retain as its agent one who is obligated to a union.

The certification of 17 RNs as an employee-bargaining unit in *NLRB v. American Medical Services*[16] was shown to be improper. The nursing home contended that a very low ratio of supervisors to employees would occur if the NLRB's decision was upheld. Substantial evidence had been presented to the court showing that the nurses exercised substantial supervisory powers, including the authority to issue work assignments and discipline employees.

The Taft-Hartley Act as applied in this case illustrates the importance of balancing the rights of both employees and employers.

> Taft-Hartley applied some brakes, so that the balance of power between companies and unions would not shift wholly to the union side. The exclusion of supervisors is one of the brakes. If supervisors were free to join or form unions and enjoy the broad protection of the Act for concerted activity, see Sec. 7, 29 U.S.C. Sec. 157, the impact of a strike would be greatly amplified because the company would not be able to use its supervisory personnel to replace strikers. More important, the company with or without a strike could lose control of its work force to the unions because the very people in the company who controlled hiring, discipline, assignments, and other dimensions of the employment relationship might be subject to control by the same union as the employees they were supposed to be controlling on the employer's behalf.[17]

AFFIRMATIVE ACTION PLAN

Health care organizations are required to comply with all applicable DHHS regulations "including but not limited to those pertaining to nondiscrimination on the basis of race, color, or national origin (45 C.F.R. part 80), nondiscrimination on the basis of handicap (45 C.F.R. part 84), nondiscrimination on the basis of age (45 C.F.R. part 91), protection of human subjects of research (45 C.F.R. part 46), and fraud and abuse (42 C.F.R. part 455). Although these regulations are not in themselves considered requirements under this part, their violation may result in the termination or suspension of or the refusal to grant or continue payment with federal funds."[18] To comply with the spirit of these regulations and Executive Order 11246, health care organizations should have an equal employment opportunity or affirmative action plan in place.

An affirmative action program includes such things as the collection and analysis of data on the race and sex of all applicants for employment, as well as a statement in the personnel policy/procedure manuals and employee handbooks that would read, for example, "Health Care Facility, Inc., is an equal opportunity/affirmative action employer and does not discriminate on the basis of race, color, religion, sex, national origin, age, handicap, or veteran status."

PATIENT RIGHTS DURING LABOR DISPUTES

Patient rights take precedence over employee and management rights when a patient's right to privacy or well-being is in jeopardy due to labor disputes.

INJUNCTIONS

An injunction is an order by a court directing that a certain act be performed or not performed. Persons who fail to comply with court orders are said to be in contempt of court. The earliest use of injunctions in labor relations was by employers to stop strikes or picketing by employees. Today, the general rule limits the availability of injunctive relief to halt work stoppages. The federal government and many states have enacted anti-injunction acts. These acts restrict the power of the courts to limit injunctions in labor disputes by setting strictly defined standards that must be met before injunctions can be granted to restrain activities such as strikes and picketing.

ADMINISTERING A COLLECTIVE BARGAINING AGREEMENT

When a collective bargaining agreement has been negotiated in good faith, it should be administered with care and good faith as well. The first-line supervisors are responsible for administering the agreement at the grassroots level. They should familiarize themselves with the provisions of the agreement. Educational programs should be provided by the organization. Special emphasis should be placed on the use of corrective discipline, as provided under the contract, and on how to respond to grievances. The organization's management, through its human relations department, maintains the ultimate responsibility in the facility for the fair and effective administration of its union contract(s).

Maintaining propitious records of all grievances, grievance meetings, and grievance resolutions is the responsibility of supervisors and management. Regardless of whether a grievance is meritorious and settled by management or whether it is spurious and therefore denied, clear and complete records should be maintained. The ability to document resolutions of particular problems, as well as management's approach to grievances, is especially important if arbitration is required to settle a grievance.

Arbitration procedures are set in motion when the union files a demand for arbitration either with the employer or with the arbitration agency named in the contract. The arbitration hearing is a relatively informal proceeding at which labor and management frequently choose to be represented by counsel. The arbitrator's decision is binding on both parties.

The arbitrator's decision can be upset by showing any of the following:

- The arbitrator has clearly exceeded his or her authority under the collective bargaining agreement.
- The decision is the product of fraud or duress.
- The arbitrator has been guilty of impropriety.
- The award violates the law or requires a violation of the law.

DISCRIMINATION IN THE WORKPLACE

Discrimination in the workplace comes in many forms and in numerous ways, and each has its own little twist of facts: You are either too old or too young for the job; you are either overqualified or underqualified. There are laws prohibiting discrimination against any individual because of his or her race, color, religion, sex, or national origin, or to classify or refer for employment any individual on the basis of his or her race, color, religion, sex, or national origin. Unfortunately, prohibition and practice do not always match up. A variety of cases are presented in this section that describe but a few of the various forms of discrimination prohibited by law.

Age Discrimination

The Age Discrimination in Employment Act of 1967 (ADEA)[19] prohibits age-based employment discrimination against persons 40 years of age or older. The purpose of this law is to promote employment of older persons on the basis of their ability without regard to their age. The law prohibits arbitrary age discrimination in hiring, discharge, pay, term, conditions, or privileges of employment. The ADEA covers private employers with 20 or more employees, state and local governments, employment agencies, and most labor unions. The Age Discrimination and Claims Assistance Amendment of 1990 extends the suit filing period for ADEA charges that meet certain criteria. There are strict time frames in which charges of age discrimination must be filed.

According to the US Supreme Court, in *Texas Department of Community Affairs v. Burdine*, a prima facie case of age discrimination requires that evidence sufficient to support a finding for the complainant must establish all of the following:

- The complainant is in a protected age group.
- The complainant is qualified for his or her job.
- The complainant was discharged.
- The discharge occurred in circumstances that give rise to the inference of age discrimination.[20]

Disability

The Americans with Disabilities Act of 1990 (ADA) was enacted by Congress to prohibit employers from discriminating against job applicants and employees on the basis of disability.[21] It applies to employers with 15 or more employees working for 20 or more weeks during a calendar year. The ADA protects employees who are qualified individuals with disabilities capable of performing the essential functions of the job in question with or without reasonable accommodation, from discrimination by the employer.

Census data, national polls, and other studies have documented that people with disabilities, as a group, occupy an inferior status in society. The nation's proper goals regarding individuals with disabilities are to ensure equality of opportunity, full participation, independent living, and economic self-sufficiency for such individuals.

The ADA prohibits job discrimination in hiring, promotion, or other provisions of employment against qualified individuals with disabilities by private employers, state and local governments, employment agencies, and labor unions. On July 26, 1991, the EEOC issued final regulations implementing Title I of the ADA. The purpose of the ADA is to:

- Provide a clear and comprehensive national mandate for the elimination of discrimination against individuals with disabilities.

- Provide clear, strong, consistent, enforceable standards addressing discrimination against individuals with disabilities.
- Ensure that the federal government plays a central role in enforcing the standards established in the Act on behalf of individuals with disabilities.
- Invoke the sweep of congressional authority, including the power to enforce the 14th Amendment and to regulate commerce to address the main areas of discrimination faced day to day by people with disabilities.[22]

The general rule of discrimination under Title I of the act provides that "no covered entity shall discriminate against a qualified individual with a disability because of the disability of such individual in regard to job application procedures, the hiring, advancement, or discharge of employees, employee compensation, job training, and other terms, conditions, and privileges of employment."[23]

Disability Requires Reasonable Accommodation

The appellee Alley in *Alley v. Charleston Area Med. Ctr., Inc.*[24] worked for CAMC for over 17 years and suffered from epilepsy and asthma, with the asthma becoming increasingly aggravated by on-the-job exposure to certain chemicals. Alley requested a 12-week family medical leave of absence, which the hospital approved, with the agreement that the leave could be taken intermittently as needed. Alley began seeing Dr. Douglas with CAMC Physician Health Group for treatment of her asthma and epilepsy.

Alley's physician wrote a letter explaining her physical conditions and requested that Alley be allowed to work in an outpatient setting and not be exposed to people with multiple infections. Although Alley presented her request for accommodation to various CAMC supervisory personnel and to employee health services at the hospital, she was told that no accommodation would be made. The employee health services physician, Dr. Ranadive, met with Alley for 5 minutes. He did not perform any tests. Ranadive called the physician who had written the request and summarily concluded that there was no medical reason why Alley could not continue her employment and that CAMC would not accommodate her.

Alley was eventually terminated, and she filed suit against CAMC in the circuit court alleging that she had been subjected to retaliatory discharge based on physical and mental impairment. Alley claimed that CAMC refused to make reasonable accommodations for her known impairments and that this was a violation of the West Virginia Human Rights Act, and CAMC, with knowledge of Alley's asthma, exposed her to substances that exacerbated her condition.

The jury returned a verdict in favor of Alley, awarding of $325,000 in damages. On appeal, the court determined that the evidence was sufficient for a jury to find that Alley was a qualified person with a disability and that CAMC was aware of her disability and that a reasonable accommodation could have been made. The jury award was fair, considering all of the evidence and the instructions it received.

National Origin

The Immigration Reform and Control Act of 1986, 1990, and 1996 (IRCA) prohibits most employers from discriminating against employees or applicants because of national origin or US citizenship status, with respect to hiring, referral, or discharge. The act establishes penalties for employers who knowingly hire illegal aliens. Determining the legality of the employee's status is the employer's responsibility.

Pay Discrimination

The Equal Pay Act (1963)[25] is an amendment to the Fair Labor Standards Act that prohibits any discrimination in the payment of wages for men and women performing substantially equal work under similar conditions. The EPA is applicable everywhere that the minimum wage law is applicable and is enforced by the EEOC. The EPA, simply stated, requires that employees who perform equal work receive equal pay. There are situations in which wages may be unequal as long as they are based on factors other than sex, such as in the case of a formalized seniority system or a system that objectively measures earnings by the quantity or quality of production.

Pregnancy Discrimination

The Pregnancy Discrimination Act is an amendment to Title VII of the Civil Rights Act of 1964. Discrimination on the basis of pregnancy, childbirth, or related medical conditions constitutes unlawful sex discrimination under Title VII. Women affected by pregnancy or related conditions must be treated in the same manner as other applicants or employees with similar abilities or limitations by, for example, providing modified tasks, alternative assignments, disability leave, or leave without pay.

Race Discrimination

Discharge of an employee on the basis of racial bias is actionable under state and federal laws. Title VII of the Civil Rights Act of 1964 "requires the elimination of artificial, arbitrary, and unnecessary barriers to employment that operate invidiously to discriminate on the basis of race."[26] An at-will employee's claim of racially motivated retaliatory discharge for filing a discrimination complaint can be actionable in tort as a violation of public policy.

In *Buckley Nursing Home v. Massachusetts Commission against Discrimination*,[27] Young, a black applicant for a nurse's aide position, filed a complaint alleging racial discrimination. Young responded to a newspaper advertisement for a nurse's aide position, filing her application on March 1, 1974, and was interviewed by the acting supervisor of nursing. The applicant called to inquire about the position on several occasions and eventually was told that the position had been filled. The advertisement ran again in the newspaper, and the applicant again called in response to the advertisement. Young was told that her application was on file and that she would be called as needed. The facility hired four full-time and one part-time nurse's aides for the evening shift between March 1, 1974, and July 1, 1974.

On the upper right hand corner of Young's application, there is a handwritten notation "no openings," even though during the relevant time periods there were openings and other persons were hired for the evening shift. That notation does not appear on any other application, and none of Buckley's witnesses could identify who wrote it or when it appeared.

Despite testimony to the contrary, the commission found that Buckley had entered discussion about Young's race and had decided not to hire her on that basis. The commission thus concluded that Buckley's reason for not hiring Young (that she was not the best qualified applicant for the job) was a pretext and that she would have been hired but for her race.

The commission awarded Young $6,986 plus interest for lost wages and $2,000 for emotional distress. Besides the monetary award to Young, the nursing facility had been instructed by the commission to develop a minority recruitment program. On appeal by the facility, the trial court upheld the commission's decision. On further appeal, the appeals court held that the evidence was sufficient to support a reasonable inference that the nursing facility's rejection of the applicant occurred after consideration of her race.

Religious Discrimination

Discrimination based on religion is valuing a person or group lower because of their religion, or treating someone differently because of what they do or don't believe. While many religious and secular authorities tend to stress that religion is something personal, the highly social nature of most religions makes conflicts between religious groups, and thus discrimination, still very probable. Reasonable accommodations should be made for an employee's religious beliefs.

Sex Discrimination

In *Jones v. Hinds General Hospital*,[28] a prima facie case of sex discrimination was established by evidence showing that a hospital laid off female nursing assistants while retaining male orderlies who performed the necessary functions. The court, however, held that Title VII of the Civil Rights Act was not violated by the hospital's use of gender as a basis for laying off employees. Gender was a bona fide occupational qualification for orderlies because a substantial number of male patients objected to the performance of catheterizations and surgical preparation by female assistants.

Sexual Harassment

Section 703 of Title VII and the EEOC defines sexual harassment in employment as unwelcome sexual advances, requests for sexual favors, and other verbal or physical conduct of a sexual nature when this conduct explicitly or implicitly affects an individual's employment; unreasonably interferes with an individual's work performance; or creates an intimidating, hostile, or offensive work environment.

Sexual conduct becomes unlawful only when it is unwelcome by the victim. The victim must not have solicited or invited the actions and must have considered the conduct undesirable or offensive. To determine if the victim may have solicited or encouraged the claimed sexual harassment, a court may assess the victim's sexual aggressiveness or consistent use of sexually oriented language in the work environment. Of course, indications of an employee's sexually aggressive nature will not necessarily negate a claim of sexual harassment, just as voluntary participation in sexual conduct by the victim will not necessarily negate the claim. An employee may participate in sexual conduct for fear of repercussions, thus each claim must be examined individually to determine whether the particular conduct complained of was unwelcome.

Unwelcome sexual conduct becomes harassment when it creates a working environment that is unreasonably intimidating or offensive. A reasonable person must find the work environment offensive, and the complaining employee must have perceived the conduct as offensive.

When sexual conduct is determined to be unwelcome, the court must evaluate its level of interference with the employee's job, and whether the harassment created a hostile work environment. The court will consider the type of harassment (verbal, physical, or both), as well as the frequency of the harassment. A hostile work environment usually requires a pattern of conduct that has a repetitive effect. An isolated incident of physical advance is more likely to constitute a hostile environment (such as unwanted touching of the intimate body parts) than would a single case of verbal advance. In the same respect, sexual flirtation or vulgar language will not often constitute a hostile work environment as readily as would pervasive and continuous proliferation of pornography and demeaning comments.

An employer may be held liable for harassment inflicted by a supervisor, which results in a tangible employment action, or a significant change in the victim's employment status. Such tangible employment action may fall under categories such as: hiring, firing, promotion, demotion, undesirable reassignment, decision causing a significant change in benefits, compensation decisions, and work assignment. The victim of sexual harassment as well as the harasser may be a man or woman. The harasser can be the victim's supervisor, an agent of the employer, a supervisor in another area, a coworker, or a nonemployee. The victim does not have to be the person harassed but could be anyone affected by the offensive conduct. Unlawful sexual harassment may occur without economic injury.

An employee who claims harassment based upon a hostile work environment must demonstrate that the conduct complained of was sufficiently severe and/or pervasive to alter the conditions of employment and create a work environment that would qualify as hostile or abusive to employees because of their sex. An employer, however, will not always be held liable for sexual harassment that occurs in the workplace if the employer can prove: (1) it had in place an antiharassment policy with an effective complaint procedure; (2) it promptly took action to prevent and correct any harassment; and (3) that the employee unreasonably failed to avoid further harm by complaining to management. If the harassment is committed by a nonsupervisor, the lower courts have held that the employer will only be liable if it knew or should have known about the conduct and failed to take appropriate corrective action.

Notes

1. 29 U.S.C. § 151.
2. NLRA § 2 (14) (1974).
3. NLRB v. Shelby Mem'l Hosp. Ass'n, 1 F.3d 550 (7th Cir. 1993).
4. 436 F.3d 843 (C.A. 8, Mo. 2006).
5. Norris-LaGuardia Act 29 U.S.C. ch. 6 (1932).
6. United States v. Hutcheson, 312 U.S. 219 (1941).
7. Labor-Management Reporting and Disclosure Act of 1959, Pub. L. No. 86-257 (29 U.S.C. ch. 11).
8. Fair Labor Standards Act of 1938, 29 U.S.C. ch. 8.
9. Equal Employment Opportunity Act of 1972, 42 U.S.C. § 2000e et seq.
10. OSHA's Mission, Occupational Safety and Health Administration, US Department of Labor, http://www.osha.gov/oshinfo/mission.html.
11. Occupational Safety and Health Act of 1970, 29 U.S.C. § 651.
12. PUB. L. NO. 91-596, § 2, 84 Stat. 1590 (Dec. 29, 1970); see also 29 U.S.C.A. § 651 (1990).
13. Rehabilitation Act of 1973, 29 U.S.C. ch. 14.
14. 641 N.W.2d 525 (Iowa 2002).
15. 676 P.2d 922 (Or. Ct. App. 1984).
16. 705 F.2d 1472, 1474-75 (7th Cir. 1983).
17. NLRB v. Res-Care, Inc., 705 F.2d 1461, 1465 (7th Cir.1983).
18. 42 C.F.R. § 483.75 (1989).
19. Age Discrimination in Employment Act of 1967, 29 U.S.C. ch. 14, as amended.
20. 450 U.S. 248, 253 (1981).
21. Americans with Disabilities Act of 1990, PUB. L. NO. 101-336, 104 Stat. 327 (July 26, 1990).
22. Id. at 329.
23. Id. at 331–332.
24. No. 31591 (W.Va. 2004).
25. Equal Pay Act of 1963, 29 U.S.C. ch. 8.
26. Griggs v. Duke Power Co., 401 U.S. 424 (1971).
27. 478 N.E.2d 1292 (Mass. App. Ct. 1985).
28. 666 F. Supp. 933 (D. Miss. 1987).

20

EMPLOYMENT, DISCIPLINE, AND DISCHARGE

Fairly balancing the rights of the employee and the needs of the organization is an extremely complex objective. This chapter provides some direction in this balancing act.

For the health care worker, an unexpected termination may mean a significant setback in career progression, financial hardship, and loss of self-esteem. For the organization and its community, a termination means a lack of stability in the management structure and possible disruption and realignment of services provided. A growing consensus is that high turnover rates are unhealthy and provide a disservice to an industry already plagued with cost constraints and other pressures.

Wrongful discharge claims are difficult, time consuming, and expensive lawsuits to defend. Employers who experience favorable court decisions in wrongful discharge claims often have unfavorable repercussions because of bad press and the negative effects a discharge has on employee morale.

EMPLOYMENT AT WILL

An at will prerogative without limits could be suffered only in an anarchy, and there not for long; it certainly cannot be suffered in a society such as ours without weakening the bond of counter balancing rights and obligations that holds such societies together.

Sides v. Duke Hospital[1]

The common-law employment-at-will doctrine provides that employment is at the will of either the employer or the employee, meaning that employment may be terminated by the employer or employee at any time for any or no reason, unless there is a contract in place that specifies the terms and duration of employment. Historically, termination of employees for any reason was widely accepted. However, contemporary thinking does not support this concept.

> In recent years the rule that employment for an indefinite term is terminable by the employer whenever and for whatever cause he chooses without incurring liability has been the subject of considerable scholarly debate and judicial and legislative modification. Consequently, there has been a growing trend toward a restricted application of the at-will employment rule whereby the right of an employer to discharge an at-will employee without cause is limited by either public policy considerations or an implied covenant of good faith and fair dealing.[2]

In *Sides v. Duke Hospital*, the North Carolina Court of Appeals found it to be an

> obvious and indisputable fact that in a civilized state where reciprocal legal rights and duties abound, the words "at will" can never mean "without limit or qualification," as so much of the discussion and the briefs of the defendants imply; for in such a state the rights of each person are necessarily and inherently limited by the rights of others and the interests of the public.
>
> • • • •
>
> If we are to have law, those who so act against the public interest must be held accountable for the harm inflicted thereby; to accord them civil immunity would incongruously reward their lawlessness at the unjust expense of their innocent victims.[3]

The concept of the employment-at-will doctrine is embroiled in a combination of legislative enactments and judicial decisions. Some states have a tendency to be more employer oriented, such as New York, whereas others, such as California, emerge as being much more forward thinking and in harmony with the constitutional rights of the employee.

> The employment-at-will common law doctrine is not truly applicable in today's society, and many courts have recognized this fact. In the last century, the common law developed in a laissez-faire climate that encouraged industrial growth and improved the right of an employer to control his own business, including the right to fire without cause an employee at will. . . . The twentieth century has witnessed significant changes in socioeconomic values that have led to reassessment of the common law rule. Businesses have evolved from small- and medium-size firms to gigantic corporations in which ownership is separate from management. Formerly there was a clear delineation between employers, who frequently were owners of their own businesses, and employees. The employer in the old sense has been replaced by a superior in the corporate hierarchy who is himself an employee.[4]

As discussed here, exceptions to the employment-at-will doctrine involve contractual relationships, public policy issues, defamation, retaliatory discharge, and fairness. It would seem that the doctrine has little applicability in modern society.

PUBLIC POLICY ISSUES

The public policy exception to the employment-at-will doctrine provides that employees may not be terminated for reasons that are contrary to public policy. Public policy originates with legislative enactments that prohibit, for example, the discharge of employees on the basis of disability, age, race, color, religion, sex, national origin, pregnancy, union membership, and/or filing of safety violation with various governmental agencies. Any attempt to limit, segregate, or classify employees in any way that would tend to deprive any individual of employment opportunities on these bases is contrary to public policy.

Public policy also can arise as a result of judicial decisions that address those issues not covered by statutes, rules, and regulations. "[I]t can be said that public policy concerns what is right and just and what affects the citizens of the state collectively. It is to be found in the state's constitution and statutes and, when they are silent, in its judicial decisions."[5]

In those instances in which state and federal laws are silent, not all courts concur with the use of judicial decisions as a means for determining public policy. A California court determined that a public policy exception to the at-will employment doctrine must be based on constitutional or statutory provisions rather than judicial policy making.[6]

Nurse Suggests Patient Change Physician

The patient began losing weight and having hallucinations. A nurse documented the patient's difficulties and attempted on several occasions to call the patient's physician, however, the physician failed to return the nurse's calls. Because of the patient's deteriorating condition, the family contacted the nurse. After the nurse advised the patient's family as to her concerns, a member of the patient's family asked her what they should do. The nurse advised that she would reconsider their choice of physicians. The nurse was terminated by the nursing facility because she advised the patient's family to consider changing physicians.

The nurse brought a lawsuit for wrongful discharge in violation of public policy. The complaint was dismissed by a trial court and the nurse appealed.

The language in the Nursing Practice Act (NPA) of North Carolina and regulations of the board of nursing describes the practice of nursing as assessing a patient's health, which entails a responsibility to communicate, counsel, and provide accurate guidance to clients and their families. The nurse's comments that resulted in her termination were made in fulfillment of these responsibilities.

The North Carolina Court of Appeals held that the nurse stated a claim for wrongful discharge in violation of public policy. Although there may be a right to terminate at-will employment for no reason, or for an arbitrary or irrational reason, there can be no right to terminate such employment for an unlawful reason or purpose that contravenes public policy.

The North Carolina Court of Appeals gave considerable attention to language in the NPA and the regulations that recognized nursing to include teaching and counseling about a patient's health care and of providing information to patients and their families, including making referrals to appropriate resources.[7]

Reporting Patient Abuse

An employer may not discharge an employee for fulfilling societal obligations or in those instances in which the employer acts with a socially undesirable motive.[8] A tort claim for wrongful discharge was stated in *McQuary v. Air Convalescent Home*[9] by allegations that the plaintiff was discharged wrongfully from her position at the nursing facility in retaliation for threatening to report to state authorities instances of alleged patient mistreatment. Such mistreatment purportedly involved violation of a patient's rights under the Nursing Home Patient's Bill of Rights. To prevail, the discharged employee was not required to prove that patient abuse actually had occurred but only that she acted in good faith.

> This conclusion is consistent with established Oregon law. Statutes which protect employees against retaliation do not require that the alleged violation which the employee claims be ultimately proved. See, e.g., ORS 652.355 (protects an employee who merely consults an attorney or agency about a wage claim); ORS 654.062(5) (protects any employee who makes a complaint under the Oregon Safe Employment Act); ORS 659.030(1)(f) (prohibits discrimination against an employee who filed a civil rights complaint); ORS 633.120(3) (prohibits discrimination against an employee for filing an unfair labor practices complaint). We have, in fact, upheld

> awards for retaliation despite holding that the original complaint did not show discrimination.
>
> • • • •
>
> Similar considerations of public policy lead to our conclusion that an employee who reports a violation of a nursing home patient's statutory rights in good faith should be protected from discharge for that action.[10]

This case, which had been dismissed in the lower court, was reversed and remanded for trial.

Whistle-Blowing

A whistle-blower is one who reveals wrongdoing in the organization to a public entity or someone in authority. This often occurs when one believes that the public interest overrides the interest of the organization and can involve illegal or fraudulent activities. A whistle-blower provides information he or she reasonably believes evidences violation of any law, rule, or regulation; gross mismanagement; a gross waste of funds; an abuse of authority; a substantial and specific danger to public health; and/or a substantial and specific danger to public safety.[11]

Paving Her Way to Heaven

The nurse–plaintiff was employed as a charge nurse with supervisory duties. A short time after one of her patients had been admitted to the hospital, the charge nurse determined the patient was suffering from toxic shock syndrome. Knowing that death would result if left untreated, the charge nurse assumed that the physician would order antibiotics. After a period of time passed without having received such orders, the charge nurse discussed the patient's condition with the nursing director. She was informed by the director to document, report the facts, and stay out of it.

The charge nurse discussed the patient's condition and lack of orders with the chief of staff. Although the chief of staff took appropriate steps to treat the patient, the patient died. The nursing director was informed by a member of the patient's family that the charge nurse offered to obtain the medical records and was later told that the charge nurse was heard to say that the physician was paving the patient's way to heaven. As a result, the charge nurse was terminated.

The trial court entered a summary judgment for the defendant–hospital, stating that there were no triable issues of fact, and there was no public policy exception to the charge nurse's at-will termination. The court could not find any law or regulation prohibiting the hospital from discharging her as a nurse.

The Missouri Court of Appeals reversed the granting of summary judgment and remanded the case for trial, holding that the Nursing Practice Act (NPA) provided a clear mandate of public policy that nurses had a duty to provide the best possible care to patients. Therefore, if the plaintiff refused to follow her supervisor's orders to stay out of a case where the patient was dying from a lack of proper medical treatment, there would be no grounds for her discharge under the public policy exception to the employment-at-will doctrine. Her persistence in attempting to get the proper treatment for the patient was her absolute duty. The hospital could not lawfully require that she stay out of a case that would have obvious injurious consequences to the patient.[12]

RETALIATORY DISCHARGE

There is a tendency for some people in positions of power to abuse that power through threats, abuse, intimidation, and retaliatory discharge, all of which are cause for legal action. Employees who become the targets of a vindictive supervisor often have difficulty proving a bad-faith motive. In an effort to reduce the probability of wrongful discharge, some states have enacted legislation that protects employees from terminations found to be arbitrary and capricious.

The burden of proof for establishing some hidden motive for discharge from employment rests on discharged employees.

> The National Labor Relations Act and other labor legislation illustrate the governmental policy of preventing employers from using the right of discharge as a means of oppression. . . . Consistent with this policy, many states have recognized the need to protect employees who are not parties to a collective bargaining agreement or other contract from abusive practices by the employer. . . . Those states have recognized a common law cause of action for employees-at-will who were discharged for reasons that were in some way "wrongful." The courts in those jurisdictions have taken various approaches: some recognizing the action in tort, some in contract.[13]

The court in *Khanna v. Microdata Corp.*[14] held that substantial evidence supported a finding that the employer fired the employee in bad-faith retaliation for bringing a lawsuit against the employer, thus violating an implied covenant of good faith and fair dealing.

> Under the traditional common-law rule, codified in section 2922 of the [California] Labor Code, an employment contract of indefinite duration is in general terminable at the will of either party. During the past several decades, however, judicial authorities in California and throughout the United States have established the rule that, under both common law and the statute, an employer does not enjoy an absolute or totally unfettered right to discharge even an at-will employee.[15]

FAIRNESS: THE ULTIMATE TEST

"Is it fair?" is the ultimate question that a supervisor must ask when considering a termination. In general, bad-faith and inexplicable terminations are subject to the scrutiny of the courts. Some courts and legislative enactments have overturned the view that employers have total discretion to terminate workers who are not otherwise protected by collective bargaining agreements or civil service regulations. Montana legislation grants every employee the right to sue the employer for wrongful discharge. The mere fact that an employment contract is terminable at will does not give the employer an absolute right to terminate it in all cases.

There is an implied covenant of good faith and fair dealing in every contract that neither party will do anything that will injure the right of the other to receive benefits from the agreement. An employee in *Pugh v. See's Candies*[16] was found to have shown a prima facie case of wrongful termination in violation of an implied promise that the employer would not act arbitrarily in dealing with the employee. The employer's right to terminate an employee is not absolute. It is limited by fundamental principles of public policy and by expressed or implied terms of agreement between the employer and the employee.

Procedural issues are as important as issues of discrimination. In *Renny v. Port Huron Hospital*,[17] the Michigan Supreme Court found, as did the jury, that the employee's discharge hearing was not final and binding because it did not comport with elementary fairness. The court found that there was sufficient evidence for the jury to find that the employee had not been discharged for just cause. The existence of a just-cause contract is a question of fact for the jury when the employer establishes written policies and procedures and does not expressly retain the right to terminate an employee at will. That the hospital followed the grievance procedure with the plaintiff is evidence that a just-cause contract existed on which the plaintiff relied.

The employee handbook provided for a grievance board as a fair way to resolve work-related complaints and problems. This was not a mandatory procedure to which the hospital's employees had to submit. The employee was not bound by the grievance board's determination that her discharge was proper because evidence supported a finding that she was not given adequate notice of who the witnesses against her would be.

She was not permitted to be present when the witnesses testified, and she was not given the right to present certain evidence.

There was sufficient evidence for the jury to conclude that the plaintiff had suffered damages. Evidence presented indicated that her subsequent professional employment did not equal her earnings before discharge and that she experienced increased expenses because of the loss of her health insurance as well as other financial losses that she suffered as a result of her discharge.

Defending a Claim of Unfair Discharge

An employee who believes that he or she has been unfairly discharged will most likely seek access to the following information in defense of his or her claim:

- minutes of pertinent meetings
- written reports, typed or handwritten
- personnel file
- tapes
- letters, cards, and handwritten notes written on the employee's behalf from the public
- personnel handbook
- personnel and departmental policies and procedures books
- oral testimony from fellow employees and supervisors

Employers must document carefully and fairly any disciplinary proceedings that might be subject to discovery by a disgruntled employee; failure to do so could place the organization or supervisor at a disadvantage should a complaint reach the courts.

TERMINATION

A decision to terminate an employee should be reviewed carefully by a member of management who is familiar with the issues of wrongful discharge. Oral counseling, written counseling, written counseling with suspension, and written counseling with termination are the textbook responses to disciplinary action and discharge. Whatever form of discipline is used, it should be designed to produce a more effective and productive employee.

The employer's right to terminate an employee is not absolute. It is limited by fundamental principles of public policy and by express or implied terms of agreement between the employer and the employee.

> Formulating a standard for substantive fairness in employee dismissal law requires accommodating a number of different interests already afforded legal recognition. The legal interest of employees to be protected against certain types of unfair and injurious action . . . are at the core of any employee dismissal proposal. Arrayed against these interests are employer and societal interests in effective management of organizations, which require that employees not be shielded from the consequences of their poor performance or misconduct and that supervisors not be deterred from exercising their managerial responsibilities by the inconvenience of litigating employees' claims.[18]

Before termination of an employee, the employer should ask: was the termination:

- a violation of public policy
- a violation of any policy or procedure outlined in an administrative manual, the employee handbook, the human resource department's policies and procedures, or any other health care facility policies and procedures or regulations
- retaliatory in nature (e.g., refusal to perform an illegal act or a questioning of a management practice)
- arbitrary and capricious

- discriminatory on the basis of age, disability, race, creed, color, religion, gender, national origin, or marital status
- a violation of any contract, oral or written
- consistent with the reasons for discharge
- discriminatory against the employee for filing a lawsuit
- fixed before any appeal actions can be taken
- an interference with an employee's rights as secured by the laws or Constitution of the United States (e.g., right to freedom of speech)

Employment Disclaimers

A disclaimer is the denial of a right that is imputed to a person or that is alleged to belong to him or her. Although a disclaimer is often a successful defense for employers in wrongful discharge cases, it should not be considered a license to discharge at will and at the whim of the supervisor in an arbitrary and capricious manner.

Employers can help prevent successful lawsuits for wrongful discharge that are based on the premise that an employee handbook or departmental policy and procedure manual is an implied contract by incorporating disclaimers in published manuals, such as that described in *Battaglia v. Sisters of Charity Hospital*,[19] in which a personnel manual could not be interpreted to limit the hospital's power to terminate an at-will employee. Language in the manual indicated that the personnel manual was not a contract; that it could be modified, amended, or supplemented; and that the hospital retained the right to make all necessary management decisions for the delivery of patient care services and the selection, direction, compensation, and retention of employees.

Handbooks that do not contain disclaimers can alter an employee's at-will status. An appeals court in *Trusty v. Big Sandy Health Care Center*[20] noted that the handbook did not contain any disclaimer or any other language that employment was at will. The court held that there was sufficient evidence to establish that the handbook had altered the employee's at-will status and determined that the employee could bring a wrongful discharge suit.

The employer's disclaimers were considered to be clear in *Simonson v. Meader Distribution Co.*,[21] in which an employee filed a breach of contract suit alleging that a dismissal was outside company-adopted disciplinary guidelines. The court held that the company could and did reserve the discretion to discipline employees outside adopted guidelines. The policy manual contained the following three specific reservations of management discretion:

> (1) management reserves the right to make any changes at any time by adding to, deleting, or changing any existing policy; (2) the rules set out below are as complete as we can reasonably make them, however, they are not necessarily all-inclusive because circumstances that we have not anticipated may arise; and (3) management may vary from the above policies if, in its opinion, the circumstances require it.[22]

Health care organizations can be successful when confronted with wrongful discharge suits based on breach of contract by placing similar language in their personnel manuals.

Termination for Cause

A termination-for-cause-only clause in an employment contract is binding. An employment contract in *Eales v. Tanana*[23] that provided that an employee hired up to retirement age could be terminated only for cause was upheld by the court.

Termination and Financial Necessity

No breach of employment contract occurred in *Wilde v. Houlton Regional Hospital*[24] when, because of financial difficulties, a hospital terminated the employment of two nurses, a ward clerk, and a dietary supervisor. Even if the employees were correct in contending that their indefinite contracts of employment had been modified by virtue of a dismissal for cause provision in the employee's handbook and by management's oral assurances that they were permanent, full-time employees whose jobs were secure so long as they performed satisfactorily, the employees' discharge for financial or other legitimate business reasons did not offend the employment contracts as thus modified. A private employer had an essential business prerogative to adjust its workforce as market forces and business necessity required, and the layoffs in question violated no compelling public policy.

Hostile Attitude

The chief X-ray technician in *Paros v. Hoemako Hospital*[25] was dismissed because of a chronic argumentative and hostile attitude inconsistent with the performance of supervisory duties. The trial court entered a summary judgment in favor of the hospital and the administrator. On appeal, the appeals court held that the discharge was properly based on good cause and precluded recovery for breach of contract and wrongful discharge.

Poor Work Performance

In *Yerry v. Ulster County*,[26] a nurse's aide had been terminated from a county infirmary for misconduct. Among other things, she failed to report, in a timely manner, bumping and injuring a resident's leg, failed to feed a resident properly as ordered by the resident's physician, and, on another occasion, fed a resident food that burned the resident's mouth. The court held that eyewitness testimony and believable hearsay were sufficient to sustain the findings of the hearings officer who recommended her termination.

> As to the imposition of discipline, when the petitioner's serious performance deficiencies were considered in light of her experience and the grave responsibility that her work demanded in caring for helpless and dependent patients, the court found that the penalty imposed was not disproportionate to the offenses. She showed an insensitivity and a lack of ability that made her unsuitable for the work, and this constituted a danger to the well-being of the infirmary's elderly residents.[27]

The plaintiff in *Silinzy v. Visiting Nurse Association*[28] brought an action claiming racial discrimination and retaliatory discharge. The court granted a motion for summary judgment by the defendant–employer. The district court held that the plaintiff failed to establish a prima facie case of racial discrimination and retaliatory discharge. The plaintiff's poor job performance was the reason for her discharge. The defendant was found to have produced ample evidence that the plaintiff was not performing her job adequately. Numerous complaints regarding her negative attitude and poor job performance, from a variety of sources, were documented.

Alcoholism

Discharge of an employee because of alcoholism is not necessarily a discriminatory practice. The hospital's discharge of a staff physician for alcoholism in *Soentgen v. Quain & Ramstad Clinic*[29] was found not to be a discriminatory practice. The physician had been discharged on a bona fide occupational qualification reasonably necessary for a physician.

Insubordinate Behavior

Substantial evidence supported a finding that the claimant's employment as a certified nurse's aide in a residential health care facility was terminated due to misconduct where the record indicated that the nurse's aide had been terminated after she refused to attend a meeting to discuss her job performance. She did this despite the request of her supervisor, who had warned her that she would be discharged if she did not attend the meeting. Although the nurse's aide asserted that her refusal was because she was upset and feared she might say something prompting her termination, her insubordinate conduct in failing to comply with her employer's reasonable request constituted disqualifying misconduct.[30]

EFFECTIVE HIRING PRACTICES

The best way for the human resources manager to prevent negligent hiring litigation for the employer is to become familiar with the risks and avoid hiring workers who are likely to become problematic employees. The organization should:

- Develop clear policies and procedures on hiring, disciplining, and terminating employees.
- Include appropriate language in the organization's policies and procedures reserving the right to add, delete, and/or revise the same.
- Develop an application that realistically determines an applicant's qualifications before hiring.
- Take appropriate precautions to prevent the hiring of those who might be a hazard to others.
- Review each applicant's background and past work behavior.
- Become familiar with any state laws that might be applicable when hiring an individual with a past criminal record.
- Develop an effective interview system for screening applicants. (The interviews should be conducted first by an appropriately trained member of the human resources department and then by the supervisor of the service to which the applicant is applying.)
- Solicit references with the applicant's permission using a release form, and follow up with a telephone call for further information.
- Provide an employee handbook and present a job description to each new employee. (Signed documentation should be maintained in the employee's personnel folder indicating that the employee received, read, and understood the employee handbook and job description.)
- Develop constructive performance evaluations that reinforce good behavior, and provide instruction in those areas needing improvement. (The performance evaluation should include a written statement regarding the employee's performance.)
- Develop a progressive disciplinary action policy.
- Provide in-service education programs for supervisors on such subjects as interviewing techniques, evaluations, and discipline. (Various colleges, universities, and consultants provide in-service education programs for employers.)
- Be mindful of the importance of developing appropriate employment contract language.

CLEAR COMMUNICATIONS

Employers must communicate clearly to prospective employees that their employment is at will and can be terminated at any time by either the employer or the employee. During the course of employment, handbooks and personnel manuals must provide fair and unambiguous standards for employee discipline and termination.

Notes

1. 328 S.E.2d 818 (N.C. Ct. App. 1985).
2. 44 A.L.R. 4th 1136 (1986).
3. Supra Note 1.
4. Pierce v. Ortho Pharm. Corp., 417 A.2d 505, 509 (N.J. 1980).
5. Palmateer v. International Harvester Co., 421 N.E.2d 876, 878 (Ill. 1981).
6. Gantt v. Sentry Ins., 824 P.2d 680, 687–688 (Cal. 1992).
7. Deerman v. Beverly Cal. Corp., 518 S.E.2d 804 (N.C. App. 1999).
8. Delaney v. Taco Time Int'l, 681 P.2d 114 (Or. 1984). This case involved an employer found liable by the Oregon Supreme Court for the

wrongful discharge of an at-will employee who was discharged for fulfilling a societal obligation because he refused to sign a false and arguably tortious statement that cast aspersions on the work habits and moral behavior of a former employee.

9. 684 P.2d 21 (Or. Ct. App. 1984).
10. Id. at 24.
11. Whistle-blowing, US Office of Special Counsel, http://www.osc.gov/documents/pubs/post_wb.htm.
12. Kirk v. Mercy Hosp. Tri-County, 851 S.W.2d 617 (Mo. Ct. App. 1993).
13. Pierce v. Ortho Pharm. Corp., 417 A.2d 505, 509 (N.J. 1980).
14. 215 Cal. Rptr. 860 (Cal. Ct. App. 1985).
15. Id. at 865.
16. 171 Cal. Rptr. 917 (Cal. Ct. App. 1981).
17. 398 N.W.2d 327 (Mich. 1986).
18. H. H. PERRITT, EMPLOYEE DISMISSAL LAW AND PRACTICE 354 (1984).
19. 508 N.Y.S.2d 802 (N.Y. App. Div. 1986).
20. No. 89-CA-2272-MR (Ky. Ct. App. Mar. 22, 1991).
21. 413 N.W.2d 146 (Minn. Ct. App. 1987).
22. Id. at 147.
23. 663 P.2d 958 (Alaska 1983).
24. 537 A.2d 1137 (Me. 1987).
25. 681 P.2d 918 (Ariz. Ct. App. 1984).
26. 512 N.Y.S.2d 592 (N.Y. App. Div. 1987).
27. Id. at 593.
28. 777 F. Supp. 1484 (E.D. Mo. 1991).
29. 467 N.W.2d 73 (N.D. 1991).
30. Daniul v. Commissioner of Labor, 807 N.Y.S.2d 477 (N.Y. App. Div. 2006).

21

Managed Care and Organizational Restructuring

The declining trust in the nation's ability to deliver quality health care is evidenced by a system caught up in the morass of managed care companies, which have in some instances inappropriately devised ways to deny health care benefits to their constituency. In addition, the continuing reporting of numerous medical errors serves only to escalate distrust in the nation's political leadership and the providers of health care.

Gp

Managed care organizations (MCOs) represent a major shift away from the domination of the fee-for-service system toward networks of providers supplying a full range of services. *Managed care* is the process of structuring or restructuring the health care system in terms of financing, purchasing, delivering, measuring, and documenting a broad range of health care services and products. Managed care is nothing new to the US health care delivery system; it has been around in some form for decades.

The two major and objected-to constraints of MCOs are their (1) limitations on the choice of providers by the consumer and (2) requirements for prior authorization to obtain services. As reviewed in this chapter, managed care comes in a variety of packages.

COMMON MODELS OF MANAGED CARE ORGANIZATIONS

There are a wide variety of managed care models that integrate financing and management with the delivery of health care services to an enrolled population. The following sections describe some of the common models.

Health Maintenance Organizations

HMOs are organized health care systems that are responsible for both the financing and the delivery of a broad range of comprehensive health services to an enrolled population. They are the most highly regulated form of MCOs. HMOs act both as insurer and provider of health care services. They charge employers a fixed premium for each subscriber. An independent practice association (IPA)-model HMO provides medical care to its subscribers through contracts it establishes with independent physicians. In a staff-model HMO, the physicians would normally be full-time employees of the HMO. Individuals who subscribe to an HMO are often limited to the panel of physicians who have contracted with the HMO to provide services to its subscribers.

Preferred Provider Organizations

Preferred provider organizations (PPOs) are entities through which employer health benefit plans and health insurance carriers contract to purchase health care services for covered beneficiaries from a selected group of participating providers. Most states have specific PPO laws that directly regulate such entities. Common characteristics of PPOs include:

- select provider panel
- negotiated payment rates
- rapid payment terms
- utilization management (programs to control utilization and cost)
- consumer choice (allow covered beneficiaries to use non-PPO providers for an additional out-of-pocket charge [point-of-service option])

In PPOs, a payer, such as an insurance company, provides incentives to its enrollees to obtain medical care from a panel of providers with whom the payer has contracted a discounted rate.

Exclusive Provider Organizations

Exclusive provider organizations (EPOs) limit their beneficiaries to participating providers for any health care services. EPOs use a gatekeeper approach to authorize nonprimary care services. The primary difference between an HMO and an EPO is that the former is regulated under HMO laws and regulations, whereas the latter is regulated under insurance laws and regulations. Characteristics of EPOs include:

- Primary care physicians are reimbursed through capitation payments or other performance-based reimbursement methods.
- Primary care physicians act as gatekeepers.

Point-of-Service Plans

Point-of-service (POS) plans use primary care physicians as gatekeepers to coordinate and control medical care. Subscribers covered under POS plans may decide whether to use HMO benefits or indemnity-style benefits for each instance of care. In other words, the member is allowed to make a coverage choice at the POS. A patient who chooses a provider outside the plan is responsible for higher copayments.

Experience-Rated HMOs

Under experience-rated benefit options, an HMO receives monthly premium payments much as it would under traditional premium-based plans. Typically, to arrive at a final premium rate, there is a settlement process in which the employer is credited with some portion or all of the actual utilization and cost of its group. Then refunds or additional payments are calculated and made to the appropriate party.

Specialty HMOs

Specialty HMOs provide limited components of health care coverage. Dental HMOs, for example, have become more common as an option to indemnity dental insurance coverage.

Independent Practice Associations

An independent practice association (IPA) is a legal entity composed of physicians organized for the purpose of negotiating contracts to provide physician services. For example, an IPA might contract with an HMO or a physician-hospital organization (PHO). The physicians maintain their own practices and do not share services, such as claims, billing, scheduling, accounting, and so forth.

Group Practice

A physician group that has only one or a small number of service delivery locations is a group practice. It is completely integrated economically, sharing costs and revenues. Group practices often are either specialty or primary-care dominated.

Group Practice Without Walls

A group practice without walls is a physician organization formed for the purpose of sharing some administrative and management costs while physicians continue to practice at their own locations rather than at a centralized location.

Physician–Hospital Organizations

A PHO is a legal entity consisting of a joint venture of physicians and a hospital. It is formed to facilitate managed care contracting, to improve cost management and services, and to create new health care resources in the community.

Medical Foundations

In a medical foundation, the foundation employs or contracts with physicians to provide care to the foundation's patients.

Management Service Organizations

A management service organization (MSO) is an entity that provides administrative and management services to physicians. The organization performs services, such as practice management, marketing, managed care contracting, accounting, billing, and personnel management. The MSO can be hospital affiliated, a hospital–physician joint venture, physician owned, or investor owned.

Vertically Integrated Delivery System

A vertically integrated delivery system (IDS) is any organization or group of affiliated organizations that provides physician and hospital services to patients. The goal of hospital–physician integration is to provide a full range of services to patients. A vertically IDS achieves this goal, providing services ranging from primary outpatient care to tertiary inpatient care. More elaborate systems provide additional services, such as home health care, long-term care, rehabilitation, and mental health care.

HORIZONTAL CONSOLIDATIONS

A horizontal merger involves similar or identical businesses at the same level of the market. There is no single qualitative or quantitative factor from which it can be determined whether such a group merger is permissible. Recognizing a congressional intent to preserve competition by preventing undue market concentration, the courts have focused primarily on the possibility that consolidation will substantially lessen competition.

FEDERALLY QUALIFIED HMOs

Many HMOs are federally qualified. Federal qualification, which is entirely voluntary, requires HMOs to meet federal standards for legal and organizational status, financial viability, marketing, and health service delivery systems, as delineated in the federal HMO act and its implementing regulations. The disadvantage of federal qualification—beyond the fees involved—is that a federally qualified HMO has less flexibility in its benefits package and in developing premium rates.

Federally qualified HMOs must provide or arrange for basic health services for their members as needed and without limitation as to time, cost, frequency, extent, or kind of services actually provided. Basic health services include:

- physician services, including consultant and referral services by a physician
- inpatient and outpatient services, including short-term rehabilitation services and physical therapy
- medically necessary emergency health services
- 20 outpatient visits per member per year for short-term, evaluative, or crisis intervention mental health services
- medical treatment and referral services
- diagnostic laboratory and diagnostic and therapeutic radiology services
- home health services
- preventive health services, including immunizations and well-child care from birth

STATE LAWS

Most states have enacted comprehensive HMO laws that are often based on the National Association of Insurance Commissioners' Model HMO Act. State laws generally specify what type of entities can apply for a certificate of authority to operate an HMO. Typically, the state insurance department is the primary regulatory body.

Generally, state HMO laws require that an application for a certificate of authority be accompanied by a description of the proposed marketing plan that the regulator must approve. HMO laws generally specify that a schedule of charges and amendments must be filed and approved by the commissioner.

The majority of state HMO laws requires that the provision of basic health services includes emergency care, inpatient care, physician care, and outpatient care. State HMO laws contain several provisions designed to protect enrollees in the event that the HMO becomes insolvent. These include deposit, capital, reserve, and net worth requirements. State laws pertaining to HMOs generally require that:

- The HMO cannot cancel or refuse to renew an enrollee solely because of the individual's health.
- If an individual terminates employment or membership in a group, that person must be permitted to convert to a direct-payment basis.
- Grievance procedures must be in place.

CASE MANAGEMENT FIRMS

Case management firms assist employers and insurers in managing catastrophic cases. They identify cases that will become catastrophic, negotiate services and reimbursement with providers who can treat the patient's condition, develop a treatment protocol for the patient, and monitor the treatment.

THIRD-PARTY ADMINISTRATORS

A third-party administrator (TPA) is a firm that provides services for employers and associations that have group insurance policies. The TPA acts as a liaison between the employer and the insurer. The TPA performs administrative activities, such as claims processing, certifying eligibility, and a preparation of reports required by the staff.

UTILIZATION REVIEW

Utilization review (UR) is a process whereby a third-party payer evaluates the medical necessity of a course of treatment. Managed care organizations use a utilization review process to compare a patient's request for care with what treatment doctors commonly practice in similar medical circumstances. Medical care is considered to be necessary when it is needed to prevent, diagnose, and treat a patient's medical condition. Generally, UR is performed prospectively, concurrently, or retrospectively.

- Prospective review: The payer determines whether to pay for treatment before the treatment is initiated. If the review reveals that the treatment is not medically necessary, the payer then indicates its decision not to pay for the medical care.
- Concurrent review: This review is performed during the course of treatment. Concurrent review entails monitoring whether medical care continues to be appropriate and necessary. If it is not, the payer will discontinue payment for additional care.
- Retrospective review: This type of review is performed after treatment has been completed. If the review indicates that medical care was not necessary, the insurer can deny the claim.

Most insurance companies and MCOs rely on prospective and concurrent UR to determine if care is necessary, as well as what level of care is appropriate. Utilization review has become an accepted and essential part of cost containment.

Case management is an increasingly important aspect of utilization management. It involves identifying at an early stage those patients who can be treated more cost effectively in an alternative setting or at a lower level of care without negatively affecting the quality of care. Case management usually is employed in catastrophic or high-cost cases.

Utilization Management Firms

Utilization management firms perform utilization management activities for managed care entities, insurers, or employers. Mental health and dental care are two common types of such firms. In recent years, the regulation of utilization by private review agents or utilization review organizations (UROs) has increased dramatically.

Just as health care entities have a corporate duty to select and monitor physicians carefully, they also have a duty to carefully select the URO with which they contract. That duty entails investigating the URO before contracting with it to ensure that its procedures are adequate and its personnel are qualified to perform UR activities.

Negligent UR Decisions

MCOs that perform UR may be found liable for undesirable patient outcomes because of defects or failures in the UR process or because of a negligent UR decision. The first reported case involving liability for UR was *Wickline v. State of California*.[1] In that case, the court stated that a third-party payer of health care services can be held legally accountable when medically inappropriate decisions result from defects in the design or implementation of cost-containment mechanisms. Liability in the UR process can arise from several sources, including failure to gather information adequately before making a decision as to medical necessity, failure to initiate a meaningful dialogue between UR personnel and the treating physician, failure to inform members of their right to appeal an adverse UR decision, and failure to issue a timely UR decision.

LIABILITY FOR NONPARTICIPATING PHYSICIANS

MCOs may be liable for the medical malpractice of nonemployee participating physicians under an ostensible or apparent agency theory if (1) the patient reasonably views the entity rather than the individual physician as the source of care and (2) the entity engages in conduct that leads the patient reasonably to believe that the source of care is the entity or that the physician is an employee of the entity.

The doctrine of corporate negligence clearly applies to staff-model HMOs in which the HMO employs the physicians and provides the facility within which they offer care. If an HMO employs physicians, such as in a staff-model HMO, the HMO can be held liable for the negligence of its employees under the doctrine of respondeat superior.

EMPLOYEE RETIREMENT INCOME SECURITY ACT

Congress enacted the Employee Retirement Income Security Act of 1974 (ERISA). It was designed to ensure that employee welfare and benefit plans conform to a uniform body of benefits law. ERISA sets minimum standards for most voluntarily established pension and health plans in private industry to provide protection for individuals in these plans. ERISA requires plans to provide participants with plan information including important information about plan features and funding; provides fiduciary responsibilities for those who manage and control plan assets; requires plans to establish a grievance and appeals process for participants to get benefits from their plans; and gives participants the right to sue for benefits and breaches of fiduciary duty.

The law does not, however, regulate the contents of the welfare benefit plans. For example, it does not mandate that specific benefits be provided to beneficiaries. To qualify as an employee benefit plan, the plan must be maintained by an employer or employee organization for the benefit of its employees. ERISA requires that every plan (1) describe procedures for the allocation of responsibilities for its operation and administration and (2) specify the basis on which payments are made to and from the plan.

The Consolidated Omnibus Budget Reconciliation Act (COBRA) included an amendment that expanded benefits, providing some workers and their families with the right to continue their health coverage for a limited time under certain circumstances, such as the loss of a job. Another amendment to ERISA is contained in the Health Insurance Portability and Accountability Act (HIPAA), which provides protection for employees and their families who have preexisting medical conditions or might otherwise suffer discrimination in health coverage based on factors that relate to an individual's health. In general, ERISA does not cover group health plans established or maintained by governmental entities, churches for their employees, or plans that are maintained solely to comply with applicable workers' compensation, unemployment, or disability laws.

HEALTH CARE QUALITY IMPROVEMENT ACT OF 1986

The Health Care Quality Improvement Act of 1986 (HCQIA) was enacted in part as a response to numerous antitrust suits against participants in peer-review and credentialing activities. Congress passed the act to encourage continued participation in these activities. The purpose of the HCQIA is to provide those persons giving information to professional review bodies and those assisting in review activities limited immunity from damages that may arise as a result of adverse decisions that affect a physician's medical staff privileges. The immunity does not extend to civil rights litigation or suits filed by the United States or an attorney general of a state.

MANAGED CARE AND LEGAL ACTIONS

The following cases describe but a few of the many legal actions involving managed care.

Failure to Disclose Financial Incentives

The patient in *Shea v. Esensten*[2] died after suffering a heart attack. Although the patient had recently visited his primary-care physician and presented symptoms of cardiac problems, including a family history of cardiac trouble, the physician did not refer the patient to a cardiologist. The patient's widow sued the HMO for failing to disclose the financial incentive system it provided to its physicians to minimize referrals to specialists. The US Court of Appeals for the Eighth Circuit agreed that knowledge of financial incentives that affect a physician's decisions to refer patients to specialists is material information requiring disclosure, and it reversed a lower court's dismissal of the claim.

Financial Incentives Disclosed

In 1996, Dr. Linda Peeno, featured in Michael Moore's 2007 film *Sicko*, testified before Congress to discuss her prior work as a medical reviewer for Humana.

Her testimony included the following remarks after which she embarked on a journey to become one of the best-known whistleblowers about HMOs and the health care industry.

> I am here primarily today to make a public confession. In the spring of 1987, as a physician, I denied a man a necessary operation that would have saved his life and thus caused his death. No person and no group has held me accountable for this, because in fact, what I did was I saved a company a half a million dollars for this.

Dr. Peeno, now a physician in Louisville, Kentucky, remains unsanctioned by her peers and unpunished by the justice system for the act described above and others she admitted to committing because the medical profession remains self-regulating, and the medical licensing boards are comprised mostly of physicians. Moreover, courts are generally reluctant to get involved with the internal affairs of a professional society unless any sanctions they impose violate public policy.

Recently, the medical community has turned its attention to the authority of state medical boards to police improper physician expert testimony in medical malpractice actions. The discussion has been broadened to consider whether or not the presentation of testimony constitutes the carrying out of the practice of medicine. Depending upon the state, some cases have held that the "carrying out" requirement means that the medical judgment must affect or have the possibility of affecting the patient. For example, in *Murphy v. Board of Medical Examiners*[3] an Arizona court held that a physician performing prospective utilization review was practicing medicine because his decisions "could affect" a patient's health. Dr. Peeno was engaging in prospective utilization review. However, several federal courts have held that neither prospective nor retrospective review constituted the practice of medicine.[4]

The public has the right to expect expert physicians to be accurate and truthful when giving testimony. If the profession cannot police itself, then the states will be forced to intervene to protect the public from other unrepentant Dr. Peenos.

Open Enrollment

Federal HMO regulations require federally qualified HMOs to hold an open enrollment period of not less than 30 days per year during which the HMO must accept individual applicants for coverage regardless of their health status. Not all state HMO laws require open enrollment periods.

Emergency Care

HMOs can refuse benefit coverage to patients if they determine retrospectively that a patient's condition did not require emergency care. Of course, hindsight is 20/20. Determining whether one's chest pains are because of diet or a coronary condition requires expensive testing. To refuse a patient care before determining the etiology of a patient's condition could be financially disastrous to an organization. In addition, federal law prohibits hospital emergency departments from turning away patients seeking emergency care. Unfortunately, retrospective denial places the burden on the provider to seek reimbursement from the patient if the insurer denies the charges.

Benefit Denials

The California Supreme Court has ruled that insurers must inform beneficiaries of their right to contest a benefit denial. The court, in *Davis v. Blue Cross of N. California*,[5] held that the insurer breached its duty of good faith and fair dealing by failing to adequately apprise an insured of his rights under the policy's arbitration clause.

The insured in *Katskee v. Blue Cross/Blue Shield*[6] brought action against the health insurer for breach of contract. In January 1990, on recommendation of her gynecologist, Dr. Roffman, the appellant consulted with Dr. Lynch regarding her family's history of breast and ovarian cancer, and particularly her health in relation to such a history. After examining the appellant and investigating her family's medical history, Lynch diagnosed her as suffering from a genetic condition known as breast–ovarian carcinoma syndrome. Lynch then recommended that the appellant have a total abdominal hysterectomy and bilateral salpingo-oophorectomy. Roffman concurred with Lynch's diagnosis and agreed that the recommended surgery was the most medically appropriate treatment available.

Initially, Blue Cross/Blue Shield sent a letter to the appellant and indicated that it might pay for the surgery. Two weeks before surgery, Dr. Mason, the chief medical officer for Blue Cross/Blue Shield, wrote to the appellant and stated that Blue Cross/Blue Shield would not cover the cost of the surgery. Nonetheless, the appellant had the surgery. She filed an action for breach of contract, seeking to recover $6022.57 in costs associated with the surgery. Blue Cross/Blue Shield filed a motion for summary judgment. The district court granted the motion. It found that there was no genuine issue of material fact and that the policy did not cover the appellant's surgery. Specifically, the court stated that:

1. The appellant did not suffer from cancer, and although her high-risk condition warranted the surgery, it was not covered by the policy.
2. The appellant did not have a bodily illness or disease that was covered by the policy.
3. Under the terms of the policy, Blue Cross/Blue Shield reserved the right to determine what is medically necessary.

The appellant filed a notice of appeal to the Nebraska Court of Appeals contending that the district court erred in finding that no genuine issue of material fact existed and in granting summary judgment in favor of appellee. Blue Cross/Blue Shield denied coverage because it concluded that appellant's condition did not constitute an illness, and thus the treatment she received was not medically necessary.

An insurance policy is to be construed, as any other contract, to give effect to the parties' intentions at the time the contract was made. The issue was whether the insured's breast–ovarian carcinoma syndrome was an illness, defined as a bodily disorder or disease within meaning of the health insurance policy.

The Nebraska Supreme Court held that the insured's breast–ovarian carcinoma syndrome was an illness within meaning of the health insurance policy, notwithstanding the insurer's contention that the syndrome was merely a predisposition to cancer. The court found that whether a policy is ambiguous is a matter of law for the court to determine. A general principle of construction, which the courts apply to ambiguous insurance policies, holds that an ambiguous policy will be construed in favor of the insured. The language used in the policy at issue in the present case was not reasonably susceptible to differing interpretations and thus not ambiguous. The issue then becomes whether appellant's condition—breast–ovarian carcinoma syndrome—constituted an illness.

Blue Cross/Blue Shield argued that the appellant did not suffer from an illness because she did not have cancer. Blue Cross/Blue Shield characterized the appellant's condition only as a predisposition to an illness. The record on summary judgment included the depositions of Lynch, Roffman, and Mason. According to Lynch's testimony, some forms of cancer occur on a hereditary basis. Breast and ovarian cancer are such forms of cancer. Women diagnosed with the syndrome have at least a 50% chance of developing breast and/or ovarian cancer, whereas unaffected women have only a 1.4% risk of developing breast or ovarian cancer. Generally, by the time ovarian cancer is capable of being detected, it has already developed to an advanced stage, making treatment relatively unsuccessful. Lynch and Roffman agreed that the standard of care for treating women with breast–ovarian carcinoma syndrome ordinarily involves surveillance methods. However, for women at an inordinately high risk for ovarian cancer, such as the appellant, the standard of care may require radical surgery that involves the removal of the uterus, ovaries, and fallopian tubes. Blue Cross/Blue Shield did not provide any evidence disputing the premise that the origin of this condition is in the genetic makeup of the individual and that in its natural development it is likely to produce devastating results.

The medical evidence regarding the nature of breast–ovarian carcinoma syndrome persuaded the court that the appellant suffered from a bodily disorder or disease and, thus, suffered from an illness as defined by the insurance policy. Blue Cross/Blue Shield was, therefore, not entitled to judgment as a matter of law.

False and Misleading Statements

The plaintiff in *Drolet v. Healthsource, Inc.*[7] was a beneficiary of a health care plan administered by her employer, the Mitre Corporation. The plaintiff brought a class-action complaint alleging that Healthsource New Hampshire, Inc. and its parent corporation, Healthsource, Inc., are liable under ERISA for several materially false and misleading statements that Healthsource New Hampshire, Inc. allegedly made to the plan's beneficiaries.

The benefits provided by the plan require a member to choose a primary-care physician to be responsible for providing the member with routine medical care and coordinating the member's specialty care referrals. In defining the term "primary-care physician," the agreement emphasized that the physician has a contractual relationship with Healthsource, which does not interfere with the exercise of the physician's independent medical judgment. The plaintiff contended that the physician–patient relationship was compromised by various undisclosed financial incentives that are provided to the plan's physicians to reduce expenditures on specialty care services. Among these incentives, the plaintiff alleged, are referral funds that permit a physician to earn up to 33% in additional income by minimizing the use of specialty services such as diagnostic tests, referrals, and hospitalizations.

If Healthsource New Hampshire made material misrepresentations in the group subscriber agreement and other plan documents, it can be enjoined under ERISA to prevent further breaches of its fiduciary duty. Regulations do not authorize Healthsource New Hampshire, as a fiduciary, from making misrepresentations to beneficiaries.

Price Fixing

Price fixing is considered a per se violation of the antitrust laws. Price fixing occurs when two or more competitors come together to decide on a price that will be charged for services or goods. The per se rule applies to restraints in trade that are so inimical to competition and so unjustified that they are presumed to be unreasonable and, therefore, are illegal. Examinations of per se violations include price fixing, horizontal market allocation, tying, and group boycotts.

The provider-controlled MCO is at significant antitrust risk when setting provider reimbursement and bargaining with payers. There is a danger that provider-controlled organizations will be viewed as a horizontal conspiracy between competitors that acts as a mechanism for price fixing.

One of the leading cases involving price fixing is *Maricopa County Medical Society v. Arizona University*,[8] a US Supreme Court case that involved the exercise of provider control over the level of physician reimbursement. Because the physicians had no financial stake in the success of the plan, the Supreme Court found that the maximum fee schedule set by the physicians constituted illegal price fixing.

In *Maine v. Alliance Healthcare, Inc.*,[9] an entity composed of four hospitals and their affiliated physician groups was formed to contract with managed care plans. The state attorney general charged that the entity was engaged in price fixing because it allegedly forced HMOs to pay physicians on a fee-for-service basis instead of a capitation basis. In the resulting consent decree, the entity agreed to cease collectively negotiating prices for its members.

Market Power

Whenever an MCO possesses significant market power or deals with a group that has significant market power, antitrust implications should be considered. To determine market power, it is necessary first to identify the market in which the entity exercises power. For antitrust purposes, the relevant market has two components: (1) a product component and (2) a geographic component.

Product Market

The relevant product market involves the product or service at issue and all substantially acceptable substitutes for it. The relevant product market for MCOs is the market for health care financing. Broadly defined, this market includes traditional insurers, HMOs, PPOs, IPAs, and so on, and their subscriber members.

Market power results from the ability to cut back the market's total supply and then raise prices because of consumer demand for the product. Generally, the market in health care financing is competitive because the customers can switch companies readily, new suppliers can enter the market quickly, and existing suppliers can expand their sales rapidly.

Geographic Market

The relevant geographic market is the market area in which the seller operates and to which the purchaser can practically turn for supplies. The primary factors that courts have examined to determine the geographic scope of the market for hospital services are:

- patient flow statistics
- location of physicians who admit patients
- determinations of health planners
- public perception

Patients Have Rights

Although ERISA preempts state law affecting employee benefit plans, the following case illustrates that there are circumstances under which ERISA will not preempt state law. Ms. Moran, in *Rush Prudential HMO, Inc. v. Moran*[10] sought treatment from Dr. LaMarre, her primary physician under her HMO plan (Rush Prudential HMO, Inc.) because of numbness, pain, and decreased mobility in her right shoulder. During a series of physiotherapy treatments under LaMarre, Moran obtained the name of an out-of-network physician, Dr. Terzis, and submitted a request to Rush for a referral to consult with this physician. Her request was denied. Moran had the consult anyway and was diagnosed with plexopathy and thoracic outlet syndrome. Terzis recommended a more involved and expensive surgery. Two plan physicians recommended a less-complicated surgery. LaMarre formally asked Rush to approve Terzis's recommended surgery. Rush denied approval of the surgery. Moran made a written demand to Rush seeking its compliance with the Illinois Health Maintenance Organization Act, Section 4-10, which requires

HMOs to provide an independent physician review when a patient's primary care physician disagrees with an HMO about the medical necessity of a proposed treatment. Moran eventually decided to undergo the surgery with Terzis at her own expense. She later submitted the bill to Rush and sought a court order requiring Rush to comply with Section 4-10. Rush moved the case to a federal court citing the statute's conflict with ERISA. The district court agreed with Rush that ERISA preempted Moran's claims and granted summary judgment to Rush.

The case eventually reached the US Supreme Court, which upheld Section 4-10 of the Illinois HMO Act, which provides a mechanism whereby insured patients can enforce their rights under insurance plans.

Notes

1. 239 Cal. Rptr. 810 (Cal. Ct. App. 1986).
2. 107 F.3d 625 (8th Cir. 1997).
3. 949 P2d 530, 535 (Ariz. Ct. App. 1997).
4. Adnan Varol, M.D., P.C. v. Blue Cross Blue Shield of Mich., 708 F. Supp. 826 (E.D. Mich. 1989); Corcoran v. United Health Care, 956 F.2d 1321 (5th Cir. 1992).
5. 600 P.2d 1060 (Cal. 1979).
6. 515 N.W.2d 645 (Neb. 1994).
7. 968 F. Supp. 757 (D.C. N.H. 1997).
8. 457 U.S. 332 (1982).
9. 1991-1 Trade Cas. (CCH)¨ 69,339.
10. 536 U.S. 355 (2002).

22

Tort Reform and Risk Reduction

The tort system has proven to be inadequate in the prevention of medical malpractice. Damage awards as a deterrent to malpractice have failed to reduce the number of claims. Exorbitant jury awards and malpractice insurance premiums are costing the health care industry billions of dollars annually.

Given the difficulties in the present tort system, we often become victims of the failures of medicine as opposed to beneficiaries of its many successes. Physicians have lost in that they have changed, limited, or closed their practices after having spent the most vigorous years of their lives training for such work. Patients have lost in that the physicians of their choice, with whom they have developed trusting relationships, are no longer available to care for them. It is certain that the system requires sensible reform.

Physicians who wish to practice medicine and survive have accepted the concept of practicing defensive medicine. Defensive medicine (self-protective) is believed to be one of the most harmful effects produced by the threat of malpractice litigation. Such medicine is practiced to forestall potential litigation and provide an advantageous legal defense should a lawsuit be instituted. Defensive medicine often results in undertreatment, perhaps by avoiding high-risk tests and procedures, or overtreatment, such as the excessive use of diagnostic tests. "The message the tort system is sending to doctors is not so much deterrence, in terms of practicing good medicine, but more just 'drive defensively,' because any patient you may see may be a litigant."[1]

The various states have not ignored the need for tort reform and have and continue to legislate tort reform. This chapter reviews selected schemes for tort reform and suggested programs for coping with the malpractice crisis.

ARBITRATION AND MEDIATION

Among the many factors contributing to the malpractice crisis is the high cost of litigation. Trial by jury is lengthy and expensive. If case disputes can be handled out of court, the process and expense of a lawsuit can be significantly reduced. Arbitration and mediation are basically mechanisms for simplifying and expediting the settlement of claims.

Arbitration is the process by which parties to a dispute voluntarily agree to submit their differences to the judgment of an impartial mediation panel for resolution. It is used as a means to evaluate, screen, and resolve medical malpractice disputes before they reach the courts. Arbitration can be accomplished by mutual consent of the parties or statutory provisions. A decision made at arbitration may or may not be binding, depending on prior agreement between the parties or statutory requirements.

Mediation is the process whereby a third party, the mediator, attempts to bring about a settlement between the parties of a complaint. The mediator cannot force a settlement.

STRUCTURED AWARDS

Structured awards are set up for the periodic payment of judgments by establishing a reversible trust fund for specified risks of malpractice parts of awards due plaintiffs. The purpose of a structured award is to provide compensation during a plaintiff's lifetime. It would eliminate an unwarranted windfall to the plaintiff's beneficiaries in the event of death. Some states have sought to deal with award limitations by mandating so-called structured recoveries when awards exceed a certain dollar amount.

Structured recoveries provide that money awarded to the plaintiff be placed in a trust fund and invested appropriately so that those funds will be available to the plaintiff over a long period. The rationale behind such legislation is that an immediate award of a large sum of money is not necessary for a plaintiff to be well taken care of after suffering injuries. The prudent investment of a smaller amount of money can produce a recovery commensurate with the needs and the rights of the plaintiff. This, in turn, requires a smaller cash outlay by the defendant or the defendant's insurance company, thereby holding down the costs of malpractice insurance and the ultimate cost of medical care to the consumer.

PRETRIAL SCREENING PANELS

Pretrial screening panels are designed to evaluate the merits of medical injury claims to encourage the settlement of claims outside the courtroom. "Panels render an opinion on provider liability and, in some cases, on damages. In most states, the panel's decision on the merit of the claim is admissible in court."[2] Unlike binding arbitration, the decision of a screening panel is not binding and is imposed as a condition precedent to trial, whereas arbitration is conducted in lieu of a trial. Mandatory screenings of alleged negligence cases are useful in discouraging frivolous lawsuits from proceeding to trial.

COLLATERAL SOURCE RULE

The *collateral source rule* is a common-law principle that prohibits a court or jury from taking into account when setting an award that part of the plaintiff's damages covered by other sources of payment (e.g., health insurance, disability, and compensation). Several states have modified the collateral source rule so that evidence regarding other sources of payment to the plaintiff may be introduced for purposes of reducing the amount of the ultimate award to the plaintiff. The jury then would be permitted to assign the evidence such weight as it chooses. The award could be reduced to the extent that the plaintiff received compensation from other sources.

Imposition of the collateral source rule can result in recoveries to plaintiffs far in excess of their economic loss. Such excessive payments contribute significantly to the high cost of malpractice insurance and the high cost of health care to the public. When evidence regarding collateral sources of payment is allowed to be introduced to mitigate the damages payable to a plaintiff, excessive recoveries may be discouraged.

CONTINGENCY FEE LIMITATIONS

A *contingency fee* is payment for services rendered by an attorney predicated on the favorable outcome of a case. Payment is based on a preestablished percentage of the total award. Some states set this percentage by statute. Under a contingency agreement, if there is no award to the plaintiff, then the attorney receives no payment for services rendered.

Physicians argue that the contingency fee arrangement serves to encourage an inordinate number of lawsuits. Attorneys reason that if they or their clients must bear the initial cost of a lawsuit, only those with obvious merit will be brought forward. The contingency fee structure allows those unable to bear the cost of litigation to initiate a suit for damages. Limiting contingency fees on a sliding scale basis, with the percentage decreasing as the award to the plaintiff increases, and/or providing for a lesser fee if a claim is settled prior to trial, seems to have some merit.

COUNTERSUITS: FRIVOLOUS CLAIMS

Health care providers, in some instances, have filed countersuits after being named in what they believe to be malicious, libelous, slanderous, frivolous, and nonmeritorious medical malpractice suits. The threat of countersuits, however, has not been helpful in reducing the number of malpractice claims. Remedies for such actions vary from one jurisdiction to the next. For a physician to prevail in a suit against a plaintiff or plaintiff's attorney, the physician must show that the:

- suit was frivolous
- motivation of the plaintiff was not to recover for a legitimate injury
- physician has suffered damages as a result of the suit

There have been arguments that defendants should be allowed to recover court costs and damage awards from both the plaintiff(s) and the attorneys for frivolous claims and counterclaims. The courts thus far have not looked favorably on countersuits for frivolous and unscrupulous negligence actions.

Frivolous and unscrupulous malpractice actions have caused physicians to place limitations on their scope of practice. Many obstetricians/gynecologists, for example, have dropped the high-risk obstetrics portion of their practices to reduce their malpractice premiums. There is also an ever-increasing reluctance by physicians to perform heroic measures on accident victims because of the high risks of malpractice exposure.

JOINT AND SEVERAL LIABILITY

The *doctrine of joint and several liability* provides that a person causing an injury concurrently with another person can be held equally liable for the entire judgment awarded by a court. It is proposed by some that each defendant in a multidefendant action should be limited to payment for the percentage of fault ascribed to him or her. Some states have taken action to modify the doctrine. A Wyoming statute, for example, provides that each defendant to a lawsuit is liable only for that proportion of the total dollar amount of damages according to the percentage of the amount of fault attributed to him or her.[3] A Minnesota statute provides that a defendant whose fault is 15% or less may be jointly liable for a percentage of the whole award not greater than four times his or her percentage of fault.[4]

MALPRACTICE LIABILITY CAPS

The impetus for malpractice liability caps is due, in part, because jury awards often vary substantially from one jurisdiction to the next within the same state. As a result, negligence attorneys often prefer to try personal injury cases in those jurisdictions in which a jury is likely to grant a higher award. Different states are attempting to stem the tide of rising malpractice costs by passing laws that impose restrictions on limiting the total dollar damages allowable in malpractice actions. Although there have been challenges to statutes limiting awards, it would appear that limitations on malpractice recoveries are constitutional. The battle continues as to just how effective malpractice liability caps really are. States that have them in place are finding that the caps are from resolving the high malpractice insurance premiums paid by physicians.

NO-FAULT SYSTEM

A *no-fault system* compensates injured parties for economic losses regardless of fault. It is intended to compensate more claimants with smaller awards. A no-fault system compensates victims of medical injury whether or not they can prove medical negligence. Proponents of the no-fault approach cite as its advantages swifter and less-expensive resolution of claims and more equitable compensation for patients.

A no-fault system of compensation has its drawbacks. Opponents of the no-fault system are concerned about the loss of whatever deterrence effect the present tort system exerts on health care providers. The system's lower administrative costs can be an incentive to file lawsuits and, therefore, may not produce the desired outcome of reducing the incidence of malpractice claims.

REGULATION OF INSURANCE PRACTICES

Many believe that the regulation of insurance practices is necessary to prevent windfall profits. Both the medical profession and the legal profession believe that insurance carriers have raised premiums disproportionately to their losses and that, despite their claims of substantial losses, they have reaped substantial profits.

IMPLEMENTATION OF BEST PRACTICES

The implementation of best practices can help reduce the number of lawsuits in any given medical specialty. "Many of the specialty societies either have drafted or are drafting practice guidelines for their medical area of expertise. For example, the American Society of Anesthesiologists developed guidelines for intraoperative monitoring in 1986. During the following year, no lawsuits were brought for hypoxic injuries; in previous years hypoxic injury suits averaged six per year."[5]

RISK MANAGEMENT

The purpose of a risk-management program is to reduce the number of patient injuries and minimize the exposure of an organization to lawsuits. An effective risk-management program includes a monitoring system that identifies potential risks to patients and staff. Information gathered is used to improve patient care and treatment practices. In risk management, steps are taken on a team-effort basis to improve the quality of care and eliminate or minimize the number of accidents that become potential lawsuits. Liability insurers have been strong proponents of risk management; in many cases, insurers have cut premiums for physicians and health care organizations who adopt risk-management practices.

Risk management must include a heightened sensitivity to providing a safe environment and addressing the emotional needs of patients. The input of the provider–patient relationship cannot be overemphasized when the provider–patient relationship is intense and inescapable. Individuals, not incidents, bring lawsuits. Good relationships with patients are very important in preventing malpractice suits. Public relations for health care professionals are a challenge. It is not only good medical practice, but it is also at the very core of the problem of medical malpractice.

Increasing insurance costs and general financial constraints have pressured hospitals to assume leadership in the prevention of medically related injuries. Risk-management programs should inc[illegible]llowing components[illegible]

- a g[illegible]mechanism designed [illegible]ive as promptly and [illegible] grievances by pati[illegible]atives
- a co[illegible]spect to negative [illegible] (whether they give[illegible]
- med[illegible] mechanisms, which [illegible] committee or medi[illegible] to periodically assess [illegible]ical care being provid[illegible]
- educa[illegible] staff personnel engage[illegible]t care activities dealing with patient safety, medical injury prevention, the legal aspects of patient care, problems of communication and rapport with patients, and other relevant factors known to influence malpractice claims and suits

CONTINUOUS QUALITY IMPROVEMENT

Continuous quality improvement (CQI) is an approach to improving quality on a continuing basis. CQI is introduced here because of its value in reducing the risks of malpractice. CQI involves improving performance at every functional level of an organization's operation, using available resources (human and capital). It combines fundamental management techniques, innovative improvement efforts, and specialized technical skills in a structure focused on continuously improving processes. CQI relies on people and involves everyone. CQI is concerned with providing a quality product, getting to market on time, providing the best service, reducing costs, broadening market share, and organizational growth. The benefits of CQI are well documented and include reduced customer complaints and turnover; increased ability to attract new customers; and improved productivity, services, and quality.

The ultimate successes of CQI require commitment by the organization's leadership. In the health care setting, leadership includes the administration, governing body, medical staff, and nursing staff. From the leadership, involvement must be expanded to include the entire organization.

The organization's plan should be designed to provide a systematic and ongoing process for monitoring and evaluating patient care, identifying opportunities for improvement, and identifying high-risk areas having the potential for adverse outcomes and increased exposure to litigation.

CQI Data Collection

Data collection for improving quality performance in an organization is often categorized and based on: volume indicators, occurrence screens, focused reviews, and clinical pertinence reviews of medical records. It should be remembered that it is not just data collection that is important but the aggregation of the data in a meaningful format, such as graphs and charts. This information is then analyzed to show trends and to determine if there is a need for improving performance.

Volume Indicators

Volume indicators provide data that demonstrate the scope and frequency of services provided over time (e.g., admission/discharge data, number of procedures, and outpatient visits). Volume indicators also provide valuable information for monitoring the incidence of adverse outcomes (e.g., infection rates following surgical procedures, adverse drug reactions, and medication errors). The information and data gathered by an organization are of significant importance as they relate to budgeting, resource allocation, and strategic planning.

Clinical Indicators

Clinical indicators are used to screen the care provided to patients by clinical specialty. The screens are generally confined to those related to high-volume or high-risk problems that may be unique to the clinical specialty. Each specialty uses such indicators to aid in the identification of opportunities for improving care practices. These opportunities are identified when collected data elements cross a preestablished threshold set by the clinical department or service. When the threshold has been crossed, those cases are then examined and the reason for variation is determined.

Occurrence Screens

Occurrence screens are predetermined indicators used to signal the need for evaluation of some aspect of patient care. Screens may describe the processes in the delivery of care, clinical events, complications, or outcomes for which data can be collected to compare actual results with criteria related to the screen. Events such as unexpected deaths, returns to the surgical suite, or adverse drug reactions should prompt an investigation to determine whether the events could be traced to structural problems (e.g., availability of resources) or process problems (e.g., timeliness and skills in the delivery of health care).

Focused Reviews

Focused reviews are concentrated reviews of key areas in a department or clinical specialty determined by their high risk, high volume, or history of identified problems. Focused reviews might target a representative sample of high-volume diagnoses or procedures over a finite time period or a review of all cases of low-volume but high-risk care.

Clinical Pertinence Review of Medical Records

The clinical pertinence review of medical records is a CQI process that monitors and evaluates the clinical pertinence, completeness, accuracy, timeliness, and legibility of documentation as reflected in the medical record. The purpose of such a review is to identify opportunities for improvement in the record documentation process.

Successful CQI Programs

Listed here are a few of the many areas in which health care organizations have successfully implemented the CQI process:

- improving response time for thrombolytic therapy
- recognizing abnormal vital signs and changes in patient's condition
- improving response time (e.g., cardiopulmonary arrest)
- improving charting (charting objectively, descriptively, and clinically)
- providing patient–family education
- improving safety
- improving patient satisfaction
- designing and implementing clinical pathways
- providing security and confidentiality of computer-generated information
- using antibiotics effectively and efficiently
- improving pain management

The implementation of CQI in health care organizations will improve the quality of patient care and reduce the untoward events that result in lawsuits. Success will come with true commitment by each organization's leadership. Such commitment requires the full participation of all caregivers. The evolution of a truly successful CQI program involves the transition from CQI as a plan to CQI as a process, and ultimately to CQI as an organizational culture.

FAILURE MODE EFFECTS ANALYSIS

The health care industry's focus is on identification and reduction of medical errors. The approach is proactive in nature. Failure mode effects analysis has long been recognized as a method for identifying and preventing product and process problems before they occur.

ROOT CAUSE ANALYSIS

A root cause analysis (RCA) is a chronological review of an event to identify what, how, why, when, and where an unwanted event occurred to prevent reoccurrence of the event. RCAs focus on systems and processes, not individual performance.

NATIONAL HEALTH CARE REFORM

The medical malpractice crisis continues to be a major dilemma for the health care industry. Although there have been many approaches to resolving the crisis, there appears to be no one magic formula. The solution most likely will require a variety of efforts, including tort reform.

The ever-increasing proliferation of regulations by policy makers, which have been designed to control costs and improve the quality of care, has alienated health care providers and added fuel to the practice of defensive medicine.

Physicians who are on the front lines often have been excluded from the decision-making processes that threaten their autonomy and financial security. A concerted effort must be made to include them in policy development and implementation. The present system of punishment for all because of the inadequacies of the few has proven to be costly and far from productive. The key to improving quality and controlling costs is cooperation, not alienation. Policy makers have failed in this arena and must return to a commonsense approach to policy development by including those who are on the front lines of medicine.

Notes

1. THE ROBERT WOOD JOHNSON FOUNDATION, The Tort System for Medical Malpractice: How Well Does It Work, What Are the Alternatives? ABRIDGE, Spring 1991, at 2.
2. THE ROBERT WOOD JOHNSON FOUNDATION, Legal Reform, ABRIDGE, Spring 1991, at 3.
3. WYO. STAT. § 1-1-109 (1986).
4. MINN. STAT. § 604.02 (1988).
5. THE ROBERT WOOD JOHNSON FOUNDATION, Preventing Negligence, Abridge, Spring 1991, at 8.

23

Patient Safety and Zero Tolerance

The Institute of Medicine (IOM) of the National Academies was chartered in 1970 as a component of the National Academy of Sciences. The November 1999 IOM report, "To Err Is Human: Building a Safer Health System," indicated that at least 44 thousand and perhaps as many as 98 thousand people die in hospitals each year as a result of preventable medical errors. Such figures rank medical errors as the eighth leading cause of death in the United States, ahead of deaths from motor vehicle accidents, breast cancer, or AIDS.

Both health care organizations and accrediting bodies are adopting a zero-tolerance policy toward poor judgment and careless mistakes by focusing on processes and not individuals. Strides are being made to ensure that desired outcomes are more closely aligned with predictability. More focus on how to do things right the first time will lessen the likelihood of having to ask why things went wrong after a medical error occurs.

This chapter focuses on the development of a corporate culture of safety with emphasis on national patient safety goals. A self-evaluation process, including a variety of safe practices, is also presented on the following pages.

DEVELOPING A CULTURE OF SAFETY

Organizations are encouraged to create and maintain a culture of safety to reduce the risks of patient injuries and deaths due to common mistakes. Patients expect hospitals to provide a safe environment for medical care. Although health care organizations are aware of where systems often break down, evidence suggests that they have been ineffective in preventing patient injuries that are often the result of human error or just plain carelessness.

Implementation of the following suggestions will help hospitals move toward a culture of safety:

- Ensure that accountability and responsibility have been assigned for monitoring an organization's safety initiatives.
- Involve the medical staff in the development and implementation of systems that are designed to create a culture of safety.
- Educate all staff members as to their individual roles in establishing and maintaining a safe environment for patients.
- Encourage patients to question their care. Provide guidelines in patient handbooks as to the kinds of questions that they should ask caregivers (e.g., Is this a new medication? I don't recognize it. What is this medication for? Did you wash your hands [before changing my surgical dressing]?).
- Establish a patient safety committee with responsibility for oversight of the organization's patient safety program.
- Set up a dedicated safety hotline.
- Participate in the Institute for Healthcare Improvement's 100K Lives Campaign by committing to the implementation of its six life saving initiatives: (1) establishment of a rapid response team; (2) improvement of care for myocardial infarctions; (3) prevention of adverse drug events; (4) prevention of central-line–associated bloodstream infections; (5) prevention of surgical site infections; and (6) prevention of ventilator-associated pneumonia.
- Utilize the online tools released by the Agency for Healthcare Research and Quality (AHRQ) to assist organizations in evaluating and improving safe care.

National Patient Safety Goals

The Joint Commission is striving to improve patient safety by identifying national patient safety goals in its accreditation process. Some of these goals include improving the accuracy of patient identification; effective communications among caregivers; safe use of high-alert medications; elimination of wrong-site, wrong-patient, wrong-procedure surgery through the development of universal protocols; safe and effective use of clinical alarm systems; and reduction in the frequency of health care–acquired infections.

Periodically, The Joint Commission introduces national patient safety goals into its survey process. The Joint Commission surveyors evaluate organizations at the time of an organization's accreditation survey, determining compliance with patient safety goals. The goals encourage compliance with safe practices in the delivery of patient care and are designed to reduce the likelihood of medical errors in the delivery of patient care. Due to the frequency of questions asked as to interpretation and implementation of the goals, along with the periodic introduction of new goals to the survey process, The Joint Commission, on its Web site at www.jointcommission.org, clarifies existing goals and describes new goals.

Patient Complaint Process

The Joint Commission has implemented a patient complaint process that requires that the health care organizations it accredits educate employers and employees as to their right to report safety or quality concerns to The Joint Commission. The Joint Commission policy forbids accredited organizations from taking retaliatory actions against employees for having reported quality of care concerns to The Joint Commission. Patient complaints may be reported by:

- Online: www.jointcommission.org/GeneralPublic/Complaint/
- Fax: Office of Quality Monitoring at (630) 792-5636
- Written correspondence: Office of Quality Monitoring, The Joint Commission, One Renaissance Boulevard, Oakbrook Terrace, IL 60181
- Telephone: (800) 994-6610 for questions about how to file a complaint

National Quality Forum

The National Quality Forum (NQF) is a private, nonprofit, public-benefit corporation created for the purpose of developing and implementing a national strategy for health care quality measurement and reporting. NQF is a unique public–private partnership representing all sectors of the health care industry, including consumers, employers, insurers, and health care providers. The NQF has identified 30 safe practices that it recommends for adoption in health care settings to reduce the risks of harm to patients. For complete information on the activities and functioning of the NQF, visit the corporation's Web site at www.qualityforum.org/.

Agency for Healthcare Research and Quality

The Agency for Healthcare Research and Quality (AHRQ) is the lead federal agency within the Department of Health and Human Services charged with improving the quality, safety, efficiency, and effectiveness of health care. Information from AHRQ's research helps people make more informed decisions and improve the quality of health care services. AHRQ collaborated with the National Quality Forum in identifying the 30 safe practices just noted. Evidence shows that such practices can prevent or reduce the number of medical errors.

Institute for Healthcare Improvement

The Institute for Healthcare Improvement (IHI) is a not-for-profit organization whose mission is to improve health care throughout the world. The IHI was founded in 1991 and is based in Cambridge, Massachusetts. To reduce medical errors, health care organizations are becoming more proactive by implementing safe practices. Some hospitals have joined the IHI 100K Lives Campaign, which has a goal of saving 100 thousand lives annually. For complete information on the activities and functioning of the IHI, visit the corporation's Web site at www.IHI.org/.

The Leapfrog Group for Patient Safety

The Leapfrog Group and its members work together to reduce preventable medical mistakes and improve the quality and affordability of health care. The Leapfrog Group promotes improvements in the safe delivery of health care by collecting and providing the necessary information for health care consumers to make informed health care decisions. For complete information on the activities and functioning of The Leapfrog Group, visit its Web site at www.leapfroggroup.org/.

ECRI

ECRI (formerly the Emergency Care Research Institute) is a nonprofit health services research agency and a collaborating center of the World Health Organization (WHO). It is designated as an evidence-based practice center by the AHRQ. ECRI is widely recognized as one of the world's leading independent organizations committed to advancing the quality of health care. ECRI's mission is to promote the highest standards of safety, quality, and cost effectiveness in health care to benefit patient care through research, publishing, education, and consulting. For complete information on the activities and functioning of ECRI, visit its Web site at www.ecri.org/.

EVALUATING SAFE PATIENT CARE

A tool for evaluating the safe delivery of patient care is presented throughout the remainder of the chapter. Each statement is meant to assist the practicing professional in evaluating a health care organization. This tool has been developed to apply to a variety of health care organizations. Each bulleted statement is meant to encourage the reader to ask more—who, how, what, why, when, and where.

Leadership

- The organization's mission, vision, and values have been identified.
- There is a strategy that charts the direction of the organization in response to community need.
- The planning process identifies the organization's strengths and opportunities for improvement.
- Patient input is solicited to improve services through, for example, patient satisfaction surveys and focus groups.
- A process for setting priorities has been established.
- The governing body has adopted a conflict-of-interest policy.
- Care is not based on ability to pay.
- A corporate compliance program has been developed and implemented.
- The governing body monitors the effectiveness of the organization's leadership.

Credentialing Licensed Practitioners

- There is a process for credentialing licensed health care practitioners.
- The National Practitioner Data Bank is utilized in the credentialing process.
- There is ongoing evaluation of each professional.
- Delineation of clinical privileges includes: a description of the privileges requested; relevant education, training, and experience; limitations on privileges requested; evidence of competency in performing requested privileges; verification of current licensure; relevant references; and evaluation of current competency.

Human Resources Process

- Job descriptions reflect each staff member's duties and responsibilities.
- The technical skills of each position have been determined.
- The organization has the appropriate competencies, mix, and numbers of employees.
- Recruitment, retention, development, and recognition programs have been implemented.
- There is a department-specific orientation program for employees, agency and contracted staff, and volunteers.
- The education and training needs of staff are assessed.

Patient Education

- The patient's first contact with a staff member involves the establishment of trust, which emanates from patient recognition that the caregiver is knowledgeable and competent.
- Greetings, gestures, manner of taking information, and attitude are important ingredients in establishing a good relationship with the patient.
- There is evidence of patient/family education in the patient's record.
- An assessment of the patient's readiness/willingness, ability, and need to learn is conducted.
- Education is conducted in all settings (e.g., inpatient, ambulatory, emergency department, home care) on a collaborative basis.
- Education includes medication safety; nutrition; medical equipment use; access to community resources; how to obtain further care if necessary; and responsibilities of the patient and family.
- The patient understands the care instructions.

Communications

- Abbreviations are discouraged. Where abbreviations are permitted, they have one meaning.
- A process is in place for validating the correct interpretation of illegible medication orders.

Critical Tests

- Critical test results and values are reported on a timely basis.
- Data are collected to measure and assess the success of timely reporting.
- Action is taken, when necessary, to improve the reporting process.

Emergency Services

- Adequate staff is available to care for patients.
- Medical records are maintained for each patient treated.
- Patients are triaged, assessed, and treated within a reasonable period of time.
- Criteria for admission and discharge have been established.
- Response time by on-call physicians is timely.
- The organization has a mechanism for obtaining consultations.
- All patients are assessed and treated by a physician prior to discharge.
- The records of patients treated in other settings within the organization (e.g., ambulatory care settings) are readily available.
- Patient education is provided in the emergency department (ED) prior to discharge.
- Documentation is complete.
- There is a procedure in place for reading X-rays and other imaging studies when there is no radiologist readily available.

Security

- Security issues have been addressed throughout the organization.
- Sensitive areas have been identified.
- Newborns are footprinted.
- An organization-approved identification band is attached to mothers and infants.
- Identification badges for mother and infant match.
- All staff members have current color photo identification badges.
- Staff and parents are educated as to security procedures.
- Infant abduction drills are conducted.
- An electronic security alarm system has been installed.
- Security cameras and monitors have been installed.

Emergency Preparedness

- The organization has an emergency preparedness plan for both internal and external disasters.
- The plan has been developed in cooperation with local and national emergency preparedness programs.
- The organization identifies its vulnerabilities (e.g., equipment, supplies, staff, communications) and implements improvements.
- The plan is periodically practiced to determine the organization's readiness for a variety of disasters (e.g., earthquake, hurricane, act of terrorism).

Patient Identification

- The patient's wristband is checked for identification prior to rendering treatment.
- Two identifiers are noted prior to treatment (patient's name, birth date, medical record number, etc.) and match the information on the wristband to the patient's medical chart.
- A patient's room number or bed location within a room is never used as a patient identifier.

Infection Control

- Hand hygiene protocols have been developed.
  - Use recommended soaps.
  - Use alcohol-based hand rubs.
- Appropriate temperature and humidity levels are maintained.
- Patients at risk for developing pressure ulcers are assessed.

  - Protocols to prevent development of pressure ulcers are followed.
- Food products are labeled as to contents and expiration dates.
- Infection-control policies and procedures include gowning, masks, and glove changes between patients.
- Furniture, equipment, and toys are disinfected with appropriate germicidal solutions.

Laboratory Services

- Critical lab values are reported promptly.
- Therapeutic ranges are closely monitored.
- Blood levels for toxicity are closely followed.
- Test results that do not fit a patient's clinical picture or expected outcomes are addressed by the patient's physician(s).

Surgical Specimens

- Second reads are conducted as appropriate.
- Procedures are implemented to reduce the risk of surgical specimen mix-ups.
- Specimens are properly jarred and labeled at the surgical table.
- All specimens, including blood, do not leave one's possession until labeled.
- A strict chain of custody for each specimen is maintained.
- Pre- and postoperative pathology report discrepancies are addressed.

Medication Safety

- Drugs are safely stored, ordered, and distributed.
- Potentially dangerous look-alike, sound-alike drugs are separated in the pharmacy to prevent mix-ups.
- All medications are labeled including the drug, dosage, and expiration date.
- A process is implemented for obtaining and documenting a complete listing of a patient's current medications upon admission to the organization.
- A determination as to which medications should be continued during the patient's stay is made by the attending physician.
- Upon discharge, the attending physician instructs the patient as to which drugs should be continued or discontinued.
- A complete list of drugs is made available to the next provider when the patient is transferred to another setting, service, practitioner, or level of care within or outside the organization.
- Risk-reduction activities are in place to reduce the likelihood of adverse drug reactions and medication errors.
- There is a mechanism for monitoring the effect of medications on patients.
- Responsibility for ensuring the integrity of crash carts has been assigned.
- The organization maintains the appropriate medications and equipment on crash carts for treating both children and adults.
- Staff members are appropriately trained in the testing and use of equipment contained in or on the crash cart.
- Staff members who participate in codes are periodically tested for competency.
- High-risk drugs are easily identified and standardized when feasible.
- There is a mechanism in place for approving and overseeing the use of investigational drugs.
- Investigational drug protocols and criteria have been developed and approved.
- Look-alike medications are repackaged or relabeled, as necessary, in the pharmacy.
- Causes and trends of medication errors are tracked.
- Educational processes have been implemented to reduce the likelihood of medication errors.

Patient Assessments

- There is a process for assessing patient care needs.
- The organization has a policy for conducting screenings and assessments.

- Second opinions are obtained as necessary; literature is searched; and other resources are used to provide current, timely, and accurate diagnoses and treatment of patients.
- The criteria for nutritional screens have been developed and approved.
- Nutritional screens and assessments are performed by a dietitian or an appropriately trained nurse.
- Patients on special diets are monitored to ensure that they have the appropriate food tray.
- Functional screens have been developed and implemented.

Surgery and Invasive Procedures

- Patients are informed of the risks, benefits, and alternatives to anesthesia, surgical procedures, and the administration of blood or blood products.
- Consent forms are executed and placed in the patient's record.
- Responsibility has been assigned for ensuring that appropriate equipment, supplies, and staffing are available prior to the administration of anesthesia.
- A pertinent and thorough history and physical have been completed and reviewed prior to surgery.
- A process exists by which there is a correlation of pathology and diagnostic findings.
- A preanesthesia assessment has been conducted.
- The surgeon has been credentialed to perform the surgical procedure that he or she is about to perform.
- Vital signs, airway, and surgical site assessments are continuously monitored.
- A procedure for instrument and sponge counts prior to closing the surgical site has been implemented.
- Surgical equipment is properly cleaned and stored following each procedure.

Assuring Correct Patient/Correct Site Surgery

- A process has been implemented to clearly mark the correct surgical site.
- If the actual site cannot be marked, a mark is placed in close proximity of the surgical site.
- Both the operating physician and patient are involved in the preoperative marking process.
- The patient's medical record is available to help determine the correct site prior to the start of surgery.
- Imaging studies are available for review prior to surgery to help determine the correct surgical site.
- There is verbal verification of the correct site by each member of the team in the operating room prior to induction of anesthesia.
- Observation confirms that the correct site has been marked, with the patient's participation.
- Anesthesia is not administered until the operating surgeon is in the operating suite.
- The surgical team (all disciplines) conducts a documented "time out" prior to the start of surgery to confirm the correct patient, correct site, and correct procedure.

Spiritual Care Services

- The spiritual needs of patients are addressed.
- Patients know such services are available and how to access them.
- Organizational policies and procedures address the psychosocial, spiritual, and cultural variables that influence one's understanding and perception of illness.
- Referrals are made by caregivers for spiritual assessment, reassessment, and follow-up.
- Documentation is placed in the patient's medical record to indicate that the patient's spiritual needs have been addressed.

24

Worldwide Search

Knowledge is of two kinds. We know a subject ourselves, or we know where we can find information upon it.

Samuel Johnson (1709–1784)
English author and lexicographer

This chapter is designed to assist the reader in conducting a worldwide search of ethics health care and law-related topics through the effective use of the Internet. "The World Wide Web (WWW) is the universe of network-accessible information, an embodiment of human knowledge," according to the organization that Web inventor Tim Berners-Lee helped found, the World Wide Web Consortium.

This chapter provides helpful Web sites to readers searching for best practices. It is a journey to the far corners of the earth in search of answers to difficult issues. This chapter is written for those individuals unwilling to accept an end without a fight; it recognizes that the answers to difficult disease processes may lead the reader to exotic lands in search of a remedy. Sometimes the issue(s) may be so overwhelming that it would seem easy to give up. Don't do it; the answer may be a click away.

This is the beginning of a new adventure. Enjoy the trip by first taking a comfortable journey to the National Library of Medicine's Web site at www.nlm.nih.gov/. The library, located on the grounds of the National Institutes of Health in Bethesda, Maryland, is the world's largest medical library. There are more than six million items in its collection, including books, journals, photographs, and images.

Before the journey begins, consider the following observations made during travels to hospitals throughout the nation.

TREATMENT OPTIONS

Patients are not always aware of the various treatment options for their medical conditions. Unique experiences and successes of physicians and hospitals from different parts of the country often remain unnoticed. Thus, physicians are left in the dark as to who is doing what and where. Varying combinations of treatment programs might be helpful in treating their patients. For example:

- In Florida, a physician described a case in which a muscular dystrophy (MS) patient needing wound care came to the hospital in a wheelchair. After 42 wound care treatments in a hyperbaric chamber, the patient left with a cane, not in a wheelchair.
- In New Jersey, a physician described how he developed a "cocktail of medications" for MS patients.
- In New Hampshire, a physical therapist described equipment that has helped both MS patients and stroke victims learn to walk again without the assistance of a cane.

These observations may not lead to a formula for the successful treatment of MS patients, but the message is unmistakable; there needs to be a repository for the compilation and sharing of unexpected successful outcomes.

EVALUATING WEB SITES

When evaluating health care Web sites on the Internet, look for the symbol of the HON code of conduct for health care at the bottom of Web pages. Health On the Net Foundation is the leading organization promoting and guiding the deployment of useful and reliable online medical and health information and its appropriate and efficient use. Created in 1995, HON is a nonprofit, nongovernmental organization, accredited to the Economic and Social Council of the United Nations. For more information on the HON Foundation, go to www.hon.ch.

SEARCH ENGINES

A search engine is a program that searches the World Wide Web for Web sites and creates a catalog of information about those sites. The search engine that one chooses to use will search its catalog for the occurrences of the text being searched. A majority of search engines are subject and keyword engines. Not all search engines access all possible Internet Web sites; therefore, it may be necessary to use different search engines to conduct a successful search. Listed here are some of the more popular search engines in use:

Altavista
 www.altavista.com/
America Online
 www.aol.com/
Ask Jeeves
 www.ask.com/
Dogpile
 www.dogpile.com/
Excite
 www.excite.com
Google
 www.google.com/
InfoSpace
 www.infospace.com/
Internet Explorer
 www.microsoft.com/windows/ie/default.asp
Lycos
 www.lycos.com/
Mamma
 www.mamma.com/
Medscape
 www.medscape.com
Northern Light
 www.northernlight.com
WebMD
 www.webmd.com/
Yahoo
 www.yahoo.com/

SEARCH TIPS

The following tips provide helpful information when conducting Web searches.

- Review the search tips that various search engines provide.
- Use quotion marks around phrases to ensure adjacency of words.

- Use a variety of search engines if you are having difficulty locating a particular topic.
- Domain names describe the location of the server where the information being sought is stored.
  - Knowing domain names where files are stored is helpful when conducting random searches for information. Domain Web sites include the following:

    .com: commercial organizations (businesses)

    .edu: educational organizations

    .gov: government agencies

    .mil: military

    .org: miscellaneous organizations

    .net: network providers

A path name follows the domain name and identifies the location of an item on the server.

TELEMEDICINE

Telemedicine is the delivery of health care services by means of telecommunications technology (e.g., fax, telephone, Internet, interactive audiovisual transmissions). It is a means for connecting remote areas of the nation and world with various forms of modern communications. The use of telemedicine brings modern health care to remote areas of the nation and the world. Telecommunications links the United States with the world. It includes teleradiology, the interpretation of imaging procedures at a site remote from the patient and where the diagnostic procedure was performed. Telepathology involves the interpretation of slides at a location far from where the slides are prepared. EEGs and EKGs can also be transmitted almost anywhere in the world. Teleeducation is a tremendous learning tool for linking lectures and formal education programs to multiple sites.

The possibilities of telemedicine are endless. The benefits include improving access to high tech care in remote areas of the nation and the world as well as reducing the transportation hardships for patients. Patients can remain in their communities and still have access to the marvels of modern medicine. Global telemedicine has arrived to provide worldwide medical consultations; continual access to updated physiological data about patients in remote areas; electronic medical records; remote review of imaging studies; remote examination of patients; and remote consultations.

Telemedicine Web Sites

AMD Telemedicine
www.amdtelemedicine.com/

American Telemedicine Association
www.atmeda.org/

Association of Telehealth Service Providers
www.atsp.org/

Biohealthmatics.com
www.biohealthmatics.com/healthinformatics/telemedicine/telemed.aspx

Personal MD
www.personalmd.com

QUACKWATCH

Quackwatch (www.quackwatch.com) is a Web site guide to health care fraud, quackery, and intelligent decisions. It includes questionable products, services, advertisements, and theories. It also covers education, consumer protection, research, additional links to other Web sites, and legal and political activities, as well as sources not recommended for health advice.

ETHICS-RELATED WEB SITES

Bioethics
www.bioethics.net

EthicsWeb.ca
http://www.ethicsweb.ca/resources/bioethics/

Ethics Resource Center
http://www.ethics.org/

Markkula Ctr for Applied Ethics
http://www.scu.edu/ethics/practicing/focusareas/medical/

TransWeb.org
www.transweb.org

LEGAL-RELATED WEB SITES

American Bar Association
www.abanet.org/
American Society of Law, and Ethics
www.aslme.org
Answers to Your Legal Questions
www.legalscholar.com
Federal Law
www.thecre.com/fedlaw/default.htm
FindLaw
www.findlaw.com
Guide to Law
www.loc.gov/law/guide
Health Law Resource
http://www.netreach.net/~wmanning/
Healthcare Law Net
www.healthcarelawnet.com/

(Primarily, this page is intended as a resource for health care practitioners, professionals, or anyone interested in learning more about the dynamic field of health care law, and more specifically, the regulatory and transactional aspects of health care law practice.)

InjuryBoard.com
www.injuryboard.com

(InjuryBoard is a growing community of attorneys, medical professionals, safety industry experts, and local activists, committed to making a difference by helping families stay safe and avoid injury, and helping those who are injured get the assistance they need.)

Law.com
www.law.com
Legal Information
www.law.cornell.edu/soj.html
LexisNexis
www.lexisnexis.com
NoLo
www.nolo.com
U.S. Courts/Links
www.uscourts.gov/allinks.html#7th
Westlaw
www.westlaw.com

Wrong Diagnosis
http://wrongdiagnosis.com/

GOVERNMENT-RELATED WEB SITES

Agency for Healthcare Research and Quality
www.ahrq.gov
Department of Health & Human Services
www.hhs.gov/
Centers for Disease Control
www.cdc.gov
Centers for Medicare & Medicaid Services
www.cms.hhs.gov/default.asp
Clinical Trials
http://ClinicalTrials.gov
Healthfinder
www.healthfinder.gov
MedlinePlus
www.Medlineplus.gov
National Cancer Institute
http://www.cancer.gov/
National Center for Health Statistics
www.cdc.gov/nchs
National Guideline Clearing House
www.guideline.gov
National Information Center on Health Services Research & Health Care Technology
http://www.nlm.nih.gov/nichsr/

(NICHSR was created to improve the "collection, storage, anaysis, retrieval, and dissemination of information on health services research, clinical practice guidelines, and on health care technology.")

National Institute of Medicine
www.iom.edu
National Institutes of Health
www.nih.gov
Nat'l Library of Medicine
http://www.nlm.nih.gov/
National Network of Libraries of Medicine
http://nnlm.gov/
PubMed
www.ncbi.nih.gov/entrez/query.fcgi

(PubMed is an innovative Web-based literature database that provides links to full-text articles from more than 5800 journals [fees may apply]. Customer service can be reached at: custserv

@nlm.nih.gov or 1-888-FIND-NLM [1-888-346-3656].)

US Department of Justice
www.usdoj.gov/
US Food and Drug Administration
www.fda.gov

BEST PRACTICES

Advisory Board Company
www.advisoryboardcompany.com/
Agency for Healthcare Policy and Research
www.ahcpr.gov/clinic/cpgsix.htm
best4health.org
www.best4health.org
Care Plans
www.careplans.com
Centre for Evidence-Based Medicine
www.cebm.net
Clinical Pathways
www.openclinical.org/clinicalpathways.html
Health Care Professionals' Network
www.wlm-web.com/hcnet
Institute for Safe Medication Practices
www.ismp.org
MDConsult
www.mdconsult.com
American Cancer Society
www.cancer.org
Association of Cancer Online Resources
www.acor.org
Cancer Links
www.cancerlinks.org
Clinical Trials Listing Service
www.centerwatch.com
NCI Clinical Trials
http://www.cancer.gov/clinicaltrials
Rarediseases.com
www.rarediseases.com
Disaster Center
www.disastercenter.com

HOSPITAL AND PHYSICIAN FINDERS

American Board of Medical Specialities
www.abms.org
AMA DoctorFinder
www.ama-assn.org/aps/amahg.htm
Best Hospitals
www.usnews.com/usnews/health/best-hospitals/tophosp.htm
Besthospitals.com
www.besthospitals.com
HealthGrades.com
www.healthgrades.com
Hospital Connect
www.hospitalconnect.com
National Practitioner Data Bank
www.npdb-hipdb.com

HEALTH CARE RESOURCES

Alternative Medicine
www.askdrweil.com
American Academy of Pain Medicine
www.painmed.org
American Library Association
http://www.ala.org/

(The American Library Association is the oldest and largest library association in the world, with more than 65,000 members.)

American Hospital Association
http://www.aha.org/aha_app/index.jsp
American Medical Association
http://www.ama-assn.org/
American Pain Foundation
www.painfoundation.org
Directory of Open Access Journals
http://www.doaj.org/

(This service covers free, full-text, quality controlled scientific and scholarly journals, covering all subjects and languages. There are now 3231 journals in the directory. Currently, 1036 journals are searchable at the article level.)

FamilyDoctor.org
http://familydoctor.org/online/famdocen/home.html

(Health information for the whole family from the American Academy of Family Practitioners.)

HealthWorld Online
www.healthy.net

InteliHealth
www.intelihealth.com
Library Spot
www.libraryspot.com
Life Extension Foundation
www.lef.org
MayoClinic.com
http://www.mayoclinic.com/

(One of the nation's finest clinics provides information on: (1) diseases and conditions; (2) drugs and supplements; (3) treatment decisions; (4) healthy living; (5) ask a specialist; (6) health tools; (7) slide shows; (8) video; and, blogs and podcasts.)

Virtual Library Pharmacy
www.pharmacy.org
MDChoice.com
www.mdchoice.com/pt/index.asp
Medscape
www.medscape.com
DaySpring
www.dayspring.com/ (Search "Hospital Spiritual")
Virtual Hospital
http://www.uihealthcare.com/vh/

(Link to a wealth of patient information.)

INTERNATIONAL MEDICAL-RELATED WEB SITES

Cancer Index
www.cancerindex.org/clinks5o.htm
International Clinical Trial Mgm't
www.medisearch-int.com/ictm.html
International Union Against Cancer
www.uicc.org
World Health Organization
www.who.int
World Medical Association
http://www.wma.net/e/

25

Journey to Excellence

Excellence can be attained if you . . .
Care more than others think is wise.
Risk more than others think is safe.
Dream more than others think is practical.
Expect more than others think is possible.

Author Unknown

THE JOURNEY

The *Journey to Excellence* begins with a vision by an organization's leadership to continuously improve the way care is provided in multiple settings. Leadership must be committed to providing more, charting new waters, and improving patient care.

A room designated for planning new directions should be available to all departments within the organization. Such a room could be designated the *health care war room*. It is a room designed for and dedicated to brainstorming, strategizing, and storyboarding courses of action. The war room encourages far-reaching dreams with the belief that they can become reality.

In the war room ideas are formed, prioritized, and assigned to a team member who accepts and champions new ideas and takes a leadership role in making them happen. The champion has the vision and passion to turn a dream into reality.

The doors of the war room are always open to all departments within the organization. Resources are readily available to aid in making positive changes. In the war room, caregivers have a unique opportunity to present ideas that otherwise may never have been taken seriously.

IDEAS FOR GETTING STARTED

The journey to excellence is not an easy path to follow:

> There is nothing more difficult to take in hand, more perilous to con-

duct, or more uncertain in its success, than to take the lead in the introduction of a new order of things. Because the innovator has for enemies all those who have done well under the old conditions, and lukewarm defenders in those who may do well under the new. This coolness arises partly from fear of the opponents, who have the laws on their side, and partly from the incredulity of men, who do not readily believe in new things until they have had a long experience of them.

Niccolo Machiavelli
(*The Prince*, 1513)

The ideas that follow are but a few of the many to help get the war room up and running. They are offered as agenda items for the first war room's leadership meeting, and they include some practices that have been implemented successfully by other organizations. They are not the end—they are merely the means to a new beginning.

Ambassadors Worldwide

The structure of world peace cannot be the work of one man, or one party, or one nation. . . . It must be a peace which rests on the cooperative effort of the whole world.

Eleanor Roosevelt

Eleanor Roosevelt's words apply to the world of health care. A first class health care system is not the work of one man or one nation. It must be a system that depends on the cooperative effort of the world community. Leaders should encourage employees to contact other caregivers in their discipline from around the world. Employees could begin by inquiring about the way in which another professional addresses a specific issue. From there, a professional relationship may ensue. This gives the two a type of informal partnership to learn what works in one another's country and how to best apply the treatments and procedures in their home countries. Such sharing of information will create worldwide ambassadors for health care, leading to a melding of resources and knowledge for the most effective care of patients.

Hospitals that implement such a program should then share the program's findings with their local community by publishing a hospital newsletter highlighting the most interesting and informative results.

Professional Exchange Program

This concept involves an exchange program whereby international host families would sponsor a health care professional in their home for 2 or more weeks. The professional would work in a foreign university hospital setting to learn the practices used in that health care setting, while also sharing with the host hospital best practices from his or her hospital. Thus, the program would provide a different cultural environment in which caregivers can share best practices.

Partners in Education

Partners in health care education programs, created by hospital–school partnerships, support and enrich student learning by introducing students to opportunities in the health care professions. Partners in education can take the form of a school lunch program whereby health care professionals (e.g., nurses, pharmacists, physical therapists, physicians) from a local community hospital are matched with students from a local middle school or high school who have an interest in a particular health career. Hospital employee volunteers are matched with one or more students for a semester and have lunch with them during a set day and time each week. Students may even choose to learn about a different discipline the following semester. The earlier this process begins, the greater the opportunity a student has to discover a successful career path.

Best Practices

The journey to excellence involves searching for best practices worldwide. It is a journey to the far corners of the earth in search of answers to difficult health care issues. It is the "worldwide search" to improve the quality of life on a global basis. It involves providing information to those individuals unwilling to accept an end without a fight. It recognizes that the answers to complex disease processes may lead the reader to exotic lands in search of a remedy. Although many issues may seem overwhelming, the answer to many health care issues may be a click away (see Chapter 24).

Focus on Preventative Medicine

Hospitals and physicians are often so busy treating symptoms, diseases, conditions, and injuries that preventative care is often not addressed. By committing more time to preventative medicine, the risks of early onset of disease can be reduced.

Information Technology

Health care organizations need to improve their information technology systems to reduce the tremendous amount of paperwork required of caregivers, allowing more time for direct patient care. The medical record has become a cumbersome compilation of illegible notes from many health care disciplines. It has become an unfriendly and far-from-effective communications tool in the care and treatment of patients. Its purpose has shifted from being a useful communications tool between caregivers to becoming a tool for satisfying regulatory bodies. The proverbial wheel is broken, so reinventing the "medical record" wheel is a must, requiring serious attention by the health care industry and regulatory bodies, to provide patients with increased bedside care.

ADOPT A HOSPITAL

Highways and rivers are adopted, why not *Adopt a Hospital*? Creating change on a grand scale requires financial backing by mission-driven individuals and corporations willing to adopt hospitals and provide funding for their capital needs for new or expanded programs and services. With fewer than 6,000 hospitals and numerous for-profit corporations in the United States, the health care system would be able to continuously grow and provide quality services with an Adopt a Hospital sponsorship from the nation's wealthiest people and corporations such as General Electric, Johnson and Johnson, Google, IBM, Intel, and Microsoft. In such a program, hospitals would be matched with corporations based on size and needs.

FUNDING YOUR DREAMS

> *The way to predict the future is to create it. Vision is the gift to see or do what others only dream.*
>
> Author Unknown

To help make a dream become reality, it is important for others to see and understand the dream. This can be accomplished effectively by visually displaying the vision on an electronic dream board (e.g., plasma screen TV) and making it easily visible to all who pass by. The dream board could be placed, for example, in high-traffic areas such as the hospital lobby or in the emergency department, intensive care, oncology, and rehabilitation waiting areas. It is important to remember that there can be multiple dreams displayed in various locations within the organization.

Dreams fulfilled should be displayed in what might be termed the "Hall of Dreams," celebrating the successes of those who worked hard to achieve them.

Glossary

Abandonment: Unilateral severance by the physician of the professional relationship between him- or herself and the patient without reasonable notice at a time when the patient still needs continuing care.

Abortion: Premature termination of pregnancy at a time when the fetus is incapable of sustaining life independent of the mother.

Admissibility (of evidence): Refers to the issue of whether a court, applying the rules of evidence, is bound to receive or permit introduction of a particular piece of evidence.

Advance directives: Written instructions expressing one's health care wishes in the event that he or she becomes incapacitated and is unable to make such decisions.

Adverse drug reaction: Unusual or unexpected response to a normal dose of a medication; an injury caused by the use of a drug in the usual, acceptable fashion.

Affidavit: A voluntary statement of facts, or a voluntary declaration in writing of facts, that a person swears to be true before an official authorized to administer an oath.

Agent: An individual who has been designated by a legal document to make decisions on behalf of another individual; a substitute decision maker.

Americans with Disabilities Act (ADA): Federal act that bars employers from discriminating against disabled persons in hiring, promotion, or other provisions of employment.

Appellant: Party who appeals the decision of a lower court to a court of higher jurisdiction.

Appellee: Party against whom an appeal to a higher court is taken.

Artificial nutrition and hydration: Providing food and liquids when a patient is unable to eat or drink, such as intravenous feedings.

Assault: Intentional act that is designed to make the victim fearful and produces reasonable apprehension of harm.

Attestation: Act of witnessing a document in writing.

Autonomy: Right of an individual to make his or her own independent decisions.

Battery: Intentional touching of one person by another without the consent of the person being touched.

Beneficence: Describes the principle of doing good, demonstrating kindness, and helping others.

Best evidence rule: Legal doctrine requiring that primary evidence of a fact (such as an original document) be introduced or that an acceptable explanation be given before a copy can be introduced or testimony given concerning the fact.

Borrowed servant doctrine: Refers to a situation in which an employee is temporarily placed under the control of someone other than his or her primary employer. It may involve a situation in which an employee is carrying out the specific instructions of a physician. The traditional example is that of a nurse employed by a hospital who is "borrowed" and under the control of the attending surgeon during a procedure in the operating room. The temporary employer of the borrowed servant can be held responsible for the negligent acts of the borrowed servant under the doctrine of respondeat superior. This rule is not easily applied, especially if the acts of the employee are for the furtherance of the objectives of the employer. The courts apply a narrow application if the employee is fulfilling the requirement of his or her position.

Captain-of-the-ship doctrine: A doctrine making the physician responsible for the negligent acts of other professionals because he or she had the right to control and oversee the totality of care provided to the patient.

Cardiopulmonary resuscitation: A lifesaving method used by caregivers to restore heartbeat and breathing.

Case citation: Describes where a court's opinion in a particular case can be located. It identifies the parties in the case, the text in which the case can be found, the court writing the opinion, and the year in which the case was decided. For example, the citation *Bouvia v. Superior Court* (Glenchur), 225 Cal. Rptr. 297 (Ct. App. 1986), is described as follows:

- *Bouvia v. Superior Court* (Glenchur) identifies the basic parties involved in the lawsuit.
- 225 Cal. Rptr. 297 identifies the case as being reported in volume 225 of the California Reporter at page 297.
- Ct. App. 1986 identifies the case as being in the California Court of Appeals in 1986.

Case law: Aggregate of reported cases on a particular legal subject as formed by the decisions of those cases.

Certiorari: Writ that commands a lower court to certify proceedings for review by a higher court. This is the common method of obtaining review by the US Supreme Court.

Charitable immunity: Legal doctrine that developed out of the English court system that held charitable institutions blameless for their negligent acts.

Civil law: Body of law that describes the private rights and responsibilities of individuals. The part of law that does not deal with crimes; it involves actions filed by one individual against another (e.g., actions in tort and contract).

Clinical privileges: On qualification, the diagnostic and therapeutic procedures that an institution allows a physician to perform on a specified patient population. Qualification includes a review of a physician's credentials, such as medical school diploma, state licensure, and residency training.

Closed-shop contract: Labor–management agreement that provides that only members of a particular union may be hired.

Common law: Body of principles that has evolved and continues to evolve and expand from court decisions. Many of the legal principles and rules applied by courts in the United States had their origins in English common law.

Complaint: In a negligence action, the first pleading that is filed by the plaintiff's attorney. It is the first statement of a case by the plaintiff against the defendant and states a cause of action, notifying the defendant as to the basis for the suit.

Congressional Record: Document in which the proceedings of Congress are published. It is the first record of debate officially reported, printed, and published directly by the federal government. Publication of the Record began March 4, 1873.

Consent: See informed consent.

Criminal negligence: Reckless disregard for the safety of others. It is the willful indifference to an injury that could follow an act.

Defamation: Injury of a person's reputation or character caused by the false statements of another made to a third person. Defamation includes both libel and slander.

Defendant: In a criminal case, the person accused of committing a crime. In a civil suit, the party against whom the suit is brought, demanding that he or she pay the other party legal relief.

Demurrer: Formal objection by one of the parties to a lawsuit that the evidence presented by the other party is insufficient to sustain an issue or case.

Deposition: A method of pretrial discovery that consists of statements of fact taken by a witness under oath in a question-and-answer format as it would be in a court of law with opportunity given to the adversary to be present for cross examination. Such statements may be admitted into evidence if it is impossible for a witness to attend a trial in person.

Directed verdict: When a trial judge decides either that the evidence and/or law is clearly in favor of one party, the judge may direct the jury to return a verdict for the appropriate party. The conclusion of the judge must be so clear and obvious that reasonable minds could not arrive at a different conclusion.

Discharge summary: That part of a medical record that summarizes a patient's initial complaints, course of treatment, final diagnosis, and suggestions for follow-up care.

Discovery: To ascertain that which was previously unknown through a pretrial investigation; it includes testimony and documents that may be under the exclusive control of the other party.

Do not resuscitate (DNR): Directive of a physician to withhold cardiopulmonary resuscitation in the event that a patient experiences cardiac arrest.

Durable power of attorney: Legal instrument enabling an individual to act on another's behalf. In the health care setting, a durable power of attorney for health care is the authority to make medical decisions for another.

Ethical dilemma: A situation that forces a person to make a decision that involves breaking some ethical norm or contradicting some ethical value. The effect of an action may put others at risk, harm others, or violate another person's rights.

Ethicist: One who specializes in ethics.

Ethics: A set of principles of right and wrong conduct; a theory or system of moral values, of what is right and what is wrong. Ethics is a system of values that guides behavior in relationships among people in accordance with certain social roles.

Ethics committee: A committee created to deal with ethical problems and dilemmas in the delivery of patient care.

Euthanasia: A Greek word meaning "the good death." It is an act conducted for the purpose of causing the merciful death of a person who is suffering from an incurable condition, such as providing a patient with medications to hasten his or her death.

Evidence: Proof of a fact, which is legally presented in a manner prescribed by law, at trial.

Expert witness: Person who has special training, experience, skill, and knowledge in a relevant area and who is allowed to offer an opinion as testimony in court.

Futility: Having no useful result. Futility of treatment, as it relates to medical care, occurs when the physician recognizes that the effect of treatment will be of no benefit to the patient. Morally, the physician has a duty to inform the patient when there is little likelihood of success.

Good Samaritan laws: Laws designed to protect those who stop to render aid in an emergency. These laws generally provide immunity for specified persons from a civil suit arising out of care rendered at the scene of an emergency, provided that the one rendering assistance has not done so in a grossly negligent manner.

Grand jury: Jury called to determine whether there is sufficient evidence that a crime has been committed to justify bringing a case to trial.

Grievance: The process undertaken to resolve a labor–management dispute when there is an allegation by a union member that management has failed in some way to meet the terms of a labor agreement.

Guardian: Person appointed by a court to protect the interests of and make decisions for a person who is incapable of making his or her own decisions.

Health: According to the World Health Organization, "[a] state of complete physical, mental, and social well-being and not merely the absence of disease or infirmity."

Health Care Financing Administration (HCFA): Federal agency that coordinates the federal government's participation in the Medicare and Medicaid programs.

Health care proxy: Document that delegates the authority to make one's own health care decisions to another, known as the health care agent, when one has become incapacitated or is unable to make his or her own decisions.

Hearsay rule: Rule of evidence restricting the admissibility of evidence that is not the personal knowledge of the witness.

Holographic will: A will hand written by the testator.

Home health agency: An agency that provides home health services. Home health care involves an array of services provided to patients in their homes or foster homes because of acute illness, exacerbation of chronic illness, and disability. Such services are therapeutic and/or preventative.

Home health care: Home health care is an alternative for those who fear leaving the secure environment of their home. Such care is available through home health agencies. These agencies provide a variety of services for the elderly living at home. Such services include part-time or intermittent nursing care; physical, occupational, and speech therapy; medical social services, home health aide services, and nutritional guidance; medical supplies other than drugs and biologicals prescribed by a physician; and the use of medical appliances.

Hydration: Intravenous addition of fluids to the circulatory system.

Incompetent: Individual determined by a court to be incapable of making rational decisions on his or her own behalf.

Independent contractor: One who agrees to undertake work without being under the direct control or direction of an employer.

Indictment: Formal written accusation presented by a grand jury, charging a person therein named with criminal conduct.

Informed consent: Legal concept that provides that a patient has the right to know the potential risks, benefits, and alternatives of a proposed procedure prior to undergoing a particular course of treatment. Informed consent implies that a patient understands a particular procedure or treatment, including the risks, benefits, and alternatives; is capable of making a decision; and gives consent voluntarily.

Injunction: Court order either requiring a person to perform a certain act or prohibiting the person from performing a particular act.

In loco parentis: Legal doctrine that permits the courts to assign a person to stand in the place of parents and possess their legal rights, duties, and responsibilities toward a child.

Interrogatories: List of questions sent from one party in a lawsuit to the other party to be answered under oath.

Judicial notice: An act by which a court, in conducting a trial or forming a decision, will of its own motion and without evidence, recognize the existence and truth of certain facts bearing on the controversy at bar (e.g., serious falls require X-rays).

Jurisdiction: Right of a court to administer justice by hearing and deciding controversies.

Larceny: Taking another person's property without consent with the intent to permanently deprive the owner of its use and ownership.

Liability: As it relates to damages, an obligation one has incurred or might incur through a negligent act.

Libel: False or malicious writing that is intended to defame or dishonor another person and is published so that someone other than the one defamed will observe it.

Life support: Medical intervention(s) designed to prolong life (e.g., respirator, kidney dialysis machine, tube feedings).

Living will: A document in which an individual expresses in advance his or her wishes regarding the application of life-sustaining treatment in the event that he or she is incapable of doing so at some future time. A living will describes in advance the kind of care one wants to receive or does not wish to receive in the event that he or she is unable to make decisions for himself or herself. A living will takes effect when a person is in a terminal condition or permanent state of unconsciousness.

Malfeasance: Execution of an unlawful or improper act.

Malpractice: Professional misconduct, improper discharge of professional duties, or failure to meet the standard of care of a professional that results in harm to another; the negligence or carelessness of a professional person, such as a nurse, pharmacist, physician, or accountant.

Mandamus: Action brought in a court of competent jurisdiction to compel a lower court or administrative agency to perform—or not to perform—a specific act.

Medicaid: Medical assistance provided in Title XIX of the Social Security Act. Medicaid is a state-administered program for the medically indigent.

Medicare: Medical assistance provided in Title XVIII of the Social Security Act. Medicare is a health insurance program administered by the Social Security Administration for persons aged 65 years and older and for disabled persons who are eligible for benefits. Medicare Part A benefits provide coverage for inpatient hospital care, skilled nursing facility care, home health care, and hospice care. Medicare Part B benefits provide coverage for physician services, outpatient hospital services, diagnostic tests, various therapies, durable medical equipment, medical supplies, and prosthetic devices.

Misdemeanor: Unlawful act of a less-serious nature than a felony, usually punishable by a jail sentence for a term of less than 1 year and/or a fine.

Misfeasance: Improper performance of an act.

Negligence: Omission or commission of an act that a reasonably prudent person would or would not do under given circumstances. It is a form of heedlessness or carelessness that constitutes a departure from the standard of care generally imposed on members of society.

Non compos mentis: "Not of sound mind"; suffering from some form of mental defect.

Nonfeasance: Failure to act, when there is a duty to act, as a reasonably prudent person would in similar circumstances.

Nuncupative will: Oral statement intended as a last will made in anticipation of death.

Ombudsman: Person who is designated to speak and act on behalf of a patient/resident, especially in regard to his or her daily needs.

Opined: To give or express as an opinion.

Perjury: Willful act of giving false testimony under oath.

Plaintiff: Party who brings a civil suit seeking damages or other legal relief.

Privileged communication: Statement made to an attorney, physician, spouse, or anyone else in a position of trust. Because of the confidential nature of such information, the law protects it from being revealed even in court. The term is applied in two distinct situations. First, the communications between certain persons, such as physician and patient, cannot be divulged without the consent of the patient. Second, in some situations, the law provides an exemption from liability for disclosing information for which there is a higher duty to speak, such as statutory reporting requirements.

Probate: A judicial proceeding that determines the existence and validity of a will.

Probate court: A court with jurisdiction over wills. Its powers range from deciding the validity of a will to distributing property.

Process: A series of related actions to achieve a defined outcome.

Prognosis: Informed judgment regarding the likely course and probable outcome of a disease.

Proximate: In immediate relation with something else. In negligence cases, the careless act must be the proximate cause of injury.

Real evidence: Evidence furnished by tangible things (e.g., medical records and equipment).

Rebuttal: Giving of evidence to contradict the effect of evidence introduced by the opposing party.

Release: Statement signed by one person relinquishing a right or claim against another.

Remand: Referral of a case by an appeals court back to the original court, out of which it came, for the purpose of having some action taken there.

Res gestae: "The thing done"; all the surrounding events that become part of an incident. If statements are made as part of the incident, they are admissible in court as res gestae despite the hearsay rule.

Res ipsa loquitur: "The thing speaks for itself"; a doctrine of law applicable to cases in which the defendant had exclusive control over the thing that caused the harm and where the harm ordinarily could not have occurred without negligent conduct.

Res judicata: "The thing is decided"; that which has been acted on or decided by the courts.

Respondeat superior: "Let the master answer"; an aphorism meaning that the employer is responsible for the legal consequences of the acts of the servant or employee who is acting within the scope of his or her employment.

Slander: False oral statement, made in the presence of a third person, that injures the character or reputation of another.

Standard of care: Description of the conduct that is expected of an individual in a given situation. It is a measure against which a defendant's conduct is compared.

Stare decisis: "Let the decision stand"; the legal doctrine that prescribes adherence to those precedents set forth in cases that have been decided.

Statute of limitations: Legal limit on the time allowed for filing suit in civil matters, usually measured from the time of the wrong or from the time when a reasonable person would have discovered the wrong.

Statutory law: Law that is prescribed by legislative enactments.

Stipulation: Agreement, usually in writing, by attorneys on opposite sides of an issue as to any matter pertaining to the proceedings. A stipulation is not binding unless agreed on by the parties involved in the issue.

Subpoena ad testificandum: Court order requiring one to appear in court to give testimony.

Subpoena duces tecum: Court order that commands a person to come to court and to produce whatever documents are named in the order.

Subrogation: Substitution of one person for another in reference to a lawful claim or right.

Summary judgment: Generally, an immediate decision by a judge, without jury deliberation.

Summons: Court order directed to the sheriff or other appropriate official to notify the defendant in a civil suit that a suit has been filed and when and where to appear.

Surrogate decision maker: Individual who has been designated to make decisions on behalf of an individual determined incapable of making his or her own decisions.

Testimony: Oral statement of a witness given under oath at trial.

The Joint Commission: A not-for-profit independent organization dedicated to improving the quality of health care in organized health care settings. The major functions of The Joint Commission include developing organizational standards, awarding accreditation decisions, and providing education and consultation to health care organizations.

Tort: Civil wrong committed by one individual against another. Torts may be classified as either intentional or unintentional. When a tort is classified as a criminal wrong (e.g., assault, battery, and false imprisonment), the wrongdoer can be held liable in a criminal and/or civil action.

Tort-feasor: Person who commits a tort.

Trial court: Court in which evidence is presented to a judge or jury for decision.

Union–shop contract: Labor–management agreement making continued employment contingent on joining the union.

Venue: Geographic district in which an action is or may be brought.

Verdict: Formal declaration of a jury's findings of fact, signed by the jury foreperson and presented to the court.

Waiver: Intentional giving up of a right, such as allowing another person to testify to information that ordinarily would be protected as a privileged communication.

Will: Legal declaration of the intentions that a person wishes to have carried out after death concerning property, children, or estate. A will designates a person or persons to serve as the executor(s) responsible for carrying out the instructions of the will.

Witness: Person who is called to give testimony in a court of law.

Writ: Written order that is issued to a person or persons requiring the performance of some specified act or giving authority to have it done.

Wrongful birth: Applies to the cause of action of the parents who claim that the negligent advice or treatment deprived them of the choice of aborting conception or of terminating the pregnancy.

Wrongful life: Refers to a cause of action brought by or on behalf of a defective child who claims that but for the defendant (e.g., a laboratory's negligent testing procedures or a physician's negligent advice or treatment of the child's parents), the child would not have been born.

Case Index

Index